A History of Medicine in
the Early U.S. Navy

Harold D. Langley

A History of Medicine in the Early U.S. Navy

The Johns Hopkins University Press
Baltimore and London

This book has been brought to publication with the generous assistance of
the Smithsonian Institution.

The Johns Hopkins University Press
2715 North Charles Street
Baltimore, Maryland 21218-4319
The Johns Hopkins Press Ltd., London

ISBN 0-8018-6672-3
Library of Congress Cataloging-in-Publication Data will be found
at the end of this book.

A catalog record for this book is available from the British Library.

To my wife Patricia,
who has lived with this project
for some time

Contents

List of Illustrations ix

Preface xi

Secretaries of the Navy, 1798–1843 xix

1 The Health, Welfare, and Safety of Seamen 1

2 The Quasi-War with France 19

3 Medicine and Health in the Quasi-War 53

4 The Barbary Wars 79

5 New Orleans 107

6 Medical Care Ashore: Boston 125

7 Naval Health Care in the North and South 141

8 Washington, D.C. 161

9 The War of 1812 at Sea 175

10 The War of 1812 Ashore 201

11 The War of 1812 on the Lakes 219

12 Toward a More Professional Service 241

13 Health Care and Hospitals, 1816–1829 267

14 Continuing Reform Efforts 291

15 Health Problems, 1829–1842 315

16 The Growth of Professionalism 335

17 Establishment of the Bureau of Medicine and Surgery 351

Abbreviations 361

Notes 363

Bibliography 407

Index 427

Illustrations

First Marine Hospital as It Appeared in 1930   9

Map of the West Indies during the Quasi-War   28

Commission of Surgeon William Graham of Maryland, 1799   36

Sick Bay of the USS *Constitution* as It Appeared in 1914   41

Sailors in Hammocks on the Gun Deck of a Warship, circa 1840   55

Eighteenth-Century English Medical Chest of the Type Used in the U.S. Navy   57

Map of the Mediterranean Region during the Barbary Wars   82

Surgeon Jonathan Cowdery in His Later Years   98

Surgeon Lewis Heermann   121

Surgeon Lewis Heermann's Naval Hospital at New Orleans   123

Dress Uniform Coat of Surgeon James M. Taylor, 1805–1807   147

Surgeon William P. C. Barton   152

Sailors Scrubbing a Deck, circa 1840   170

Surgeon Edward Cutbush   172

Surgeon's Instruments from the USS *Constitution*   178

Detail of Surgeon's Instruments from the USS *Constitution*   179

Cockpit of the British Frigate *Macedonian*   181

Death of Captain Lawrence in the *Chesapeake*   184

Map of the Atlantic and Gulf Theaters during the War of 1812   191

Map of the Chesapeake Bay Theater during the War of 1812   194

Medical Instruments from Commodore Barney's Gunboats: Cross-Legged Forceps   196

Medical Instruments from Commodore Barney's Gunboats: Dental Tooth Key   196

Medical Instruments from Commodore Barney's Gunboats: Surgical Scissors   197

Medical Instruments from Commodore Barney's Gunboats: Director and Scoop   197

Medical Instruments from Commodore Barney's Gunboats:
Pharmaceutical Bottle   198

Medical Instruments from Commodore Barney's Gunboats:
Apothecary Mixing Spatula   198

Map of the Northern Frontier in the War of 1812   220

Map of Sacket's Harbor, 1815   234

Battle of Lake Champlain, 1814   236

Surgeon Thomas Harris   254

Sailors Furling Sails, circa 1840   272

Surgeon Bailey Washington   299

Norfolk Naval Hospital as It Appeared in 1850   309

Surgeon Thomas Williamson, First Superintendent of the
Naval Hospital at Norfolk, Virginia   311

Map Showing Tracks of the U.S. Exploring Expedition, 1838–1842   330

Dress Uniform of Surgeon Bailey Washington, 1841   355

Preface

This book traces the evolution of medical practice in the U.S. Navy from the building of the first frigates in 1794 to the establishment of the Bureau of Medicine and Surgery in 1842. It grew out of an earlier study of efforts, in which some medical men were involved, to improve the lot of enlisted men in the nineteenth-century navy. Subsequent investigations led to the conclusion that the medical aspects of naval history and the contributions of various surgeons deserved to be better known to naval, medical, and social historians.

In relating the ideas behind what was the first federal health care program, it was necessary to look at developments in the merchant service which led to the establishment of marine hospitals and at how such early institutions functioned, as well as at their relationship to the men in the U.S. Navy. From the outset the navy wanted to keep control over its own sick and wounded, partly out of a desire to prevent desertion. Within the naval system itself there were separate hospital arrangements for sailors and marines. This was not necessarily the best use of men, space, or resources, but the perceived needs of the service dictated such a segregation. A number of years would pass before there were regular hospitals and the beginnings of a system that embraced the selection, training, and promotion of medical men and the procurement of, and accountability for, medical supplies. Amid all of this there were periodic discussions about the rank, pay, status, authority, and career potential for doctors in the naval service. These problems were addressed piecemeal for many years, and it was anticipated that the establishment of the Bureau of Medicine and Surgery would result in a more professional and organized way of dealing with medical questions.

Believing that the medical story should not be told without some reference to developments in the navy and the nation, where pertinent, I present the main outlines of those issues and indicate how they affected the navy and its medical branch. I hope that my non-naval readers will bear with these distractions and appreciate that contemporary concerns about those developments often delayed the consideration of medical questions.

No body of records exists from which a complete medical history of the U.S. Navy can be written. The surgeons sent quarterly reports on their practice, but most of those from the first 50 years of the navy have not survived. Medical men kept their own records, from which they prepared their reports, but they took them with them when they left the service. Only a few of the early casebooks survive. As a result the incomplete official and personal records must be pieced together to give as complete a picture as possible of the medical aspects. Hence it is inevitable that little is known about a number of questions, issues, and events that are important for this history. In such instances I have tried to present as complete an account as possible. I have occasionally noted the movement of ships, for I believe that the geographical area where a vessel operated may have had a bearing on the health of the crew even though that relationship cannot always be demonstrated. In the case of wars, the reports of the wounded and killed were made immediately after the battle and do not take into account those who later died of wounds. There is also no way to get a completely accurate account of how many men died of accidents or disease as a result of wartime activity. Therefore my attempts to arrive at figures for total casualties in various wars must be regarded as suggestive rather than definitive.

This shortage of pertinent data applies also to many of the medical personalities. There are some doctors about whom we have only the barest of biographical details. Some of the evidence that has survived is both brief and official in nature and offers little in the way of insight into a particular personality. The lack of details on the origin, education, naval experiences, and subsequent careers of many of the early navy doctors is a source of much disappointment. As this study evolved, it soon became obvious that I could not trace the development of medicine in the navy and provide a profile of the medical corps in the same volume. The latter aspect deserves a study in itself. In this study I have noted some general trends and personalities that are a part of the larger professional profile. Additional research in geneologies may eventually help to fill in details on some. But there is enough detail on others to give us some idea of their lives, their medical attainments, and the disappointments and rewards of naval service.

Despite the problem of incomplete sources, enough survives to give both the main outlines of the story and some colorful and fascinating details. At the same time there are several aspects of the naval medical story that cannot be fully treated even in a work as long as this. These include such topics as the drug supply of the navy, the acquisition and preparation of food, and the professional training and development of individual medical officers. I hope to enlarge upon some of these topics at a later date. I also hope that medical historians may find material in this work which will shed light on what was taking place in a special part of American society. Though usually out of sight and mind of most of the populace and generations of historians, navy doctors were involved in important efforts to upgrade and professionalize their part of the medical world. They were concerned about the quality of the care given to the men in their charge and about the responsibilities of their superiors and the Congress for health matters. While attached to navy yards in major cities, navy doctors not only cared for the servicemen, their families, and the workmen attached to the installation but also, on their own time, provided medical expertise to the surrounding civilian community. Through their duty assignments and travel, navy doctors were exposed to a variety of climates, societies, and health problems that were well beyond the experience of most civilian practitioners. They had knowledge of the state of public health in many parts of the world and the relationships of medical men to it, and in articles and books they wrote of their experiences and insights for medical colleagues at home. Those who left the service to begin civilian practice had acquired considerable professional expertise. Thus navy doctors had both direct and indirect influence on medicine in the country at large.

Research on this book has consumed a number of years, and in the process I have incurred many intellectual debts.

My research really began with a visit to the Navy Surgeon General's Library, where the librarian, the late Catherine O'Connell, showed me some articles that bore on the subject of my inquiry. In more recent years, Jan Herman, the historian of the Bureau of Medicine and Surgery, has been most helpful in making available for research some intriguing items.

One of the earliest supporters of this project was James H. Cassedy, historian, History of Medicine Division, National Library of Medicine, Bethesda, Maryland, who encouraged me to apply for a grant to explore the feasibility of this work by searching for manuscript materials. Subsequently a Public Health Service grant allowed me to visit several manuscript depositories and examine their holdings on medical men who had served in the U.S. Navy. From this research I was able to determine to what degree I could use personal papers to supplement the official record in the National Archives. Another early supporter at the History of Medicine Division was Manfred J. Wasserman, who also showed me the results of his own research on a surgeon of the American Revolution. Both he and Dr. Cassedy encouraged me to organize my preliminary findings and present them to a group of local medical historians for comment and reaction. As my work progressed, I became increasingly familiar with some of the holdings of the History of Medicine Division, and my labors there were assisted by Dorothy Hanks, Margaret Kaiser, Betty Tunis, and Carol Clausen of the library staff.

My efforts to produce a medical history of the early navy might never have come to fruition had it not been for the continuous encouragement of Robert R. T. Joy, M.D., professor and chairman of medical history at the Uniformed Services University of the Health Sciences, Bethesda, Maryland. He saw the need for such a study and was familiar with some of my work on the navy. There is scarcely a paragraph in this book that has not come under his critical eye and provoked some kind of comment. If the final work does not include all the colorful language and medical information he hoped for and contains more naval material than he wanted, it was not that he did not try. I have learned a great deal from his comments and suggestions for additional research. He encouraged me to present some preliminary findings at a meeting of the Washington Society for the History of Medicine. His colleague at the Uniformed Services University, Dale C. Smith, Ph.D., has also helped me and given me information on the results of his own research. Both Dr. Joy and Dr. Smith have contributed much to my understanding of the nature of medical practice in the army and navy and to the interpretation of some specific cases. Another physician who offered his insights into nineteenth-century medicine was the late Peter D. Olch, then the deputy chief of the History of Medicine Division of the National Library of Medicine.

No historian with an interest in late-eighteenth- and early-nineteenth-century medicine can afford to ignore the works of J. Worth Estes, M.D., professor of pharmacology at the School of Medicine, Boston University. In the course of my research and writing he has been most patient and outgoing in helping me to understand and write about early medical practices. I have profited from all his criticisms and suggestions, and I hope that at least some of the text reflects this.

Over the years I have been helped by the staffs of many libraries and manuscript depositories. These include the National Archives and Records Service, the Library of Congress, the Navy Library, the Naval Historical Center, the Marine Corps Historical Center, the Library of the National Museum of American History, Smithsonian Institution, and the National Library of Medicine; the Massachusetts Historical Society and the New England Genealogical Society, Boston; the Harvard University Archives; the American Antiquarian Society, Worcester, Massachusetts; the Rhode Island Historical Society and the John Hay Library, Brown University, Providence; the Beinecke Library, Yale University; the Warren Hunting Smith Library, Hobart and William Smith Colleges, Geneva, New York; the Franklin D. Roosevelt Library, Hyde Park, New York; the New York Historical Society, the New York Public Library, and the Medical Library of the College of Physicians and Surgeons, Columbia University; the New Jersey Historical Society, Newark; the Princeton University Library; the

Historical Society of Pennsylvania, the Library of the College of Physicians of Philadelphia, the American Philosophical Society, the Free Library of Philadelphia, the archives of the Pennsylvania Hospital, the Rare Book Room and the Archives of the University of Pennsylvania, and the Academy of Natural Sciences, Philadelphia; the Franklin and Marshall College Library, Lancaster, Pennsylvania; the Maryland Historical Society, Baltimore; the special collections of the Nimitz Library and the Museum of the U.S. Naval Academy, Annapolis, Maryland; the Alderman Library of the University of Virginia, Charlottesville; the Earl Gregg Swem Library of the College of William and Mary, Williamsburg, Virginia; the Virginia Historical Society, Richmond; the Library and the Medical Center Library, Duke University, Durham, North Carolina; the University of North Carolina, Chapel Hill; the Georgia Historical Society, Savannah; the Historic New Orleans Collection; the Lilly Library, Indiana University, Bloomington; the Chicago Historical Society; the William L. Clements Library, Ann Arbor, Michigan; the Green Library, Stanford University; the Huntington Library, San Marino, California; and the Bancroft Library, University of California at Berkeley.

Special thanks are also due to Dean Allard, director of the Naval Historical Center, for courtesies and support for many years. I am deeply grateful to William S. Dudley, formerly head of the Early History Branch and now senior historian of the Naval Historical Center, and to his staff, especially Michael J. Crawford, Christine F. Hughes, and Charles E. Brodine Jr., for the use of the materials collected for the documentary volumes on *The Naval War of 1812*. Access to the microfilms of Navy Department archival materials was provided by John Vajda, then the director of the Navy Department Library, and members of his staff. Mr. Vajda also gave me access to the collection of manuscripts in the rare book room. Members of the Operational Archives staff of the center assisted me in my research in the biographical files. Charles Haberlain and Edward Finney of the Photographic Section helped me locate and obtain copies of photographs of medical men and ship interiors.

At the Marine Corps History and Museums Branch in the Washington Navy Yard, Brig. Gen. Edwin M. Simmons, USMC (Ret.), the director, and members of his staff always made me welcome and helped me whenever they could. I owe a special debt of gratitude to Richard Long, formerly head of special projects and now the head of oral history, for information and comments on the early history of the Marine Corps and for his continuous support for my book. I am also obliged to Denny J. Crawford, head of the Reference Section, and his assistant, Robert J. Aquilina, for useful information on marine casualties.

Past and present officials at the Smithsonian Institution have supported this project. Brooke Hindle, Otto Mahr, and Roger G. Kennedy, former directors of the Museum of History and Technology, now the National Museum of American History, and Spencer Crew, the present director, provided me with opportunities for research. Roger G. Kennedy supported my application for a Smithsonian research opportunities grant, which enabled me to complete my work in libraries and historical societies far from Washington. David Challinor, a former assistant secretary for science, administered a fund that made it possible for me to explore additional leads. Thanks to the efforts of Assistant Secretaries Thomas L. Freudenheim and Robert S. Hoffman and endorsements from my supervisors at the museum, I received the necessary funds to publish this book. Robert D. Selim, director of the Publications Division, handled the paperwork and coordination with the Johns Hopkins University Press to implement that decision. My research over the years has been supported by James Hutchins, curator/supervisor of the Armed Forces History Division; the late Edward C. Ezell, who formerly held that position; Philip K. Lundeberg, a former curator/supervisor of the Division of Naval History; and Bernard S. Finn, Arthur P. Molella, and Ramunas Kondratas, former chairmen and the present acting chairman, respectively, of the Department of the History of Science and Technology. Audrey Davis and Ramunas Kondratas of the museum's Division of Medical Sciences lent me books and journals and answered queries. Harold W. Ellis and Joseph M. Young, museum specialists, and Frances Hainer, a collections management assistant, in the Naval History Section helped to keep things running smoothly while I was engaged in research. Kevin J. Crisman, a former Smithsonian Institution fellow and now on the faculty of Texas A&M University, provided useful information on naval vessels in the War of 1812 and on Sacket's Harbor, New York. Volunteers in the Armed Forces History Division have saved me time and energy at critical moments: Slator Blakiston Jr. and John Prokos Jr. ran down leads and references in the Library of Congress and the National Archives and supplied me with photocopies of pertinent documents; H. Paul Mullis carefully copied the details of service of a large number of medical officers. Mary Ellen McCaffrey and her colleagues in the Office of Printing and Photographic Services helped me to get fine quality prints.

My research has taken me to many interesting places, including Lake Erie, where I participated in a cruise to commemorate the naval battle there in 1813. The day was made memorable in part through the efforts of Gerard T. Altoff, the supervisory park ranger at Perry's Victory and International Peace Monument, Put-in-Bay, Ohio, who also made available to me his then unpublished work on the soldiers who served as sailors in Commodore Oliver H. Perry's ships. While cruising on Lake Erie, I also had the opportunity to review the role of Surgeon's Mate Usher Parsons in that battle in discussions with his biographer, Seebert J. Goldowsky, who later gave me information on Parsons which was discovered after his book was published. Research on the War of 1812 on the lakes later brought me in contact with Patrick Wilder, then of the Sacket's Harbor Battlefield, Sacket's Harbor, New York, who located the site of the hospital and gave me a copies of maps of that wartime base.

For much useful biographical information on medical officers who served between 1794 and 1815 and clarification of doubtful points, as well as continuous personal and professional support, I am most grateful to Christopher McKee, librarian of Grinnell College, Grinnell, Iowa. His knowledge of the early navy and its colorful personalities is unsurpassed, and he has been most generous in giving me the benefit of it.

Others who have been very helpful in supplying specific information include Robert J. Taylor and Richard Alan Ryerson, former and present editors in chief of the Adams Papers, Massachusetts Historical Society; James Roan, reference librarian, National Museum of American History; William Dunne, who is writing a biography of Captain Stephen Decatur; John McCusker, Trinity University, San Antonio, Texas; Linda Maloney, Berkeley, California; William J. Rooney, New Orleans; John Pascandola, formerly of the History of Medicine Division, National Library of Medicine; Paul Sifton, a former member, and John McDonough a current member of the staff of the Manuscript Division of the Library of Congress; Bart Greenwood, former director of the Navy Library; Comdr Tyrone G. Martin, USN (Ret.), a former captain of the USS *Constitution* and a historian of the ship; Henry Merriman, Waterbury, Connecticut; Mark N. Brown, curator of manuscripts, Brown University Library; Thomas A. Horrocks, director of the Library for Historical Services, College of Physicians of Philadelphia; Alice Creighton, head of special collections, Nimitz Library, U.S. Naval Academy; Margaret Klapthor, former curator of political history and chair of the Department of National and Military History at the Smithsonian's Museum of History and Technology; Toby Gearhart, the Historical Society of Pennsylvania; John D. Stinson, manuscripts specialist, New York Public Library; Terry Alford, Fairfax, Virginia; and Alan M. Richman, Stephen F. Austin State University, Nacogdoches, Texas. My son, David, introduced me to the world of word processors and has been active in trying to keep me abreast of the latest developments in that technology.

For permission to reproduce maps or photographs, I am grateful to

Carole Le Faivre, American Philosophical Society; Tamatha Kuenz, Philadelphia Museum of Art; Ann Grimes Rand, curator of the USS *Constitution* Museum; Richard J. Wolfe, curator of rare books and manuscripts, Francis A. Countway Library of Medicine, Harvard University; John C. Dann, director, William L. Clements Library, Ann Arbor, Michigan; Jeff D. Goldman, Maryland Historical Society; Robert J. Hurry, registrar, Calvert Marine Museum, Solomons, Maryland; Joseph M. Judge, curator, Hampton Roads Naval Museum, Virginia; Jan Herman, historian, U.S. Navy Bureau of Medicine and Surgery; Michael Crawford, head of the Early History Branch, and Charles Haberlain of the Photographic Section, Naval Historical Center; Robert U. Massey, editor, *Journal of the History of Medicine and Allied Sciences;* and Terrence J. Gough, historian, U.S. Army Center of Military History, Washington, D.C.

All this might have been for naught had not George F. Thompson, then acquisitions editor with the Johns Hopkins University Press, expressed an interest in what I was doing. This lead to a contract and a regular writing schedule. Along the way there were delays, discouragements, and pitfalls, but through it all Jacqueline Wehmueller, my editor, was positive, patient, and supportive. Copy-editing was done with great skill and much stamina by Irma F. Garlick. Karen Poirier coordinated the effort to get good photographs, clear maps, and proper permissions, as well as guidelines for their placement. Barbara B. Lamb, the managing editor of the press, kept everybody on track and mindful of deadlines.

Finally, but by no means last, my thanks and gratitude go to my wife, Patricia, who has watched the evolution of this book over many years with much patience and good humor.

The time pressures of the publishing process have resulted in some oversights that I regret. Readers should be aware that it was not my intention that the terms *American* and *U.S.* be used interchangeably. The initials *U.S.* have been customarily used to denote a federal connection, especially in the nineteenth century, whereas the term *American* has a broader application. Unfortunately, it has not been possible to change all references to reflect this distinction, and I must rely on my knowledgeable readers to make the adjustments where necessary.

Secretaries of the Navy, 1798–1843

Benjamin Stoddert, June 18, 1798–March 31, 1801

Robert Smith, July 27, 1801–March 7, 1809

Paul Hamilton, May 15, 1809–December 31, 1812

William Jones, January 19, 1813–December 1, 1814

Benjamin W. Crowninshield, January 16, 1815–September 30, 1818

Smith Thompson, January 1, 1819–August 31, 1823

Samuel L. Southard, September 16, 1823–March 3, 1829

John Branch, March 9, 1829–May 12, 1831

Levi Woodbury, May 23, 1831–June 30, 1834

Mahlon Dickerson, July 1, 1834–June 30, 1838

James K. Paulding, July 1, 1838–March 3, 1841

George E. Badger, March 6, 1841–September 11, 1841

Abel P. Upshur, October 11, 1841–July 23, 1843

A History of Medicine in
the Early U.S. Navy

Chapter 1

The Health, Welfare, and Safety of Seamen

Long before there was a U.S. Navy or a medical service for it, there was a concern among some Americans about the health, welfare, and safety of seamen, especially those in foreign ports. One indication of this came at the end of the American Revolution when a committee of the Continental Congress consisting of Thomas Jefferson of Virginia, Elbridge Gerry of Massachusetts, and Hugh Williamson of North Carolina responded to letters from U.S. ministers in Europe concerning a number of pending questions.

Among them was a suggestion that the Congress acknowledge the services of John Baptist Pecquet, a French consular agent at Lisbon, for his work among the suffering American sailors who were carried into that port as prisoners of war by the British during the American Revolution. Benjamin Franklin and John Adams found Pecquet in Paris and in need of money. He was given 10 guineas. Franklin, Adams, and Jay recommended that the United States pay him 150 guineas, or 4,000 *livres,* and send him a letter expressing the gratitude of the Congress for his services. On December 20, 1783, the committee recommended that Pecquet be indemnified for his losses and rewarded for his zeal. Subsequently, Pecquet received the thanks of the United States and a monetary reward for his services. Pecquet was also hoping that either he or his son would be appointed as the U.S. agent at Lisbon, but Franklin and his colleagues told him that this would have to be done by the Congress.[1] That body was already considering what to do about commercial relations with various powers, but as things worked out, there was no place for Pecquet or his son. Before any permanent appointments were made, it was necessary to establish the framework of commercial relations by treaties.

1

In May 1784, Congress instructed the U.S. diplomatic representatives in Europe to negotiate treaties of amity and commerce with a number of countries. At this time treaties were already in force with France (1778), the Netherlands (1782), and Sweden (1783). Congress was trying to establish a system that would govern U.S. trade with all nations. Among other things, a model treaty provided for the protection of American property and citizens in foreign lands. Model treaties were subsequently negotiated with Prussia (1785) and Morocco (1787). In the latter case, the intercession of the Spanish government made it possible to come to terms with the sultan. The treaty provided that in the event of war, captives would not be enslaved but treated as prisoners of war. Friendly commercial relations were established between the two countries. Included in this treaty was an arrangement whereby, in the event of disputes between U.S. citizens residing in Morocco, the U.S. consul would decide between them and if necessary, his government would enforce his decision. Efforts by U.S. diplomats to extend the model treaties to the other Barbary States and Turkey, Austria, and Denmark failed because of the growing inability of the government under the Articles of Confederation to enforce its treaties on the 13 states.[2] This need for a stronger central government led to the Constitutional Convention and to a new form of government under the Constitution in 1787.

Meanwhile there was an appreciation in commercial circles that on a day-to-day basis there was an urgent need to appoint consuls in certain foreign ports. These were the men who handled the paperwork associated with the sale and shipment of cargoes and who had the most contact with captains and sailors. Responding to this need, and in anticipation of the action of Congress, President Washington in 1790 appointed 12 consuls and 5 vice consuls at various ports. For the most part, these were Americans who were or planned to be engaged in trade in the ports. In places where no Americans were available, foreigners were appointed. Consuls received no salary; their remuneration was from the fees they collected for their services. These officials met the immediate needs of those engaged in foreign commerce while Congress struggled to form a permanent consular establishment.[3]

The difficulty was that while the Constitution provided for the appointment of consuls, there was no law or regulation establishing a system or defining their powers and duties. In the absence of legislation, Secretary of State Thomas Jefferson issued a circular on August 26, 1790, setting forth their duties. These included sending a report every six months of the U.S. vessels that entered or cleared their port, commercial informationy, and news of military preparations. In the event of imminent war, it was their duty to warn U.S. merchants and vessels in their area. Consuls were given the authority to appoint consular agents to smaller ports within their jurisdiction, thereby increasing the information to which they had access. With regard to sailors, Jefferson's instructions said only that their number was to be included along with the names of masters and owners of every U.S. ship that touched at any particular port.[4] It soon became apparent, however, that consuls had to do more than just count the seamen.

In the fall of 1791, Consul Joshua Johnson reported from London that with the discharge of crews from British warships, a number of American seamen were turned loose on the world who could not get employment. Many were starving. Johnson said that "a Man's feelings and Humanity is [*sic*] continually put to the rack, from the number of objects that present themselves to him." There was only one U.S. ship in port, and he could not get many home by that means. He said that many of the American captains demanded three to six guineas per man as well as requiring them to work their passage home. Most of the captains wanted the cost of the man's food advanced to them as well. British captains would not take Americans because they would leave the ship when it reached the United States while their own countrymen would continue for the length of the voyage. So Johnson had many seamen on his hands whom he was helping to the best of his means. In addition, there was the problem of an insane Baltimore merchant captain. Until such time as he could find someone who would carry him to his home, Johnson was obliged to keep the unfortunate officer in a poorhouse at a cost of four shillings a week. The consul expressed the hope that the secretary of state would present these facts to Congress and that he would be reimbursed the sums advanced.[5] As things turned out, however, it was quite a while before Congress found time to consider the problem in a systematic way.

It was not until April 19, 1792, that Congress enacted the first law governing the duties and powers of consuls. It contained specific instructions concerning seamen. In cases of shipwreck, sickness, or captivity affecting mariners and seamen employed on vessels belonging to citizens of the United States, it was the duty of consuls and vice consuls to prevent the men from suffering in foreign ports. They were "to provide for them in the most reasonable manner, at the expense of the United States, subject to such instructions as the Secretary of State shall give, and not exceeding an allowance of twelve cents to a man per diem." All masters and commanders of vessels owned by U.S. citizens and destined for a U.S. port were obliged to carry such mariners and seamen thence free of charge if requested to do so by a consul or vice consul. Each master or commander had a quota of two sailors or mariners for every 100 tons burden of his ship.

The returning men were required to do duty on the ship if they were able. Thus, under the law of 1792, both the United States and private citizens had obligations to see to it that sick and distressed sailors in foreign ports were returned safely to U.S. port.[6]

Captives of Algiers

While the matter of consular regulations was being studied, a new and more serious problem arose under the heading of distressed seamen. It concerned those captured by the pirates of Algiers. As early as July 30, 1785, Richard O'Brien, captain of the *Dolphin,* sought help for himself and his crew by writing to Thomas Jefferson, then the U.S. minister at Paris. Jefferson sent an agent to redeem them, but he brought too little money. In 1787, O'Brien again called attention to the plight of his men, whose lives were endangered while they were being forced to do hard work in the port of Algiers. An epidemic, probably of bubonic plague, was raging there, and in three months 200 Christian slaves had died. O'Brien wrote that one of his crew had died and another, who had "two large buboes on him," recovered after two weeks. He reported that the Spaniards and the Neapolitans had redeemed their captives. These redemptions and the death of other captives had resulted in a shortage of slaves and the greater use of O'Brien's men. If they were not rescued soon, the captain feared they would die. O'Brien's plea was not answered quickly, and before the disease abated, 900 Christian captives died, including 6 Americans.[7]

The plight of the Americans held captive in Algiers was detailed in a report prepared by Secretary of State Jefferson which Washington sent to Congress in December 1790. In addition to O'Brien and his men, another ship's crew had been seized. There were now 21 Americans being held. In 1786 the dey of Algiers demanded $2,833 for each American, but the agent negotiating with him thought that he could get them for $1,200 each. It was pointed out that Spain had paid $1,600 a man. The United States had not been in a position to act on this offer, and with the passage of time the price had gone up. By 1790 it was estimated that each captive American would cost between $1,571 and $2,920. In his report, Jefferson said that six Americans had died in captivity and one had been ransomed by friends. The secretary left it to Congress to decide on a course of action: ransom, force, or an exchange of prisoners. While Congress considered, a new and urgent appeal was heard.[8]

The captive who had been ransomed by his friends came home and petitioned Congress for reimbursement of the price of his freedom and other expenses. This led the Senate to pass a resolution in February 1792 calling on the president to ransom the Americans still held captive and negotiate treaties with Algiers, Tunis, and Tripoli. Before this could be accomplished, the British, distracted by the wars growing out of the French Revolution, negotiated a truce with Algiers for themselves, Portugal, and the Netherlands. As a result, only the commerce of the Hansa towns of Germany and the United States was left unprotected. Algerian corsairs now sailed into the Atlantic in search of prey. By November 1793 the Algerians had captured 11 additional U.S. ships, and the number of Americans in captivity had risen to 105.[9]

Congress responded to this new threat by passing a law in March 1794 authorizing the building of a naval force. Four frigates of 44 guns and two of 36 guns were to be constructed to protect U.S. commerce. Each ship of 44 guns was to carry a captain, four lieutenants, one marine lieutenant, one chaplain, one surgeon, and two surgeon's mates. A 36-gun frigate rated the same number of officers as the larger ship except that there was only one surgeon's mate. Pay ranged from $75 a month and six rations a day for the captain to $14 a month and two rations a day for three types of petty officer. The pay of the other petty officers, as well as for the midshipmen, seamen, ordinary seamen, and marines, was to be set by the president, and they were entitled to one ration a day. A surgeon was to receive $50 a month and two rations and the surgeon's mate $30 a month and two rations a day. In addition, the act prescribed the daily ration of food and spirits for crews. The pronavy faction in Congress tried to think of everything that a future naval force might need. There were, however, some who strongly opposed the establishment of a permanent force and who saw the law as an emergency measure. They were responsible for getting into the final section of the act the proviso that if peace should prevail between the United States and Algiers, shipbuilding and other preparations for the use of naval force would cease. It was believed at the time that without this last section the bill would not have passed; it was adopted by a margin of 11 votes. The first six captains were appointed on June 5 to oversee the work of building the ships in various ports as one of the functions of the War Department. It would be some time before the ships would need the services of seamen and surgeons.[10]

Nevertheless, there is one bit of evidence that in this formative period there were some medical expenses associated with the building of the frigates. A Treasury Department official, writing to an agent for procuring supplies for the construction of the frigates, spoke of sums paid for "sundry Carpenters and Axemen employed for the purpose of cutting timber in Georgia for the Frigates, provisions for their use, including sundry expenses in getting them home, Medical assistance, etc., from September 1794, to September 1795, has been adjusted and settled at the Treasury."[11]

The assumption is that these were private physicians who were called in as needed to treat members of the work force.

Meanwhile efforts to free the men in Algerian captivity were intensified. David Humphries, the U.S. minister at Lisbon, who was in charge of the negotiations, wrote to the U.S. agent at Algiers urging him to make haste to get the men out "before they shall again be visited by that dreadful scourge of Heaven, the Plague. The early liberation of these unhappy men from their present distressing & perilous condition is considered an object too dear & too interesting to all the feelings of humanity, to admit of one moment's delay." The agent was successful, and a treaty with Algiers was signed on September 5, 1796. In return for an annual subsidy, U.S. ships were protected from molestation. The captives were released, but new complications delayed their return home.

Released with the Americans were 48 Neapolitans who wanted to return to Italy. No vessel was available to take the Americans, so Joel Barlow, the U.S. agent at Algiers, purchased the *Fortune,* which was bound for Leghorn with the Neapolitans. A few hours after the ship sailed, one of the Neapolitans came down with the plague. The captain returned to Algiers and the sick man was removed from the ship. Again the *Fortune* sailed, and this time a Neapolitan and an American were stricken with the plague and died. Contrary winds made it impossible to continue to Leghorn, and the two deaths made the captain to decide to make for Marseilles, where the ship was quarantined. The captain took what he considered to be necessary precautions to prevent the spread of the disease. Clothing belonging to the deceased men was thrown overboard and an unopened chest of clothes belonging to the dead American was taken ashore below Marseilles and burned. The ship was fumigated by burning sulphur and tarred rope yarns. Everyone on board bathed in vinegar. During the 82 days of quarantine, no new cases developed. It looked as though the ship could proceed to Leghorn. But at this point the U.S. consul at Marseilles chartered the Swedish ship *Jupiter* to carry his countrymen home without further delay. He also supplied them with woolen clothing, in anticipation of a winter crossing of the Atlantic, and other necessary items. The former captives finally reached Philadelphia early in February 1798.[12] Press coverage of their ordeal may well have given some members of Congress an additional awareness of the health perils associated with commerce on the high seas.

Problems with France

At this time, Congress was well aware that both commerce and personal safety were now at greater risk as a result of the decision of the government of Revolutionary France to seize U.S. ships. The meaning of this interference in human terms was reflected in the reports of U.S. consuls to the secretary of state. From Bordeaux, Consul Joseph Fenwicke reported that some American seamen who had been forced to serve on a French privateer had come to his door "half dead, it would wring your heart to see the distresses of our Seamen. Congress have not made sufficient provision for them. As a favor I got some into the Hospital; but they begin to grow tired of me & will receive no more; & when I offer them to American Masters, they make a thousand excuses—I cannot force them." A week later he reported that he was able to persuade the director of the French hospital at Bordeaux to admit U.S. seamen at a cost of one-half dollar per man per day. "Poetic language with all its glowing colors cannot convey to you even a faint idea of their distresses."[13]

Similar reports were received from the West Indies of men turned loose on shore without money and with no clothing but what they were wearing. As a result the government sent the brigantine *Sophia* to French and Spanish ports in the West Indies to collect the sufferers and bring them home. At Puerto Rico the captain of the *Sophia* found at least 90 men, whom he took to Santo Domingo, where they were distributed among U.S. vessels needing men. Four men were too sick for further duty and were brought to Philadelphia in late December 1797. Shortly after this the *Sophia* was ordered to carry three special ministers to France who were to try to resolve the problems with France. They were John Marshall, a Virginia Federalist, Elbridge Gerry, a Massachusetts Republican, and Charles C. Pinckney, a South Carolina Federalist who had previously been appointed minister to France but who was not recognized by that government. The stage was being set for new problems when French agents attempted to extract a bribe from the U.S. delegates. The ensuing uproar resulted in the further deterioration of relations with France. But, for the captain of the *Sophia,* the delivery of the diplomats was only one of his duties. When that was accomplished, he was to visit the ports of France and take home as many American seamen as he could. If there was not enough room in the *Sophia* for all, he was to consult with the local U.S. consuls about chartering or buying a ship for the rest of the men.[14] By the time the *Sophia* returned home, the United States was busily preparing a naval force for active duty against France, choosing officers, including medical men, acquiring medical supplies, and enlisting seamen. But before taking up that aspect, let us consider the evolution of another idea relating to the medical care of seamen.

Hospitals for Seamen

Prior to the American Revolution, colonists involved in overseas commerce were aware of the arrangements that Great Britain had for the care of its seamen. Since 1588 there had been a hospital in Greenwich for seamen of the Royal Navy which was originally supported by a tax of a sixpence a month on each seaman. Later, in 1696, the benefits of the hospital and the tax were extended to the men of the merchant service. After 1729 all seamen who were British subjects and who sailed for ports in the American colonies were taxed for the hospital. So for at least 45 years, sailors from the American colonies paid for hospital benefits that few enjoyed. When Americans were sick, they liked to be cared for close to home. This state of affairs led maritime men in Virginia to establish a marine hospital near Norfolk in 1758–59 and to try to get something larger and more permanent during the American Revolution.

In 1780, as a part of an act for the defense of its eastern frontier, Virginia authorized the establishment of a hospital for sick and disabled seamen. The cost was to paid by collecting nine pence a month in specie or equivalent money from the wages of seamen in the Virginia navy. The contribution was raised to one shilling a month in 1782 and was levied on merchant sailors as well. But it was not until December 1787 that the Assembly appointed commissioners to determine the cost of the ground, buildings, and staff of the hospital; at this time its purpose was extended to include the "aged, sick and disabled seamen." By 1788 it was agreed that the hospital would be in the town of Washington, near Norfolk, and it was to be completed by November 1789. In reality there was a shortfall in the funds collected, and the hospital was still incomplete in December 1794, at which time an appeal was made to the governor: unless something was done quickly, the work already completed would deteriorate. Meanwhile, as early as 1790, the Assembly had authorized the sale of the hospital to the federal government, but a federal law authorizing the purchase was not passed until 1798. The transfer was conditioned on the Congress paying the contractor the balance due to him. These arrangements were not completed until the fall of 1800, by which time there had been an outbreak of yellow fever in Norfolk which spread to Alexandria and Richmond. To take care of the cases in Richmond, Dr. William Fonshee asked the governor for a temporary hospital, suggesting that a merchant ship then at Richmond be purchased and its decks fitted with rooms for the sick. It is not known what became of this suggestion for what might have been the first use of a hospital ship in the United States.

While Virginia was struggling to provide for its seamen, North Carolina

8

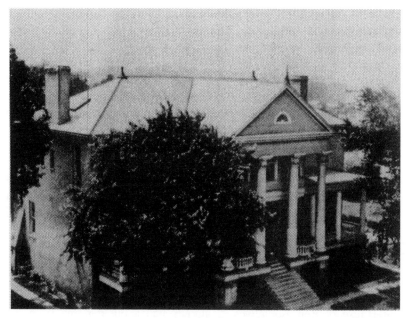

First Marine Hospital as It Appeared in 1930. Copyright 1930 by Captain Richmond C. Holcomb, MC, USN.

made its own start in 1789 by establishing a hospital fund, and similar efforts were being made on the national level.[15] During the first session of the first Congress under the Constitution, Representative William L. Smith of South Carolina presented a motion that a committee be appointed to prepare a bill "providing for the establishment of Hospitals for sick and disabled seamen and for the regulation of harbours." A committee consisting of Smith, Daniel Carroll of Maryland, and George Clymer of Pennsylvania was appointed. Although he was born in South Carolina, Smith had attended preparatory schools in England before the revolution and had received his legal training in that country. He may well have been familiar to some degree with the existence and perhaps the operation of the Royal Navy hospital at Greenwich. Pennsylvania-born George Clymer was a signer of the Declaration of Independence, and had been a member of Continental Congress and a delegate to the Constitutional Convention before being elected to the first federal Congress. Daniel Carroll received his college education in France before serving in the Continental Congress and as a delegate to the Constitutional Convention. The committee was thus made up of men of wide experience, two of whom had a knowledge of foreign countries. A bill was duly prepared which Smith presented to the

House on August 27, 1789. It provided that "hospitals shall be established and maintained in such seaport towns of the United States as the President shall direct, by a deduction from the wages of Seamen, which Captains and commanders of vessels shall pay to the officers of the customs at each entry of their vessels." The bill was read once, and then a second time the following day, before being sent to the Committee of the Whole House.

On September 15, consideration of the bill was postponed, and the following day it was deferred until the second session of the first Congress, which was to begin on January 4, 1790. The idea that such hospitals should be administered by the central government does not seem to have been challenged. Meanwhile, when the Boston Marine Society, a long-established organization of shipmasters, decided that hospitals were needed in New England and elsewhere, it also believed that the institutions should be the responsibility of the federal government.

Accordingly, a petition was drawn up, and with supporting letters it was sent to Congress in 1791. What the society had in mind was the establishment of three marine hospitals, one for the southern, one for the middle, and one for the northeastern states. When the memorial was received in the House of Representatives, it already had a bill pending from the previous session. The memorial from the Boston Marine Society was ordered to lie on the table and then, on February 7, was referred to the secretary of the Treasury, who was to examine it and to give his opinion at the next session of Congress.[16]

Before the secretary had a chance to respond, the subject came up again in a new context in 1792 when the Virginia legislature offered to sell to he federal government the marine hospital it had established in Norfolk County. This proposal was also sent to Secretary of the Treasury Alexander Hamilton for comment. Hamilton reported that the establishment of one or more marine hospitals in the United States was desirable for several reasons. First, "the interests of humanity are concerned in it, from its tendency to protect from want and misery, a very useful, and for the most part, a very needy class of the Community." Second, by affording protection and relief it would attract seamen to the country, and as a result navigation and trade would be improved. Ten cents a month could be collected from the wages of seamen to create a fund suggested by the memorial from the marine society. "The benefit of the fund ought to extend not only to disabled and decrepit seamen, but also to the widows and children of those who may be killed or drowned, in the course of their service as seamen." Hamilton also had recommendations in regard to directors who would serve without compensation for this charitable purpose. The society's memorial suggested the establishment of three hospitals, but for a considerable time one would probably do. More hospitals would mean more expense, but the additional ones would have some advantages in terms of local feelings and considerations. In the end, Hamilton left to Congress the decision on whether the offer of the Virginians should be accepted. Congress postponed its decision.

From time to time during the next five years, the question of the marine hospital would come up again in the form of a bill that would be referred to a committee, and there the matter would die, During this same five-year interval, however, Congress passed legislation relating to the duties of consuls, and this had a bearing on the care of distressed seamen overseas. The matter of reimbursing the consuls for their advances to sick and disabled seamen came up in the House in March 1797. After a brief discussion, it was decided that $30,000 would be appropriated to defray the expenses of the consuls. Discussions in the House preceding this agreement brought out the fact that under the existing circumstances, consuls were allowed to spend only 12¢ a day on the care of a seaman.[17] Another important advance took place on July 20, 1790, when Congress passed an act for the government and regulation of seamen in the merchant service.[18] This law, an attempt to put some limits and obligations on seamen, captains, and owners, is of interest for health reasons because it required every ship of 50 tons or more to carry minimum amounts of water, recently salted meat, and ship bread, and also a medicine chest. If there were any doubts in the minds of the legislators that captains would be able to use the contents of these chests effectively, they are not recorded. No doubt it seemed sufficient at the time that a ship of any size with more than a handful of sailors aboard ought to have some means of dealing with simple medical problems.

Congress was also moving slowly to consider the question of health care for seamen closer to home. In February 1797 a committee of the House of Representatives reported that a number of seamen, both native and foreign born, were arriving in U.S. ports and becoming a burden on public hospitals. Others were left to die for want of proper attention. The committee recommended that a fund be established for the relief of sick and disabled American seamen in the United States and foreign ports. Funds could be raised either by an additional tonnage duty on vessels entering U.S. ports or by a charge on the wages of the crew. It recommended that a specific sum per month be deducted from the wages of all seamen sailing from U.S. ports, to be used for the temporary relief of sick and disabled seamen and for founding hospitals for them. A bill was introduced in 1798 when Congress was concerned about the seizure of U.S. vessels by the French. By this time the proposal called for the deduction of 20¢ a month from the pay of every seaman, both American and foreign, to establish a fund for the construction of marine hospitals. The division of opinion on the issue became clear on April 10, 1798, when the bill was read for the third time in the House.[19]

Samuel Sewall of Massachusetts said that while he was unwilling to speak against the bill, its passage would bring on many inconveniences and objections. Under the heading of objections, he noted that in Massachusetts arrangements were already in place for the care of sick and disabled persons, and not just seamen, the expense being borne by everyone in the community. If the pending measure passed, Massachusetts seamen would be paying twice for the same service. Even if this were not the case, Sewall doubted the propriety of taxing only seamen for what ought to be considered a public charity. He thought that the laws of reason and charity called upon the public at large to support these men; the burden should not be laid exclusively on the seamen. Members of the House had no common feelings with them. The proposed tax would not touch any member of that body. Instead it would be placed on a small part of the community, most of whom would not derive any benefit from the measure for the next 50 years, for it would take that long to erect "large and splendid buildings" that would be exhibits to the world of public charity. There were no such buildings in Massachusetts, but no seaman, whether native born or foreign, became sick there without relief being provided. It was therefore difficult to know on what reasonable ground the seamen of his state should be asked to contribute to the fund now proposed. The only reason he had heard was that New England seamen frequently visited the southern states, and if they became ill there, there was no provision for their relief. He hoped that the southern states would take it upon themselves to supply relief to seamen, otherwise the men would have to go into the south in the same way they went into foreign countries.

Sewall went on to say that much had been made of the example of Great Britain, where similar establishments for seamen existed. But it should be noted that those British establishments began as the result of grants by individuals and that the seamen of the Royal Navy merely made contributions toward the current expenses. So the two cases, British and American, were very different, and he hoped that the pending bill would be defeated.[20]

The sentiments expressed by Sewall were not shared by Thomas Pinckney of South Carolina, who rose to answer his colleague's objections. The pending law might be thought of as being hard on Massachusetts because that state already provided for sick and disabled seamen, but it would operate for the general good of the Union. The burden on the people of Massachusetts would be lightened because they would no longer need their own system. As for Sewall's objections to taxing seamen for a general object, Pinckney thought it was only reasonable that seamen should pay for the benefits they received. In the future, he believed, the seamen's contribution would be considered as a part of his wages, and therefore a general tax that the merchant would pass on to those who purchased his merchandise. There was also the point that Sewall made about the erection of large and splendid hospitals. It was Pinckney's understanding that this was a secondary purpose of the bill. Its first was to provide relief to distressed seamen, after which, and when there was a sufficient surplus in the fund, suitable buildings would be erected as hospitals, but not large and splendid ones.

Turning next to Sewall's point about the southern states being like foreign countries as far as health care was concerned, Pinckney said that this did not apply. In the case of foreign countries, the United States had already made provision for the care of its sick and disabled seamen through its consuls, and it was planned to make them more efficient than they had been thus far. As for sailors who became sick or disabled in the South, they had "only to rely on private charity for support." But since the eastern states furnished three-fifths of the seamen of the United States, and since those states were interested in providing a more certain support for their citizens, he thought that the pending bill should be passed.

If Pinckney believed that his remarks had eliminated all objections to the bill, he was quickly disabused by Edward Livingston of New York, according to whom the arguments on the measure were based on two inequalities. The first was in regard to different parts of the Union, and the second concerned the persons it was intended to help. He thought that the objections to the first point had been answered satisfactorily, and he was sorry that they had not had that effect. He did not see how the bill could operate to the injury of any part of the Union. The president had the power to use money for the temporary relief of seamen and to reimburse Massachusetts or any other state for sums expended for this purpose. If there were any inequalities, he hoped that the objections would be waived in light of the extreme utility of the bill in other parts of the Union.

As to the inequalities on the persons helped, Livingston said that New York City already provided for the care of about 300 sick and disabled seamen a year. It was his understanding that there were similar arrangements in Philadelphia and Charleston, and he supposed that they treated a similar number of men. Seamen ought not to make any objection to the measure because they received some advantages from the Union, one of which was the bounty on their fishing vessels through a duty on the salt used to cure their fish. Sailors would not object to paying such a trifling sum as 20¢ a month for so valuable an object. "A sailor is concerned only for the present, and is incapable of thinking of, or inattentive to future welfare; he is therefore a proper object for the care of the government." It was also argued, said Livingston, that the government would be collecting a part of the sailor's wages, but the sailor himself would see no benefit from his contribution for years to come. Livingston did not believe that buildings had to be erected first, before a sailor could be treated. Rather, he felt that the fund would be properly applied. If any surplus accumulated, it would be spent "in a frugal way, so as to conduce to the happiness and comfort of this class of men and to the honour of the nation."

When Livingston took his seat, Sewall again arose to refute the arguments made against his position. On Livingston's point that this legislation would eventually save Massachusetts some money, Sewall said that the sailors in his state could not be excused from paying taxes in their home towns, so they would be paying twice for support in the case of illness. Because of his stand on the bill he had been accused of a want of benevolence, but he believed that he had a greater respect than his colleague for seamen. Seamen could take care of themselves without Livingston. Furthermore, the bill proposed erecting public hospitals, not just for U.S. citizens but also for the seamen of foreign nations. Thus U.S. seamen would be forced to support a public charity for foreigners. Very few, if any, of the Americans who contributed to the fund would derive any benefit from it. Sewall charged that Livingston had no interest in seamen or in the fisheries of the United States.

As for the points made by Pinckney, Sewall believed that New England sailors would rather take their chances about getting sick abroad than pay a tax that benefited foreigners. Large numbers of New England seamen were employed exclusively in fishing, and a few sailed to southern ports. The proposed tax would drive seamen out of the country, said Sewall, for it would fall most heavily on those with families and fixed abodes. A foreigner could afford a small deduction from his pay, but an American with a family could not. Sewall wanted measures that would help to establish harmony between the different sections of the country, but he did not favor taxing a single occupation for this purpose. He agreed with Livingston that sailors needed enough to support themselves, and he did not think that fishermen could complain. But as for their being subsidized by the duty on salt, Sewall said that the bounty on the exportation of fish was meant only as a drawback on the duty paid on the salt used to cure them. The bounty far exceeded this amount. Sewall believed that the tax would eventually fall on landlords, since they had the bulk of the seamen's money.

Josiah Parker of Virginia was the next to give his opinions. He began by saying that he was sorry that Sewall did not consider all seamen of the United States as standing on the same ground. Sewall was mistaken when he said that the bill would provide support for foreigners; it was for the relief of our own citizens. But in the present situation, when the country was threatened by war, what encouragement was there for men to enter the service if there was no asylum for them when they were sick or wounded. The British sailor knew that Greenwich hospital was available to him when his sailing days were over, and perhaps this made him more valiant. The bill under consideration would not leave U.S. sailors to the "doubtful benevolence of others" but would give them "a permanent relief" in case of sickness, debility, and old age.

More thoughts on the question were presented by Joseph B. Varnum of Massachusetts. While the bill might relieve some of the burdens of the Massachusetts taxpayer, he said, it would not exclude sailors paying to support their fellow citizens. He did not know if the United States had the power to make the proposed legislation, but the subject should be one of concern to the legislatures of the various states. If the United States thought that sailors were more important than other classes of men, the people at large ought to support them in their times of distress. If hospitals were needed, then the public and not the sailors ought to support them.

Albert Gallatin of Pennsylvania then told the House that he would vote against the bill. Before he would vote for the measure, he wanted to see some positive good arise. The bill assumed that seamen were not able to provide for themselves and therefore must be cared for. Gallatin believed that they were capable of taking care of themselves. In every community there were those who were improvident and did not make provision for their old age, but he did not believe that there were greater numbers of seamen who fitted this description than others. The kind of institution recommended in the bill was probably useful in other countries where there was a distinction between sailors and other citizens. But in the United States he had not been able to discover any such distinction. For the present he preferred to let sailors provide for themselves or be supported in the same way as the other poor, sick, and disabled. Gallatin did not favor building hospitals. He thought it would be better to have the sick dispersed throughout the country. He likewise opposed the way in which the fund was to be raised, which amounted to a tax on labor. In some instances this tax would fall upon the sailors themselves, in other cases on merchants, and in still other circumstances on the community. Since the eastern states provided two-thirds of the seamen in the country, Gallatin thought that the wishes of those states should be the deciding factor. If they were content to support seamen in the way that they had been doing, he did not know why a tax such as the proposed one should be approved. He noted that representatives from New York, Charleston, and Baltimore were in favor of the bill, but, not knowing the wishes of the people of Philadelphia, he moved for a two-day postponement. Gallatin's motion was seconded and the House voted to postpone further consideration of the bill.[21]

The lines were now clearly drawn in the House between those who believed that the sailor could provide for himself and those who argued that he should be taxed to build federal institutions that would care for him when he became ill. There were those who objected to the bill on constitutional grounds because the money would be used for foreign seamen as well as Americans, because they did not like to build hospitals along European lines, and because the tax would fall unevenly on the citizens. In the end the matter was postponed not just for two days but for two months, but in that interval a consensus emerged.

On July 16, 1798, Congress passed an act for the relief of sick and disabled seamen. It obliged the master or owner of every ship or vessel of the United States, upon arriving from a foreign port, to give the collector of the port a report of the number of seamen employed on the vessel since it last entered U.S. port. He was to pay the collector 20 cents a month for every seaman, to be deducted from the man's pay. Similar arrangements were made for sailors in the coasting trade. The collectors were to make quarterly returns to the Treasury Department. The president was authorized to use the money "to provide for the temporary relief and maintenance of sick or disabled seamen, in the hospitals or other proper institutions now established in the several ports of the United States." In ports where there were no such institutions, the president was authorized to use the money as he saw fit, except that the money collected in a given district should be used there. Any surplus was to be used under the direction of the president, together with any private donations he was authorized to receive, to invest in the stock of the United States. When the president felt that a sufficient sum had been accumulated, he was authorized to acquire ground or buildings and, when necessary, have hospitals erected "for the accommodation of sick and disabled seamen."

The president was also authorized to appoint directors of the marine hospital of the United States in such ports as he saw fit. These directors were to supervise the expenditure of the fund assigned to their port and govern the hospitals. They would hold office at the pleasure of the president, and each quarter they were to give to the secretary of the Treasury an account of monies collected and spent. No allowance or compensation was to be made to the directors "except the payment of such expenses as they may incur in the actual discharge of the duties required by this act."[22]

This law reinforced precedents that such legislation was considered to be in the province of the central government, not of the states. Nevertheless the debates in Congress underscored the desire of the New England states to care for seamen according to their own arrangements. They resented federal interference. While the law provided for the local administration of the fund, the federal regulations were regarded as violations of state's rights. The constitutional authority to pass the legislation was based on the admiralty jurisdiction of Congress as well as on its control over foreign and interstate commerce. At the same time it should be noted that this U.S. law was not as generous as that of Great Britain, which gave pensions for old age or disability and contained provisions for the wives and children of sick seamen and for widows and orphans. Thus, from the point of view of social legislation, the new law was a step backward when compared to British precedents. But it was probably the best that could have been achieved at the time. As it was, it took nine years to get it approved.

In less than a year, Congress realized the advantages of the law for the relief of sick and disabled seamen, and its provisions were extended to the navy. Under a new law, after September 1, 1799, the secretary of the navy was authorized to deduct 20 cents a month from the pay of every officer, seaman, and marine and pay the sums collected to the secretary of the Treasury. All the navy men who contributed to the hospital fund were entitled to the same benefits and privileges as the merchant seamen covered under the original act of 1798.[23]

Chapter 2

The Quasi-War
with France

President George Washington had been in office only two and a half months when a mob in Paris stormed the Bastille prison and killed its governor—actions that have ever since been popularly associated with the beginnings of the French Revolution. The progress of the revolution led to an alliance of Austria and Prussia against France and to the War of the First Coalition, 1792–97. In February 1793, France declared war on Great Britain, and in April, President Washington issued a proclamation of neutrality. The French resented the failure of the United States to honor the Franco-American alliance of 1778. They were similarly outraged by the negotiation in 1795 of the Jay Treaty, establishing a new commercial arrangement between the United States and Great Britain, which the French mistakenly interpreted as an alliance. France retaliated by seizing U.S. ships, refusing to receive the newly appointed U.S. minister, and demanding a bribe from the three U.S. commissioners sent to Paris to resolve outstanding questions. The merchants who were the victims of the French attacks on U.S. shipping reported these matters to Congress and demanded action. Members of Congress discussed the possible response, including the use of force.[1]

Earlier, when U.S. ships were being seized by Algerian pirates, Congress had authorized the War Department in 1794 to build six frigates.[2] But the law also contained a proviso that if the matter was settled peacefully, work on the ships would cease. When the Algerian problem was resolved through diplomacy, pronavy Congressmen worked to save the shipbuilding program and a compromise was struck. Under the Naval Armament Act of July 1, 1797, the frigates *United States, Constitution,* and *Constellation* were to be completed, manned, and used as the president saw fit, which meant that ultimately the services of medical men would be needed to examine those who wished to enlist and provide health care for the crews. The number, rank, and pay of the medical men assigned to the three frigates were set forth in the act of 1794 and repeated in the act of 1797.

The latter law also contained general guidelines for the compensation of any officer or enlisted man wounded or disabled in the line of duty. A commissioned or warrant officer could receive no more than half of his monthly pay, while noncommissioned officers, marines, and seamen could expect no more than five dollars a month. Lesser disabilities were to be compensated in proportion to the maximum sum. Clearly, the Congress was thinking about some of the long-range costs of war.[3]

Under the terms of the Naval Armament Act, the War Department and its agents were caught up in preparing the ships for service against the French as soon as possible. Presumably the need for medical officers would be the most urgent when the ships were ready to enlist their crews. But in Philadelphia the need for medical advice came soon after the frigate *United States* was launched on May 10, 1797. Captain John Barry, under whose supervision the ship was being built, needed information on the medical arrangements necessary for the vessel and the medicines that needed to be acquired. To help, the War Department ordered Dr. George Gillasspy to Philadelphia. Gillasspy was a New Yorker, and, it may be assumed, he had acquired his medical knowledge as an apprentice to a doctor. Whatever the extent of his medical education, it was sufficient for him to be appointed as a surgeon to the Second Infantry on March 7, 1797. His time with the army must have been brief, for he probably came to Philadelphia in the summer of 1797. It also seems likely that soon after his arrival, he began to prepare a medical chest for the *United States*.[4]

While in Philadelphia, Dr. Gillasspy decided to improve himself by enrolling in a medical course, which seems to have begun in the late fall or winter of 1797, taught by Dr. Benjamin Smith Barton at the University of Pennsylvania. In his notebook for the course, Gillasspy identified himself as "Surgeon, 2nd U.S. Regiment of Infy. & Acting Surgeon, Frigate United States." The second half of the course, begun in February 1798, was taught by Dr. Benjamin Rush, "Professor of the Practice of Physic." Gillasspy's notebook provides a fascinating insight into the medical ideas of the day. Especially interesting for naval medicine are Barton's lectures on the effects of drinking in producing diseases and Rush's views on the states of fever.[5]

Gillasspy soon found that he had to balance the intellectual demands of the courses with the need for his professional services. Some of the men who were preparing the frigate for sea became sick, and Captain Barry asked the secretary of war whether he could send Gillasspy to the ship. Secretary McHenry, a physician himself, replied on August 30, 1797, that Barry could order the doctor on board "whenever you may think proper." Presumably Gillasspy reported to the ship soon after this.[6] So it was that an army doctor began to function in his medical capacity on a war vessel.

On September 5, Lieutenant John Mullowny moved the ship to the lower end of the Kensington district and off Point Pleasant. Less than 24 hours later, yellow fever made its appearance on board. Sailing Master John Lockwood was working with a mast when he collapsed and was carried below to his berth. That night Lieutenant McRea of the marines came down with a fever. By the next morning half a dozen seamen and marines had become ill. Gillasspy treated them with emetics and bled them, in accordance with prevailing medical ideas. His energy was taxed by a bad cold, and he had more cases than he could deal with efficiently. Barry ordered Gillasspy to send anyone with the smallest complaint to the hospital on shore, but most were too sick to be moved.[7] On September 9, a marine died and three days later Lockwood passed away. Barry saw that Gillasspy was in low spirits and did not look well, so he asked Dr. Benjamin Rush to go on board to observe and make recommendations. Rush was too busy to go himself, but he sent a young assistant, who told Barry that everything that was possible was being done for the sick. Reporting the matter to the secretary of war, Barry praised Gillasspy as a man of "intellect and Great humanity." Some assistance in caring for the sick was provided by an infantry private named Jonathan Shattuck, who was assigned to the frigate as Gillasspy's "waiter." One may assume that he performed tasks similar to those associated with a loblolly boy or sick bay attendant. He was not considered a member of the ship's company, but he received his provisions there. Additional help was provided by the ship's steward, who picked up the medicines and provisions on shore.[8]

While engaged in one of these errands, the steward was accosted on a Philadelphia street by Tench Francis, the purveyor to the War Department, who threatened to stop issuing medicine and provisions because they were being misused by the doctor. About this time, Francis wrote to Barry suggesting that newly enlisted sailors and marines be kept on shore for 8–10 days before being put on board the ship. By this means he evidently hoped that disease would not be introduced onto the ship and that costs would be reduced. Before Barry could answer the letter, he had a complaint from Gillasspy about the purveyor's remarks. Edward Meade, who replaced Lockwood as the sailing master, offered the opinion that the purveyor was probably distressed that rations were not being distributed in accordance with regulations, for meat was given out on days declared banyan, or meatless, days. The reason for this was that the designated rations were not on board. The secretary and the purveyor were presumably mollified by this explanation.[9]

By this time it had become clear to Barry and others that Gillasspy needed professional assistance. Asked for a recommendation, Rush named English-born Dr. John Bullus, who had settled in New Jersey and had served an apprenticeship under Rush in 1793. Now in private practice in Reading, Pennsylvania, Bullus was restless and ready for a change. The secretary of war authorized his appointment on September 22, 1797, and soon, probably in early October, Bullus reported on board the *United States*.[10]

On October 3, Gillasspy informed Barry that there were now only two sick men on board, and only one of them was seriously ill. No new cases had appeared for several days, and he was sure the ravages of the disease were now past. Shortly after writing these words, Gillasspy was stricken with yellow fever. At the first sign, he dosed himself "and thereby overpowered it, but had nothing been done previous to the violent attack[,] bleeding would not have saved, nor all the mercury in the world have salivated me, so much was discharged with the contagion." By October 11 the worst was over. Gillasspy was not yet able to walk, but his spirits were high and he knew that he would get well.[11]

Now that the surgeon was recuperating, an assistant was on board and the crew had largely recovered, the work of preparing the ship for sea could go forward. One urgent need was for cannon. Informed by the War Department that they were available in New York and knowing that his surgeon was preparing to go there on convalescent leave, the captain asked him to investigate. Barry and Gillasspy had close personal and professional relations, so the doctor was glad to do what he could.

Gillasspy arrived at his mother's home on November 18. A few days later he went to Governors and Bedloe's islands, and on November 21 he sent Barry a report. Additional cannon were reported to be at Kinderhook, New York, on the Hudson River, and at "Salisbury furnace." Gillasspy expressed willingness to execute any additional commands during his leave, but time would be short, for he was anxious to get back to Philadelphia to see friends and attend Dr. Rush's lectures. The job of tracking down the additional cannon was given to Lieutenant Mullowney. Gillasspy apparently returned to his ship and his studies.[12]

Meanwhile, other preparations were being made in Baltimore. The 36-gun frigate *Constellation* was launched on September 7, 1797, and Captain Thomas Truxtun was anxious to put to sea as soon as possible. In a letter of instruction to Lieutenant Simon Gross, Truxtun touched on the care of the sick. The lieutenant was cautioned never to "lose sight of that humanity and Care that is due to those who may be really Sick, or otherwise stand in need of his assistance and attention." Health matters were on the captain's mind, for that fall there was an outbreak of yellow fever at Fells Point, outside Baltimore. Indeed, it was later established that many of those who went out to watch the launching of the *Constellation* came down with the fever. Truxtun doused himself twice a day to keep his bowels open and avoided all places where fever had been reported. It was not a healthy environment in which to recruit men, nor a place to find a doctor who was free to join the ship. While taking extra precautions for his own health, Truxtun sought expert advice on treating his crew. He wrote to Dr. Benjamin Rush describing the symptoms and their treatment with mercury. Rush responded that there was important information in Truxtun's letter that the doctor thought should be published in the press. "Your name will give weight to it," said Rush, "for you belong to no party or sect of Physicians." He added: "You have given in a few words the true theory of the action of mercury in the crisis [?] [of the] fever. It overcomes it by creating a less violent disease. Bloodletting acts only by weakening the force of the first poison upon the blood vessels, and thereby throws a balance of activity in favor of the mercury." If Truxtun profited from the doctor's advice, he apparently did not follow the suggestion that he publish the letter. He may well have believed that it would not help recruitment.[13] Whatever his feelings on that subject, the captain was no doubt relieved to learn that there would soon be medical advice close at hand.

To supply the needed medical men, the secretary of war drew upon the army. George Balfour of Virginia had entered the army in 1792 and had served under General Anthony Wayne in the Indian war in the Old Northwest. In February or early March 1798, Balfour took up his duties in the *Constellation*, where he was assisted by Surgeon's Mate Isaac Henry of Pennsylvania.[14] As a young doctor with a practice in Centerville, Kentucky, Henry's prospects must have seemed limited. We do know that as early as 1794, he had an interest in the new frigates and that he had been to see Congressman Alexander D. Orr of Kentucky. His efforts were rewarded and he was apparently appointed as a regimental warrant officer before formally becoming a surgeon's mate. He probably reported for duty in February or early March, about the same time as Surgeon Balfour.[15]

Now that medical men had been appointed, the secretary of war ordered Truxtun to begin recruiting men. At each recruiting rendezvous, before a sailor or marine could be signed up or paid, the surgeon or his mate was to examine him and certify to the recruiting officer that the man was "well organized, healthy, robust, and free from scorbutic and consumptive affections." Truxtun was told that it was the express orders of the president that the ship be made ready to sail on short notice.[16]

At Boston the third frigate was being readied for sea by Captain Samuel Nicholson. Here preparations were moving at a slower pace than at Philadelphia or Baltimore. According to Stephen Higginson, the navy agent at Boston, Nicholson was a rough and blustering sailor who lacked prudence, judgment, and reflection. These deficiencies were manifested also in the officers he appointed. As surgeon he chose William Read and as surgeon's mate, Charles Blake, both of Massachusetts. In Higginson's view "the Surgeon, Read, is the opposite of what he ought to be in Morals, in politics & in his profession. There is not a man in this Town who would trust the life of a dog in his hands. His second, Blake, is of the same cast of character as Read, but not so highly finished." According to Higginson, 19 of 20 of the steady citizens of Boston would agree with these characterizations.[17]

Had this devastating report arrived sooner, it might have caused Secretary McHenry to reconsider some of the medical officers. But it came too late. Orders issued on March 9, 1798, changed the status of the medical men assigned to the frigates: Gillasspy, Balfour, and Read were made surgeons in the navy in anticipation of legislation creating a separate Navy Department, while Bullus, Henry, and Blake became surgeon's mates.[18] The dual status of army surgeons was ended and the provisional appointments became permanent. All this was to the good. It was unfortunate, however that the three surgeons and the three mates all had the same date of appointment to the navy. No notice was taken of Gillasspy's seniority in office. Perhaps it was believed that the naval arm of national defense would be of only short duration. Possibly the War Department wished to sidestep that issue. But it is more likely that the officials did not think of the medical men in the same terms as the line officers, and for that matter neither did the doctors. Still, from an organizational point of view, it was unfortunate that no man was designated as the leader of his profession. As far as commissions were concerned, all three surgeons were on the same basis. No doubt few officials in the government had the time or disposition to reflect on such matters, for the deterioration of relations with France was pushing Congress to an increasingly militant stance.

On March 27, Congress appropriated additional funds and support for naval armament to complete and prepare for sea as soon as convenient the frigates *United States, Constitution,* and *Constellation.* Funds were also provided for the salaries of those in charge of the navy yards at Portsmouth, New Hampshire, Norfolk, Virginia, and New York.[19]

A month later, Congress passed an act providing for additional naval armament for the protection of U.S. trade. The president was authorized to build, purchase, or hire up to 12 vessels and have them armed and equipped. The additional officers and men were to receive the same pay and be governed by the same rules and regulations as those that applied to the frigates. Seamen and marines were to be enlisted for one year. During the recess of the Senate, the president could appoint and commission the officers needed.[20]

Another law was passed three days later which established a separate executive Department of the Navy to be headed by a secretary. Three weeks later, Benjamin Stoddert was appointed as the first secretary of the navy. Under his dynamic leadership, the work of building and manning a naval force and sending it to sea proceeded in earnest.[21]

Acting under the provisions of the law of March 27, the War Department purchased two merchant vessels, the *Ganges* and the *Hamburg Packet,* and converted them to naval use. Captain Richard Dale was ordered to command the *Ganges,* 24 guns, and in May he began recruiting men. Captain Stephen Decatur Sr. was given the command of the second ship, whose name was subsequently changed to *Delaware,* 20 guns. Since both ships were being readied at Philadelphia, it was natural that the secretary of war should call on Dr. Gillasspy to inspect their medical chests and report on their condition. He was also to confer with the surgeon of the *Ganges* and work with him in preparing an estimate of the medicines, hospital stores, and instruments needed for a three-month cruise. The surgeon of the *Ganges* was John Rush of Philadelphia, son of the famous Dr. Benjamin Rush; the surgeon's mate was John Parker. Both were commissioned on May 11.[22]

Orders issued to Captain Dale in May 1798 pointed out that since Congress had not yet declared war on France, naval operations would be limited to self-defense and the prevention of violations of national rights. Consequently, he was to cruise for three weeks between Long Island and the capes of Virginia, keeping watch over an area extending one marine league from land. Within these national waters he was to prevent any unlawful acts, defend or recapture any U.S. vessel that had been seized, and if his own ship was attacked, he was to retaliate. At the end of three weeks, he was to touch at the capes of the Delaware for further orders. So the *Ganges,* the most recent ship acquired by the navy, was the first to go to sea.[23]

Congress took the nation a step closer to war on May 28 when it authorized the seizure of any armed French vessels hovering off the coast for the purpose of committing depredations. President Adams promptly issued new orders to his captains. Dale was to proceed to Sandy Hook and convoy the barque *Adriana* to Philadelphia, after which he was to continue on to Cape Henlopen and Cape James. These were modest goals, but in pursuing them Dale found that many of the crew who had been signed on as seamen were really unskilled hands. This was a disappointment, for it would take some time to train them.[24]

While Dale struggled with his crew, Truxtun in the *Constellation* received a copy of the act of Congress and orders for sea service. He complained to the navy agent that his ship still needed food and supplies for the sick and wounded, which were being sent by the secretary. By June 19 the hospital stores were in the hands of the purser, who was to issue them to Dr. Balfour as he needed them. Truxtun put to sea and began to cruise between Cape Henry and the Georgia-Florida border. He had been at sea only a few days when he, too, complained about the number of inexperienced seamen under his command.[25]

In Philadelphia, Congress continued to take steps to prepare the United States for a conflict with France. On June 22 it authorized an increase in the Revenue Cutter Service for defense and the use of marines and navy seamen in them. The service had been the nation's first line of defense until the frigates authorized in 1797 were completed.[26] Small in size, crew, and armament, the cutters were inferior to even small privateers. By the end of 1797, only two were considered fit for service against the French. A second generation of cutters was now in the making. 10 new and larger ones were to built at eight designated ports. Most measured 180 tons, carried crews of 70, and were armed with 10 to 16 four- and six-pound guns. An exception was the *General Greene*, 11 guns, built at Baltimore. It measured 98 tons, had a crew of 34, and carried 10 four-pound cannon. Most of these new cutters were taken into the navy. On October 10, Stoddert notified the collectors of customs at the appropriate ports that henceforth designated cutters would be acting under his orders.[27]

Meanwhile on July 9, Congress had authorized the president to issue special commissions to the owners of private armed vessels, giving them the authority to seize and capture any armed French ship. Two days later a law establishing and organizing the Marine Corps was passed.[28] Given this pattern of legislative activity, it is small wonder that naval officers expected that war would be declared in the near future. It was not to be, but warlike activity was soon being reported.

The navy's first capture of a French vessel occurred on July 7, 1798, when the master of *La Croyable*, 12 guns, mistook the *Delaware* for a merchant ship and closed in for capture. When he realized his mistake, he thought he had met a British ship and sheared off and headed toward U.S. waters off Egg Harbor, New Jersey. Here the *Delaware* cornered the

French ship and forced it to surrender. The master protested the capture on the grounds that their two nations were not at war, but the captain of the *Delaware* was unmoved. Subsequently the *Delaware* was employed in more ambitious operations.[29]

On July 11, President Adams authorized the deployment of navy ships in the West Indies. Secretary Stoddert intended that a squadron consisting of the *United States*, the *Delaware*, and two other ships would cruise on the windward side of the islands of Barbados, Martinique, Guadaloupe, and Antigua. Delays prevented the two smaller ships from participating, and the *United States* and the *Delaware* departed. En route to the West Indies, Barry captured the French ship *Sans Pareil*, 10 guns, and off San Juan, Puerto Rico, the privateer sloop *La Jalouse*. In early September, Barry returned, with his two prizes, to the United States because the ship's provisions were rotten, his ship lacked ballast, the hurricane season in the West Indies was approaching, and the secretary expected him back. Stoddert was surprised and disappointed when Barry arrived at the Navy Department on September 21. Apparently he had forgotten his own earlier orders about the length of Barry's cruise. The secretary was not impressed by Barry's argument about the hurricane season, and apparently he did not consider the food situation in as serious a light as he should have.

Adding to Stoddert's disappointment was Barry's failure to act on a humanitarian problem. Barry was supposed to deliver two letters to the governor of Puerto Rico, one from the secretary of state and one from Stoddert, requesting the release of a number of American sailors who had been captured and placed on that island. Stoddert had heard that many of these men had suffered a great deal, and he believed that their relief and return ought to be matters of concern to the U.S. government and its officers. But Barry's eyes were on the capture of enemy ships and not on his unfortunate countrymen. He made no effort to contact the governor of Puerto Rico. The ultimate fate of the men is not known; presumably they were repatriated at the end of the war.[30]

Gradually the purpose of deploying ships shifted from guarding the U.S. coasts to active operations in the West Indies. Here the navy guarded convoys of merchant ships and cruised in search of prizes. By the winter of 1798–99, Stoddert had a number of ships operating in designated areas.[31]

Captain Alexander Murray in the *Montezuma*, 20 guns, learned that Stoddert expected Barry to cruise off the northern coast of South America, but since he was not doing so, Murray decided to do it on his own. He touched at Curaçao, took a convoy north and through the Mona Passage between Santo Domingo and Puerto Rico, then sailed off the northern coast of Hispaniola. Here he met the revenue cutter *South Carolina*, 12

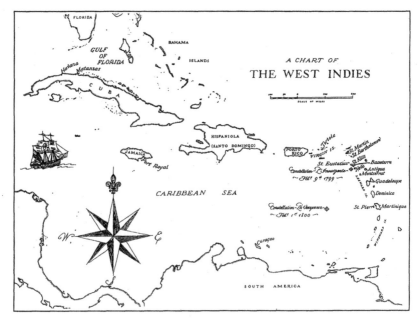

Map of the West Indies during the Quasi-War with France.

guns, under Captain James Payne, who was searching for the *Ganges.* Murray ordered Payne to join him. Together they searched the northern and western coasts of Santo Domingo for French prizes, then sailed for Kingston, Jamaica, where a convoy of merchant ships was organized. Murray sent Payne in the *South Carolina* to Havana, Cuba, to organize another convoy from that port, assisted by Captain Decatur. All was ready by the time Murray arrived off Havana with the ships from Jamaica. The combined convoys, numbering 57 ships, then sailed for the United States with their naval escort. When Murray reported his arrival off New Castle, Delaware, on April 30, 1799, he had completed one of the longest cruises during the Quasi-War. It was also a comparatively healthy one. Four marines died of fever in the West Indies; Murray had a touch of yellow fever and some of his crew were ill, possibly from the same malady.[32]

While the ship was in quarantine at New Castle, Stoddert urged Murray to give his men vegetables and fresh provisions. The secretary himself undertook to rush barrels of beef and pork to Murray, telling the navy agents at New York to give Murray as much meat as he needed. Murray was informed that the men were to be given recreation and made as comfortable as possible. These were well-deserved rewards for a crew whose commander had greatly pleased the secretary and the president.

But when the *Montezuma* was again ready for sea, Murray was too ill to go, and the command went to Lieutenant John Mullowny. By June, Murray had recovered and he was given command of a frigate.[33] These dispositions were the beginnings of Stoddert's efforts to protect U.S. commerce and bring the war to the enemy's colonial territory. As the war continued, ships were rotated and U.S. officers and seamen acquired additional experience. There were several armed clashes between French and U.S. ships, the most famous of which were the victories of the *Constellation* over the frigate *L'Insurgente* on February 9, 1799 and the frigate *La Vengeance* on February 1, 1800. But for many, the war would consist of convoy duty and relatively uneventful cruises. They are important for this study, however, for what they can tell us of the climatic conditions and health environment of the navy ships. President Adams was determined to limit the conflict, and after Napoleon came to power in France in November 1799, he too was interested in ending the undeclared war. In March 1800 a three-man U.S. peace commission began talks with their French counterparts. At the end of September, a treaty was signed, and it was ratified by the Senate in December 1801.[34]

American Medicine in the Late Eighteenth Century

A few colonists who could afford to do so went to Europe to study medicine at hospitals in London or Edinburgh, or to the University at Leyden, in the Netherlands. They might enroll in a full program of study and earn a degree or simply undertake a few months of course work or hospital experience. Those with even a small amount of European training could practice medicine back home in the same way as those with degrees. So the quantity and quality of professional medicine in the colonies was on a par with that in the mother country even though there were few practitioners with medical degrees in either setting.

This situation led a group of American medical students in London and Edinburgh during the years 1760–67 to decide that upon their return they would work to establish professional medical schools in their own country. John Morgan, William Shippen, and Arthur Lee were instrumental in persuading the College of Philadelphia (later the University of Pennsylvania) to establish a medical department, which began classes in 1765. Three years later the school awarded 10 bachelor of medicine degrees—more than the number of Americans who had graduated from Edinburgh in any single year. Meanwhile a second medical school was opened at King's College (later Columbia) in 1767. Subsequently other medical schools were established at Harvard College in 1782 and at Dartmouth in 1797.

29

Important as these educational advances were, the vast majority of physicians were still being trained by apprenticeship to a doctor. While individual contracts varied, an apprentice was usually expected to gather and compound herbs for medicines, deliver medicines to patients, collect the bills owed, and help the doctor with various tasks such as bleeding patients. Some colonial American physicians might be consulted in difficult obstetrical cases. Usually a medical practice alone was not enough to support a doctor, so he supplemented his income by keeping an apothecary shop or engaging in some other business such as the law. If he ran an apothecary shop, he sold medicines to his own patients as well as others. He was also in competition with full-time apothecaries, who sometimes acted as physicians by treating fevers and rashes, as well as with laymen and itinerant doctors, healers, and surgeon-dentists, some of whom were quacks.

In an effort to improve themselves, set fee tables, and prevent quacks and one another from competitive price cutting, doctors worked to organize professional groups. The earliest of these was the Medical Society of New Jersey, founded in 1762, which persuaded the colonial legislature to enact a law in 1772 requiring that physicians be examined by a board of medical men and licensed by the courts before practicing in the colony. Other societies were organized at the local or county level. By the late eighteenth century, the New Hampshire Medical Society forbade doctors to sell drugs.[35]

Along with improvements in the training of physicians came the establishment of new hospitals in Philadelphia in 1752 and New York in 1767, which were patterned after the hospital in Edinburgh. The U.S. hospitals provided opportunities for doctors to observe, practice, and teach, and appointments to the staff were much sought after. Those appointed were usually very able and public-spirited individuals who gave prestige to the hospital and whose own reputations were enhanced by the association with it.[36]

A medical theory dating back to the ancient Greeks held that the body was healthy when its four liquid humors—blood, phlegm, yellow bile, and black bile—were in balance. If they were not, ill health or disease would result. Those symptoms that we associate today with a "cold" would have been interpreted as representing an excess of coldness or phlegm, the evidence of which would be a runny nose and absence of a fever even in the presence of other febrile symptoms. The relationship of the humoral theory to the four seasons of the year and the four elements known to ancient peoples (fire, water, air, and earth) made it seem logical and acceptable. Advances in medical knowledge, such as the discovery of how the blood circulated, were grafted onto the earlier theory.

By the late eighteenth century, a new concept for interpreting symptoms was also being applied. This is now called solidism, to differentiate it from humoralism. It focused on the tone, strength, and elasticity of the solid portion of the blood vessels and nerves, as well as on the humors. Both arteries and nerves were considered to be hollow tubes that propel their contents through the body with forces proportional to the strength of the fibers in the tube walls. When the body was healthy, blood, urine, feces, sweat, and the fluids believed to flow through nerves were assumed to be moving freely. Obstructions to the flow of these body or nerve fluids, some of which were the humors, were thought to represent imbalances in the tone of the passageway through which they flowed, resulting in illness. Most illnesses could be interpreted simultaneously in terms of both the humoral and solidist theories. For example, a prolonged constriction of the intestines would result in constipation. Jaundice accompanied by fever might be interpreted as the result of an obstruction of the ducts through which the bile passed from the liver into the duodenum. Doctors tried to correlate their patients' symptoms and physical signs with imbalances in their humors and tones. For instance, the pulse was regarded as an index of the activity of the fibers of the cardiovascular system through which blood flows. If the pulse was slow or weak, the doctor concluded that the vascular fibers were weak or lax. If the pulse was fast, the physician deduced that the vascular fibers were hyperactive and that fever was present, for hyperactivity produced heat.

Having diagnosed his patient's problem, the doctor proceeded to treat it. He had at his disposal some 225 drugs that were prepared from about 100 different putatively active ingredients. Modern research on the therapeutic methods used by physicians in late-eighteenth-century New England (which were probably used throughout the country) shows that the most commonly prescribed drugs were cathartics, used to stimulate the intestinal tract to evacuate disease-producing materials and abnormal humors. Calomel (mercurous chloride), castor oil and jalap were among the drugs most commonly used for this purpose.

The second most commonly prescribed remedies were tonics, drugs that were thought to strengthen body tissues when they had been weakened by disease. Peruvian bark, Virginia snakeroot, and several spices were among the standard tonics. Peruvian bark, now known to contain quinine, was widely used as a tonic in the treatment of malaria as well as other types of fever.

Material that had caused the imbalance of the humors might also be eliminated by emptying the stomach with emetics, especially ipecac and tartar emetic (antimony potassium tartrate). Similarly, diuretic salt (potassium acetate) was used to increase the secretion and flow of urine. Diuretics were also used to promote the absorption of fluid by vessels throughout the body so that it could be eliminated via the kidneys. Diaphoretics such as antimony salts were drugs that stimulated increased perspiration.

The principal narcotic was opium, administered in pill form or in alcohol solutions such as laudanum. It was prescribed chiefly for the control of diarrhea, but also for pain and to induce sleep. Astringents, such as lime water, were thought to condense the solids of arteries and nerves to reduce abnormal losses of heat, fluid, and other secretions.

Patients who were severely ill might be treated with blistering agents or by bleeding. To raise a blister the physician applied an alcohol solution of cantharides (powdered Spanish flies) directly to the skin so that pus and other noxious materials, including foul humors, could escape from the body into the resulting blister fluid. Cantharides were also thought to counterirritate underlying tissues so as to neutralize the more serious naturally induced irritation that was causing pain and putrefaction. Thus cantharides were sometimes prescribed for the treatment of pneumonia accompanied by chest pain.

Another treatment for severe febrile illness was bleeding. It was usually performed only if the pulse of the patient was full and strong. The amount of blood removed at one time was between 8 and 20 ounces, the average being about 12 ounces.

Eighteenth-century physicians thus saw the body in terms of mutually dependent parts that were interconnected through the humors and the vascular and nerve fibers. They directed their attention toward regulating tensions and secretions within the body. The same diagnosis might be treated in different ways, each taking into account the changing tensions and secretions of the particular patient at hand.

New England physicians provided emergency surgical care when necessary. This included dressing wounds and reducing fractures and dislocations. Many preferred to limit themselves to simple procedures, while others chose to improve their operating skills. Surgery was just beginning to emerge as a specialty, and for those who were willing to do complex operations, several European textbooks gave detailed information on many procedures, although the abdominal and thoracic cavities were off limits until the late nineteenth century. Amputation of limbs as a result of wounds, injuries, and frostbite that had become gangrenous was not uncommon, although postoperative mortality rates ranged from 0 to 62 percent. The most newsworthy operations of the era were cataract extractions and the removal of bladder stones.

Despite the physician's best efforts, however, some of his patients died. When they did, autopsies, occasionally at the patient's own request, helped some New England physicians to determine the exact cause of death.

The most common cause of death in late-eighteenth-century America was tuberculosis, then called consumption. It accounted for 20–25 percent of the deaths in most communities on both sides of the Atlantic. Pneumonia, influenza, and other respiratory diseases resulted in another 5 percent of deaths. While yellow fever was nearly unknown in New England and malaria (then called intermittent fever) was uncommon there, both were common in the Mid-Atlantic and southern colonies. Other fevers were known, by the increasing order of their clinical severity and special signs, as slow, nervous, petechial, typhus (or ship or jail fever), and malignant fevers. Bilious fever and colic were usually accompanied by jaundice. Epidemics of smallpox killed many, especially in port cities. Diseases such as measles, scarlet fever, diphtheria, whooping cough, and croup caused the deaths of many children. Deaths that were probably due to cardiovascular diseases, stroke, or cancer were ascribed to "atrophy," the "decay of nature," or "old age," or referred to as "sudden." Accidents, such as falls, scaldings, drownings, freezings, opium overdoses, and being run over by carriages also took their toll of Americans.[37]

The first major technique for preventing any disease was given its initial largescale trial in Boston in the winter of 1721–22. Inoculation (or variolation) for smallpox was done by taking pus from the pustules on a smallpox patient and inserting it into the skin of a healthy person, who would then develop a mild case of smallpox. When the patient recovered, he or she would usually be immune to any future encounter with smallpox. Of course, much depended on how active the infecting virus was. Because there was a risk in the procedure, inoculations were usually not allowed by civil authorities unless there was an outbreak of the disease. Those physicians who gave a large number of inoculations did so in houses located on the outskirts of major towns so as not to put the entire community at risk. Persons who subjected themselves to the procedure remained under the doctor's care for six weeks, until they recovered from the disease and were no longer infective. Inoculation was so safe and effective as prophylaxis against smallpox that George Washington caused his Continental army to become the world's first military force to be protected against the predictable ravages of this disease.

In 1796, Dr. Edward Jenner began to vaccinate people in rural England with cowpox, which also made them immune to smallpox. Two years later he described his method in his book *An Inquiry Into the Causes and Effect of the Variolae Vaccine*. Dr. Benjamin Waterhouse of Boston soon received a copy, and he published a summary of it in a Boston newspaper. Jenner sent Waterhouse a supply of the cowpox vaccine, and in July 1800 he vaccinated his son and six other persons. Having satisfied himself that the new procedure worked, Waterhouse tried to establish a monopoly for distributing the vaccine in the United States in return for one-quarter of the profits derived from its use. His scheme collapsed when other U.S. physicians began receiving their own supplies from England. As the use of the vaccination procedure spread throughout the country, so did discussion of when and how it could be used in the navy.[38]

Medical Men for the Growing Navy

The rapid expansion and deployment of the naval force required the services of a number of medical officers. Between June and December 1798, nine additional surgeons, one temporary surgeon, and six more surgeon's mates were appointed.[39] The need was urgent, and it was customary for the navy agent at the port where a ship was being prepared for sea to submit to the secretary of the navy the names of doctors who were willing to serve. These were routinely approved, and commissions followed, usually after Senate confirmation. For someone seeking an appointment, a visit to the Navy Department could do wonders. Samuel Anderson called to apply for a position as a surgeon's mate. Stoddert told him that the appointment would take two or three days, by which time he would have missed the departure of the *Delaware,* to which he would be assigned. The secretary therefore suggested, "If you will immediately proceed after the Ship, & enter upon the duties of Surgeon's Mate, I can present your Name to the President for that Appointment, and there can be no doubt of your receiving it." Anderson took this advice, and his appointment dated from July 2, 1798, the day he visited the Navy Department.[40]

The service also lost two doctors during this early period of the war. Surgeon William Read, about whom Navy Agent Stephen Higginson was so concerned, was stricken by a fever and died in Norfolk on September 26, 1798. Another casualty was Surgeon's Mate John Hart, appointed September 10, who died on October 3.[41]

As the undeclared war continued, so did the demand for ships, men, and doctors. During 1799 the names of 21 surgeon's mates and 25 surgeons were added to the rolls. Among the surgeons, eight of the commissions were promotions for men who had previously served as surgeon's mates: Isaac Henry of Pennsylvania, previously of the *Constellation;* Hanson Catlett of Maryland, who had served in the *Montezuma* and the *Baltimore;* Henry Wells, whose time in the *Baltimore* marked him as a man of great merit; John Bullus, who had served in the *United States* and in the captured French frigate *L'Insurgente*, the name of which was Anglicized to *Insurgente*. The first three of these doctors were promoted in less than a year. Opportunities for advancement were also excellent for three doctors who began as surgeon's mates in 1799 and became surgeons before the year was out. Another of the men who entered as a surgeon's mate in 1798 and was now promoted was Henry Wells, who practiced in the *Baltimore,* the *Norfolk,* and the *Insurgente.*[42]

Few biographical details exist for most of the early navy doctors, and fewer still on their medical training. Among the newly recruited surgeons, however, were two who had their undergraduate training at Harvard: Hector Orr, who received his B.A. in 1792, and Benjamin Vinton, who graduated in 1795. Orr was commissioned on February 28 and served in the frigate *Essex,* 32 guns. Vinton, who was also from Massachusetts, received his commission on May 22 and served in the frigate *Boston,* 28 guns.[43] Much more is known about two of the surgeons appointed in 1799, who were veterans of the American Revolution. Peter St. Medard was born and educated in Europe and came to the United States during the Revolution, settling in Boston. Later in the war he served as a surgeon's mate in the frigate *Providence* and as a surgeon in the frigate *Dean.* He joined the U.S. Navy during the Quasi-War in response to an invitation from his old commander, Captain Samuel Nicholson, of the *Constitution.* Accepting a temporary appointment, and replacing Surgeon William Read, St. Medard began duty on December 17, 1798 and was formally commissioned on July 14, 1799. It was the beginning of a long and honorable career in the navy.[44]

Another veteran of the Revolution, whose career stands in sharp contrast to that of St. Medard, was Massachusetts-born Amos Windship. Harvard educated and with a medical apprenticeship under Dr. Ezekiel Hersey of Hingham, he practiced in Wellfleet, Nantucket, and Boston. During the Revolution he worked in a general hospital in Cambridge before becoming a surgeon's mate and then a surgeon in the state's brig-of-war, *Massachusetts.* The year 1779 found him serving as a surgeon under John Paul Jones in the frigate *Alliance.* After the war he established himself as an apothecary in Boston, then practiced medicine in Penobscot (then part of Massachusetts but now in Maine), before going back to a partnership with a wholesaler in Boston. Bad luck and poor judgment were in evidence in most of his enterprises. In 1799, at the age of 54, he entered the U.S. Navy as a surgeon and was assigned to the ship *Herald,* 18 guns. While on duty in the West Indies, he deserted and returned to Boston, pleading illness. Subsequently he was brought before a court-martialed on charges

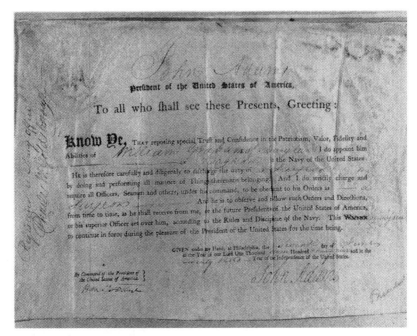

Commission of Surgeon William Graham of Maryland, 1799. The Historical Society of Pennsylvania.

of drunkenness, embezzling and selling medicines, and desertion. His case is discussed in the next section of this chapter.[45]

On the plus side of the medical ledger is the career of Philadelphia-born Edward Cutbush. At the age of 12, he entered the Philadelphia College, but two years later financial difficulties in the family forced him to drop out. His mother died in 1789 and his father a year later. Through friends of his father, he secured a position as a medical student at the Pennsylvania Hospital, where in 1793 he had the opportunity to study the treatment of the battle wounds of a number of British and French seamen. These men were the victims of an encounter between British and French ships off the capes of the Delaware during the war growing out of the French Revolution. It was an unusual and beneficial experience for a budding physician.

When Cutbush graduated from the hospital in 1794, Benjamin Rush was one of the men who signed his diploma. Cutbush opened an office in Philadelphia and began his medical practice. Soon the city and state were caught up in the excitement generated by the "Whisky Rebellion," a tax revolt by the farmers in western Pennsylvania which caused the federal government to call out the militia of several states. Cutbush was offered the position of hospital surgeon with the Pennsylvania militia, and he eagerly accepted it, later becoming the surgeon general of the Pennsylvania line. When the so-called rebellion was put down and Cutbush returned to his practice in Philadelphia, he found that his brief experience with military life had cost him the friendship and patronage of his Quaker friends. Nevertheless, he persevered and was successful enough to be able to marry in 1795. Still, it was not easy, and when the Quasi-War with France came, a new career possibility presented itself. Cutbush was quick to seize the opportunity. Appointed a surgeon on May 28, 1799, he succeeded Gillasspy in the frigate *United States* on a cruise from Hampton Roads, Virginia, to St. Mary's, Georgia, and back. So began a naval career that was to last 30 years.[46]

There were promising candidates among the 21 surgeon's mates commissioned in 1799. The first of these was Richard C. Shannon of New Hampshire, who began serving in the revenue cutter *Scammel*, 14 guns, on January 1, but whose appointment as a mate was not confirmed until July 5 of the same year. In October he became a surgeon. Promotion was rapid also for Benjamin Shurtleff of Massachusetts, who began his duties as a surgeon's mate in the *Merrimack*, 24 guns, on December 22, 1798, but was not commissioned until February 5, 1799. By the time he had served a year, he was a surgeon. A third physician who experienced a quick rise was Daniel Hughes. Assigned to the *Ganges* to succeed John Rush, he was commissioned on March 5, 1799, and the following December he became a surgeon.

Of the surgeon's mates appointed in 1799, one destined to have a long career in the navy was Samuel L. Marshall of Pennsylvania. Commissioned as a mate on May 14, 1799, he first served with Cutbush in the frigate *United States* and later in the brig *Richmond*, 18 guns, and the frigate *Congress*, 36 guns. Tobias Watkins of Maryland had a long career in medicine that included service in both the navy and the army. After graduating from St. John's College in Annapolis in 1798, he became a surgeon's mate in the navy at the age of 19 and served in the *Baltimore*. He resigned his commission in 1801 and entered the Philadelphia Medical College, from which he graduated in 1802. Adolph C. Lent of New York entered the navy in 1799 with impressive credentials: he was awarded a B.A. by Columbia in 1795 and received both M.A. and M.D. degrees from that institution in 1798. A commission as surgeon's mate was granted him on January 7, 1799, but dated from December 31 of the previous year. Lent served first in the revenue cutter *Governor Jay*, 14 guns, and later in the frigate *Adams*, 28 guns. Apparently he did not enjoy naval service and resigned his commission in August 1799.[47]

There was one other person who performed the duties of a surgeon's mate beginning in 1799 but who never received any official confirmation for such work. This was Midshipman William Dunn, who had been educated as a physician and surgeon and who had served in the British navy as a surgeon's mate. Captain Silas Talbot appointed him an acting surgeon's mate on September 3, 1799. He seems to have continued to serve in this capacity until his discharge on August 6, 1801, but there is no record of a commission as a mate.[48] Dunn's experience and an examination of some extant muster lists indicates that while the laws of 1794 and 1797 anticipated that frigates would carry one surgeon and two mates, in reality not all did so. Apparently it was not always possible to get two mates, and most frigates operated with only one.

In 1800, 3 surgeon's mates were promoted to surgeon and 3 new men were appointed as surgeons. There were also 22 new surgeon's mates appointed plus one temporary appointment to that rank. One candidate declined the appointment as a surgeon's mate.[49] Among the incoming surgeon's mates was Jonathan Cowdery of New York, son of Dr. Jabez Cowdery, who practiced in Tunbridge, Vermont, and Sandisfield, Berkshire County, Massachusetts. Jonathan was born in Sandisfield on April 22, 1767 and presumably received his medical education in some sort of quasi apprenticeship to his father. During two winters he attended lectures at Dartmouth, in Hanover, New Hampshire. He married in 1789 and for six years lived and practiced in Massachusetts, Connecticut, and New York. When his wife died in 1796, he was left with two sons under the age of seven. Leaving them in the custody of his mother, Jonathan practiced medicine in Hudson, New York, until he received his appointment as a surgeon's mate on January 1, 1800. Assigned to the frigate *Philadelphia*, he saw service in the Caribbean during the Quasi War. This was the beginning of a long career in the U.S. Navy.[50]

One of the new surgeons who had only a brief tenure during the Quasi-War but who would later become important was Walter W. Buchanan of New York. He left his appointment on the medical faculty of Columbia College for the navy. His medical knowledge was broadened by his service on the USS *Ganges*.[51]

By 1801 the end of the war appeared to be in sight, and only four surgeon's mates were added to the navy; however, one was only an acting appointment, and another was not commissioned because the war ended.[52] Of those appointed in 1801, one is especially worthy of notice: Lewis Heermann of Virginia. Born in Cassel, Germany, in 1779, he inherited a considerable estate in Hesse-Cassel. Nothing is known of his medical education in Europe, but he probably studied for a time under

Dr. John Haighton, an English physician and physiologist who lectured at St. Thomas's and Guy's hospitals in London. It is not known when he arrived in the United States, but presumably not long after this he dropped his baptismal name of Adolph Ludwig and became Lewis. Slightly more than a month after he reached the age of 22 he was appointed as a surgeon's mate, but he was not commissioned until February 8, 1802. Apparently he saw no active service at sea during the Quasi-War, but in the years that followed, he would become an influential officer.[53]

The Naval Environment

After a surgeon or mate reported to his first ship and made the acquaintance of the captain and other officers, it was usually not long before he was called upon to examine recruits. The orders were clear about the type of men wanted: healthy, robust, and "well-organized" men who were free from scorbutic and consumptive afflictions. Requirements for prospective marines were more strict. No negro, mulatto, or Indian was to be enlisted, and no foreigners unless they were clearly men of sobriety and fidelity. The men selected had to measure at least five feet six inches in their stocking feet and be between the ages of 18 and 40. A prospective marine had to be able to stand the rigors of a soldier's life. No indirect means was to be used to inveigle the men into joining, and no one was to be enlisted while intoxicated.[54]

Despite these requirements, there is no indication that navy doctors made the men remove their clothes. In the civilian world, a doctor's appraisal was based largely on what he was told and what he observed by feeling muscles and tissue through the patient's clothing. The general appearance of the body, especially the hands and face, was important, and signs of a disease might also be detected there, as well as in the patient's posture, gait, speech and breathing. The mouth and teeth were also indications of health. There is no indication that similar practices were not followed in the navy. Tattoos were a means of identification and were noted on many of the protection certificates that many seamen carried to show their nationality. It is very likely that shirts were removed to expose tattoos, but it is not clear that this was done for medical examinations, especially since the stethoscope was not common in the United States until the 1850s.[55]

Officers and men joining a ship entered a very restricted environment, and adjusting to its size must have been a problem. The ships used during the Quasi-War ranged in size from galleys and sloops to frigates, with a variety of dimensions even within the same class. For the length and beam (or width) of the early frigates, the dimensions in feet and inches ranged from 118' × 37' for the *Essex;* 124' 3" × 34' 8" for the *General Greene;* and 136' × 40 ½' for the *Constellation;* to 175' × 43 ½' for the *Constitution.* A similar range prevailed in the next larger vessels, classified as ships: the *Delaware* was 94' 9" × 28'; the *George Washington* 108' × 32 ½'; and the *Ganges* 116' 4" × 31' 4". We do not know about the interior arrangements of most of the ships used in the Quasi-War. The *Constitution* survives, and though it has been rebuilt many times, its existing configuration and plans provide a useful insight into the shipboard environment. It must be borne in mind that the *Constitution* was one of the largest ships of the Quasi-War navy and that in other vessels the living and working spaces were even more confined.[56]

When reporting on board, the surgeon or mate stepped on to the spar deck, where he would see cannon positioned at intervals along the deck and the masts, yardarms, and rigging overhead. Exposed as it was to the air, the spar deck was the place of exercise for all the ship's company. The aft part of the spar deck was partitioned off to form the captain's cabin, which was ventilated by large windows over the stern and the rear sides. On the forward part of the spar deck a triangular area was partitioned off to form the forecastle, where some of the crew lived. Forward of this, at the bow and under the bowsprit, was the exposed head, or privy, one of several on board.

In a frigate, the first deck below the spar deck was known as the gun deck. Along both sides of it cannon on wooden carriages were positioned at gun ports. Many of the crew slept here in hammocks slung adjacent to the guns. During the day they might be engaged in gun drills here or have other duties elsewhere. Hatches in the deck above provided some ventilation and light, as did the gun ports, when open. But in bad weather the gun ports and hatches would be closed and the area would become cold and damp. To help alleviate these conditions, hot coals or heated shot were placed on beds of sand in special heating pots that were hung overhead.

The next level below the gun deck was the berth deck. In ships smaller than a frigate, which had no gun deck, the berth deck was the second one down. Much of the berth deck was occupied by the crew when off duty. With no gun ports along the side, the hatchways were the principal source of ventilation, and fresh air was in short supply, especially in rough and stormy weather. In pleasant weather a captain would rig a wind sail on deck to divert air into an open hatchway. The wind sail was probably of some help in bringing air and warmth to the berth deck, but it was of little use on the orlop or next lower deck. The aft part of the berth deck was partitioned to form the wardroom, where off-duty officers relaxed and took

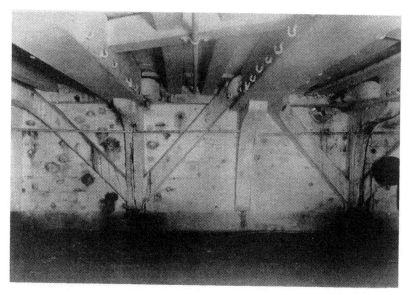

**Sick Bay of the USS *Constitution* as It Appeared in 1914. Naval Histori-
cal Center, Washington, D.C.**

their meals. Approaching the wardroom and along each side of the ship
were small staterooms for the ship's officers. In the case of the *Constitution,* the surgeon's stateroom was on the port side and measures approximately 7' × 6 ½' and there is a 6' overhead. Furnishings consisted of a
small table, a chair, and a hanging cot. A small porthole gave a little light
and some ventilation. After sundown a candle provided the only light in
the room. All the way forward on the berth deck was the sick bay, a
triangular area 18' long at the center line and 30' at the widest part, with an
overhead space of 6'.

The fourth deck down in a frigate was the orlop deck. In smaller ships it
was the space below the berth deck. This was below the waterline, dark,
and poorly ventilated. To improve the air supply, experiments were made
with primitive types of ventilator, which, at the time of the Quasi-War,
probably consisted of a system of pipes and hand-operated bellows. About
midway between the main and mizzen masts on the orlop deck was the
cockpit. In the *Constitution* this space measures 13' × 8' and has an overhead of 4' 10". It was an area less subject to motion and less likely to be
penetrated by enemy shot. When a ship was preparing for battle, nearby
mess chests would be assembled to serve as an operating table and a place
for setting out instruments. The area was lit by overhead lanterns containing as many candles as the surgeon could procure from the first lieutenant.

Wounded men were carried from the spar or gun deck down through the hatches to the cockpit for treatment. Adjacent was the dispensary or medical storeroom, which in the *Constitution* is 6' × 9 ½', with an overhead of 4' 10". On each side of the cockpit were two staterooms measuring 6 ½' × 5 ½', with the same low overhead. Two of these rooms were occupied by the surgeon's mates.

Below the orlop deck was the hold, which was used for storage. All the way aft was the powder magazine. Next came the sail room and the spirit room, where rum and later whiskey, constituting the spirit part of the ration issued to the men twice a day, was stored. Also kept in this area were the ship's supplies of molasses, vinegar, cheese, and other provisions. This was a damp and poorly ventilated area that was often infested with rats, which gnawed at the food and contaminated it with their feces and thus were a source of illness. While the *Constellation* was being prepared for sea, Truxtun wrote frequently to the secretary of the navy about the need for ventilators. These had not arrived when the frigate sailed in early June 1798. Subsequently Truxtun wrote to the secretary from Hampton Roads that the lack of ventilators had caused many stores to spoil. Had they been installed earlier, they would have saved double their costs in stores.[57]

Discipline, Courts-Martial, and Discharges

In addition to the confining atmosphere, navy doctors had to adjust to the discipline of the ship and the personalities of the captain and other officers. For some it was an easy transition. Surgeon George Gillasspy formed close and personal ties with Captain Barry very early, and no doubt this eased his relations with the other officers. Others seem to have found the adjustment more difficult. But it was essential that medical officers reach out and try to establish their personal and professional credibility with the captain. There was a clear distinction between the officers who were directly concerned with the working of the ship and those, such as the purser, the medical men, and the chaplain, whose duties were more concerned with the enlisted men. By the fourth decade of the nineteenth century, the distinctions between line and staff officers on matters of rank and precedence were creating problems for various secretaries of the navy. During the Quasi-War patterns and traditions were being established, usually in accordance with practices in the Royal Navy. Captain Thomas Truxtun had his officers dine at his table in accordance with a rigid schedule, the same group on the same night of the week.[58] Other officers may have been less rigid and less concerned about building a tradition. If more casual arrangements prevailed in some ships, the memory of them has not survived. Professional men who were older and had enjoyed some degree of prominence in their hometowns must have found the adjustment to rank and precedence a bit demeaning. Younger men who were new to the medical field and medicine had to learn to think in different ways very quickly. As Surgeon's Mate Isaac Henry wrote to his father, "I am a mere atom blown about by the breath of my Commander—I have given up all Idea of thinking or acting for myself."[59]

Under the best of captains, the nature of the naval duties in the Quasi-War could lead to boredom, frustration, and irritation. Men found relief and temporary solace in alcohol, but overindulgence could bring on other and more serious problems. One of the first surgeons to run afoul of naval discipline and be tried by a court-martial was Amos Windship. He was charged with drunkenness, selling the ship's medicines and appropriating the money for his own use, and leaving his ship in the West Indies without permission. Windship denied that he was drunk, claiming he had not had a drink in eight months. The court-martial did not find him guilty on this charge. On the matter of selling medicines, he claimed that what he did was to exchange medicines he did not need for those that were required and that in this exchange the government was the beneficiary. Two navy surgeons testified that there were no deficiencies in the contents of Windship's medical chest. Indeed, there was a slight surplus in one of the categories. As for leaving the ship, Windship said that he was in ill health and that his decision to depart from the West Indies had been endorsed by another physician. He produced certificates confirming his illness from two doctors who saw him after he returned to the United States. He went on to say that he was in trouble now because he had caught one of the junior officers taking hospital stores and had forbidden him to come to the cockpit in the future. Evidently the court did not believe him, for he was found guilty of leaving his ship without permission and of selling medical stores. He was dismissed from the navy in May 1801.[60]

Another doctor who found himself in difficulties was Hanson Catlett, surgeon of the sloop of war *Baltimore*. He was tried in 1801 for embezzlement of hospital stores, mutinous conduct, and drunkenness. According to Captain William Cowper, the surgeon purchased hospital stores without his authorization and used them for himself. The items consisted of coffee, wines, brandy, chocolate, a keg of tripe, paper, and stationery. Catlett said that these were purchased for his patients, and except for small amounts, used by them. This was confirmed in part by Surgeon's Mate Tobias Watkins. The court found that there was no proof of embezzlement.

To support the charge of mutinous conduct, the captain said that the doctor had abused and insulted him on the quarter-deck, called him a rascal, scoundrel, and similar expressions, and made several attempts to strike him. Finally the captain struck the doctor with a speaking trumpet, placed him under arrest, and had him transferred to a ship bound for the United States. Midshipman William Suggs gave the court some background on the quarrel. It seems that Surgeon's Mate Watkins and the captain's clerk were drinking wine in the wardroom and were making a great deal of noise. The captain sent a lieutenant to tell them to move to the other side of the wardroom and be quiet. They complied and were joined by Doctor Catlett, who had just left his quarters on the opposite side of the ship. At this point Captain Cowper came below and told the surgeon that he would not allow such conduct on his ship. Catlett demanded an explanation of the remark, and the captain ordered him to his cabin. Instead Catlett followed the captain to the deck, where strong words and the blow with the speaking trumpet followed. It was also stated that on an earlier occasion when Catlett was intoxicated, he had got into a fight with a marine lieutenant: knives and swords had been drawn by both parties, but according to a witness, only blows and abusive language had been exchanged. As far as the court was concerned, however, the charge against Catlett of mutinous conduct was proved.

On the charge of drunkenness, the captain stated that when a boatswain suffered a head wound during a cruise in the West Indies, Catlett was too drunk to dress the wound, and Surgeon's Mate Watkins did the job. The captain charged that the boatswain had a fractured skull, but Watkins said that the wound was only a superficial cut and not in the least dangerous. On another occasion when drunk, Dr. Catlett was accused of making a great deal of noise and of acting "in a very ungentlemanly and unofficerlike manner." Catlett reportedly said that all religion was nonsense, damned Jesus Christ, and used offensive language about the Virgin Mary that was heard by servants and members of the crew who waited on the wardroom officers. The captain tried in vain to reason with him. Witnesses did not support the captain's charges of irreligious sentiments. The court found Catlett guilty of drunkenness on only one occasion when he could not treat a patient. Therefore, on the basis of guilty findings on the charges of mutinous conduct and drunkenness, the court sentenced the surgeon to be dismissed from the service. Because of mitigating circumstances, it recommended that he receive full pay and rations and reasonable expenses until his dismissal.

When the findings of the court-martial were reviewed by President John Adams, he approved the conclusions in regard to the charges of embezzlement and drunkenness, but not that of mutinous conduct. Adams said that the evidence did not support the conclusion, adding, "The conduct of

Doctor Catlett appears to have originated more from inexperience & juvenile indiscretions, than from a litigious disposition, or disinclination to the service of his country." Adams ordered that proceedings against Catlett be ended and that he be released from arrest. Catlett was restored to duty in February 1801 but was discharged in April of that year in a reduction in force that followed the end of the Quasi-War. Captain Cowper was also discharged in April.[61]

Reference has already been made to the problems in the frigate *Congress* which took place following its damage during a severe storm. Captain James Sever nipped a mutiny in the bud, but he continued to have problems with his officers. It was in this atmosphere that Surgeon Larkin Thorndike committed suicide. His death must have come as a great shock to his colleague, Surgeon's Mate Edward Field. It also added to the burdens that Field had to take on with an injured hand. A new surgeon, Dr. Samuel R. Marshall, was sent to the ship, then in the West Indies. When he arrived, he found low morale among the officers. In January 1801, Marshall wrote to the captain requesting that he consider releasing an officer who had been in confinement for a few days. Captain Sever chose to regard this letter as improper interference, and the incident became the first in a series of charges that Sever later leveled against the surgeon.

When the bill of particulars was delivered to Marshall four months later, the surgeon found himself charged with improper interference in the arrest and confinement of an officer; using expressions on the quarter-deck that tended to excite discontent, dissatisfaction, and mutiny in the minds of the crew; sending a letter to the captain "replete with menacing, insolent, and disrespectful language"; using language in the wardroom that expressed approbation for the conduct of the crew of HMS *Hermonine,* who mutinied and killed their commander; and disobedience of the captain's orders. Marshall was arrested and confined briefly before being brought to trial.

Surgeon Marshall was a highly respected individual who was liked by the junior officers and the crew. He had no difficulty in disposing of the charges and was honorably acquitted by the court. Of special interest for our purposes are some of the points he made in his defense. Marshall said that the captain had admitted to him "that he had an aversion to all Gentlemen of the Lancet" and that this was convincing proof that his disposition toward the surgeon was "premeditatedly inimical." The surgeon asked the court: "Must we, on becoming officers, forget that we are men?" As to the matter of the *Hermonine,* Marshall said that the charge was based on a private conversation he had had in the wardroom. He had spoken with zeal because he was concerned about the persecuted sailors.

"If my sentiments on this head were erroneous; it was an error in judgment & not of the heart." Surgeon Marshall went on to a long and honorable career in the navy. Captain Sever was discharged from the service in May 1801.[62]

Medical men were not the only officers who got into trouble. Lieutenant Abraham Ludlow of the brig *Scammel* was brought to trial on charges by Surgeon Richard C. Shannon of frequently being intoxicated and abusing him without cause. The captain testified in behalf of the prisoner: Ludlow was a good officer, who got drunk only when the ship was in port. This and other favorable testimony led the court to rule that the charge of frequent intoxication had not been proved.

As for the charge of abusing a medical officer, the circumstances were as follows: When Lieutenant Ludlow returned to the ship about 8 P.M. , he appeared to be drunk, according to some witnesses. Ludlow said that he did not feel well, and having no duty, he went to his quarters, took off his coat, and returned to the deck. Here he joined the captain, his guest, and Dr. Shannon. They were already engaged in conversation and apparently directed none of it toward the lieutenant. While they were discussing the symbolism of the olive branch in the talons of the American eagle on the Great Seal of the United States, the doctor expressed an opinion. At this point Ludlow told the doctor that he had no right to say anything on the subject because it did not concern him; Shannon replied that he had the right to speak to any gentleman on the quarter-deck. The captain silenced both of them, then went to the gangway to greet some other guests who were coming on board. While the captain was gone, the lieutenant got up and struck the doctor in the face. Shannon told him not to do it again or he would resist. He then went to the captain and reported the incident, whereupon the captain ordered both to go below. A midshipman testified that he heard Ludlow say he would meet the doctor on shore with pistols the next morning for a duel. The captain's steward stated that that night, Ludlow went below, got a pair of pistols, and returned to the deck with the intention of fighting the doctor. Shannon took the pistols from him and he was sent back to his cabin. The next morning the lieutenant was in a pleasant mood and there was no further talk of duels. In his defense, Ludlow did not deny striking Shannon but claimed to have been provoked. As he told it, in view of the doctor's language to him, it was astonishing that he, Ludlow, did not go farther. The court found Ludlow guilty of abusing the doctor and sentenced him to a seven-month suspension from duty without pay or emoluments. The secretary of the navy upheld this sentence.

An interesting aspect of the case is Dr. Shannon's statement that when he first demanded the arrest of Ludlow, the captain refused. Shannon then began writing to Captain Stephen Decatur Sr. about the incident, but by the time he finished, the captain had placed Ludlow under arrest. In 1800, Shannon resigned his commission for reasons of health. As for Ludlow, he was discharged in the demobilization of 1801.[63]

There was also the case of Surgeon Charles Webb of the brig *Eagle*. He had come to the attention of his superior for allegedly sticking a dirk into the chest of a black cabin boy and flogging a seaman. When told by his commanding officer, Lieutenant M. S. Bunberry, never to inflict corporal punishment on a seaman, Webb replied that he would do as he wished. He was later charged with beating a boatswain's mate with a stick and calling Bunberry "the worst scamp in the Navy" in the presence of other officers and some members of the crew. Webb claimed he did not received orders not to flog anyone until after the affair with the boatswain. The charge that he beat and abused Joseph Anderson, who was attached to the wardroom, in a cruel and inhumane manner needed to be explained. Anderson was a black loblolly boy of about 16 who was noted for his stubbornness. He had broken the locks on the medicine chest and Webb's trunk and had taken two of his keys and some money. Webb punished him by giving him half a dozen lashes with the end of a small rope.

Webb went on to explain the incident involving a fork. When he was called to dinner, he went below for his eating utensils. Finding that his knife and fork had not been wiped, and seeing the servant, John Mattis, a distance away from him in the wardroom, the doctor "gently pitched" the utensils to Mattis for wiping. Unfortunately, the fork stuck in the servant's breast, but the injury was very small and was not done willfully or maliciously. Webb denied that he had broken a dirk over the back of this servant. Furthermore, the charges represented Mattis as a boy. He was not; he was "a stout black fellow" from Barbados.

Webb also had his version of the incident with Lieutenant Bunberry. While the *Eagle* was in St. Kitts, officers of the different ships were invited to dine with Commodore Barry on his ship. The first lieutenant and Webb went from the *Eagle*. They drank too much wine and stayed late. When the boat from the *Eagle* arrived at the flagship to take them home, the officer in charge of it was told not to inform Webb of its arrival. Webb knew that he was under orders not to stay away from the ship overnight, and fortunately another boat brought him back to the *Eagle*. In the wardroom, Webb mentioned to some officers that Bunberry had treated him like a "damned scamp" and that he did not know his duty. Six or eight days later, one of these officers reported the remark to Bunberry. The captain took no notice of it, however.

Several weeks later, Webb was informed late one evening that one of the men was dying on the berth deck. The doctor went to the man, took him in his arms, and placed him in a hammock. While he was thus engaged, a boatswain who was a favorite of the captain was descending to the berth deck, and he struck Webb in the head with his foot. The surgeon told him to mind how he came down the ladder. The boatswain gave an impertinent reply, at which Webb told him to go about his business. Instead he persisted in his impertinence, whereupon Webb took a stick the size of a man's thumb and struck the boatswain twice. The boatswain then picked up a stick the size of an arm and said that if the surgeon touched him again, he would knock him down. Webb reported the incident to the captain but received no satisfaction. Two days later, while the ship's company was mustered to witness the punishment of a cook, Bunberry told the boatswain that he would not allow any officer on board to speak to him in violent language, nor would he let the boatswain use any such words to an officer.

The surgeon was offended by this public display which seemed to afford the boatswain equality with officers. Afterward, Bunberry invited Webb to dine with him on a few occasions, but the surgeon could not bring himself to accept. Later Webb reported the conduct of the boatswain to Commodore Barry. In revenge, said Webb, Bunberry told Barry of the surgeon's remarks in the wardroom and said that Webb was intoxicated at the time. Webb was arrested that night and later brought to trial. He was found guilty of contempt, disobedience of orders of his commanding officer, and violating the 13th and 14th articles of the act for the better government of the navy of the United States. The surgeon wrote to the secretary of the navy asking him to disapprove the sentence, for the whole affair had the look of "a revengeful, hurried and summary Piece of business, and purely the effects of wine." The appeal did not move the secretary, and the sentence of the court was that Webb be dismissed from the navy. President Thomas Jefferson approved the sentence, and Webb was cashiered on July 10, 1801. Bunberry was discharged from the service that same day under demobilization procedures. He returned to the navy briefly during the War of 1812.[64]

By the time Webb's fate had been decided, the war was over. In March 1800 peace talks with France began, and at the end of September a treaty was signed. The Senate ratified it in December 1801.[65] The fall of 1800 saw a presidential election that brought Thomas Jefferson to the highest office in the land in March 1801. Before leaving office, the Federalists passed a law drastically reducing the size of the peacetime navy and the number of officers needed to sustain it. They did this in order to forestall even greater cuts or perhaps the elimination of the navy under the new Democratic-Republican administration.

Medical Officers in the Quasi-War: A Statistical Profile

Under the act of March 3, 1801, creating the naval peace establishment, only 14 surgeons and 9 surgeon's mates were to be retained.[66] The Navy Department apparently decided who was to go on the basis of reports from captains. Unfortunately many letters from this period are lost, but from those that survive, it seems that at least some officers were consulted about whether they wished to leave the service. Let us review the situation of the medical men appointed at various times.

During the Quasi-War 96 men served as medical officers in the navy, including 3 with acting or temporary appointments. Of this total the home states of 90 officers who were commissioned or warranted have been established: 25 came from Massachusetts; at least 17 and possibly 18 from Maryland; 12 from Virginia; 10 each from New York and Pennsylvania; 5 from Rhode Island; 4 from Connecticut; 3 from South Carolina; and 1 from Georgia.

Of the 12 surgeons appointed in 1798, 2 died, 1 committed suicide, and 2 resigned. One of these left after only 4 month's service and the other after 7. George Gillasspy, the first naval surgeon appointed, apparently made only one cruise. He returned to Philadelphia, formed a partnership with Surgeon's Mate Joseph C. Strong, and began supplying the navy with medicines. After February 1799, Gillasspy relinquished his pay and rations but kept his rank until discharged in April 1801. He seems to have been asked about his wishes, and he indicated that he had no desire to remain in the navy. Another former army doctor, George Balfour, who served in the *Constellation* and the *President,* was retained. Still another colleague, John Rush, had served 10 months as a surgeon when he decided he wanted to be a line officer. In March 1799 he traded his medical appointment for a commission as a lieutenant in the marines and remained in the navy until 1802. Four others, Joseph Anthony, George Wright, Jeffrey D. Shanley, and Joseph Lee, served throughout the war and were discharged in 1801.[67]

So, 5 of the 12 surgeons appointed in 1798 apparently functioned competently as doctors throughout the war, but only 2 were retained for peacetime service: John K. Read Jr. and George Balfour. Read became ill and died in 1805. Ordered to sea in 1804, George Balfour told the secretary that he needed the income from his position in a local hospital to support his family, and he could not go now. He resigned his commission in 1804. Thus all the surgeons who entered the navy in 1798 were gone by March 1805. Eleven surgeon's mates came into the navy in 1798, of whom 1 never served, 2 resigned, 2 died, and 3 were retained, 2 as surgeons and 1 as a mate. Of the 3 retained, 1 died and 1 resigned in 1802.

During 1799, 17 surgeons came into the naval service. Three of these died, and 2 others resigned in 1800, perhaps because they saw that the war would end soon. Dr. Windship left the navy in disgrace. Eight others saw the war through and were discharged in the spring of 1801. Only 4 were retained: Edward Cutbush, Peter St. Medard, George Davis, and James Wells. Of this group, George Davis began serving as the U.S. chargé d'affaires at Tunis in 1803, and three years later he became the consul there. James Wells remained active until his death in 1807. St. Medard continued until his death in 1822, but for most of that time he was more an ailing elder statesman of naval medicine than an active participant. Cutbush thus emerged as the leading personality among the early medical men of the navy, and he functioned actively until his resignation in 1829. Of the 8 surgeon's mates promoted to surgeon in 1799, only John Bullus was retained in 1801. But in 1808, Bullus left medicine for a more profitable job as a navy agent at New York. Of the 21 surgeon's mates appointed in 1799, 8 resigned, 1 retired with a disability, and 1 died. Of those who served until the end of the war, 5 were kept for peacetime duty: James Boyd, who died in 1803; Nathaniel Tisdale, who was dismissed in 1804; James Dodge, who became the U.S. chargé d'affaires at Tunis in 1805 and died the following year; Thomas Marshall, who died in 1808; and Samuel R. Marshall, who lived until 1828. Therefore, by the end of 1808, only 1 of the men who came in as a surgeon's mate in 1799 was still in the navy.

Similar stories might be noted in regard to those who entered in 1800. Only three men were appointed as surgeons. One of these, John Goddard, was retained, but he died in 1802. Walter W. Buchanan was discharged, but in 1804 he was offered a commission as a surgeon, which he turned down. Buchanan served again during the War of 1812. John Howell was appointed a surgeon, served in the *Constellation* from December 11, 1800, to May 25, 1801, and was discharged the following month. Of the 27 surgeon's mates chosen, 1 declined the appointment. One was lost at sea in the *Insurgente*. Only 1 was promoted to surgeon during the war, and this was the unfortunate Charles Webb, who was dismissed in 1801. Two of those dismissed in 1801 came back into the navy at later periods. Gershom Jacques was reappointed in 1801, promoted to surgeon in 1804, and dismissed in 1808. William Turk returned to the navy as a surgeon during the War of 1812 and remained until 1854. Following his discharge from the navy in 1801, Francis Le Barron entered the army, where he achieved some prominence in the War of 1812.

An examination of the careers of the eight surgeon's mates who were retained in the peace establishment shows that three were promoted to surgeon between 1803 and 1809. One of these, Starling Archer, died in a duel between 1805 and 1806. Another, Robert B. Starke, was promoted, stayed in the service, but was inactive by 1811. Only Jonathan Cowdery, promoted in 1804, remained in the navy until his death in 1852. Of the six who remained surgeon's mates, one died in 1806, and three others resigned in 1802, 1803, and 1806. Also, Benjamin G. Harris was serving in the *Philadelphia* in the West Indies when he decided to accept a position on shore in Monserrat and resigned his commission. Another mate, Samuel Edward Willett, was still in the navy in 1803, and then all trace of him was apparently lost.

In 1801, with the end of the war in sight, only four surgeon's mates were appointed, of whom two were promoted to surgeon in 1804. One of these, Lewis Heermann, achieved some prominence early in his career and remained in the navy until 1833. The other, Larkin Griffin, served until his death in 1814.

Hence, despite the number of men who served in the medical ranks during the Quasi-War, there was only a handful of experienced men in uniform by the end of the Barbary Wars, and even fewer by the beginning of the War of 1812.

What small medical institutional memory there was survived in the minds and experiences of Cutbush, St. Medard, Samuel R. Marshall, Cowdery, and Heermann. Yet they functioned largely as individuals: each wrote his own views on medical matters to the secretary of the navy. Even on the one professional topic of interest to all, the need for a hospital system, much of what was written to the secretary had to do with specific areas, expenditures, and needs.

Chapter 3

Medicine and Health
in the Quasi-War

At daylight the men were roused from sleep, took care of their personal needs, untied their hammocks and placed them in designated spots in the lower rigging to air, mustered, and went to breakfast. In the course of the day, they carried out various assigned duties: they loosed and furled sails, stood watches, performed gun drills, scrubbed decks or clothing, and were kept busy.

For the surgeon and his mate, the professional day began with sick call after breakfast. The doctors determined the nature of the ailment from what they were told by the men and from their own examination. They decided on treatment and whether the condition was serious enough to release the man from duty that day. A list of sick men and their ailments was presented to the captain by the surgeon usually about 10 A.M. By the time of the Quasi-War, there had been a great increase in official awareness in the British navy about what could be done to preserve the health of seamen. The writings of James Lind (1716–94) "the father of nautical medicine" and of Gilbert Blane (1749–1834), who was later made a baronet for his contributions, provided practical guidelines for public officials, naval officers, and medical men. Lind had pointed out that the diseases most common to seamen were fevers, fluxes, and scurvy and that a man was more apt to be stricken with two of these in harbor rather than at sea. The observations of Lind and Blane on the prevention of diseases in the tropics would have been of great help to U.S. medical officers and captains operating in the Caribbean, but it cannot now be ascertained to what extent the works of these authors were known and available in the United States, or which officers may have bought them.[1]

For those ailing enlisted men who had been admitted to the sick bay, a roughly triangular area in the bow of the ship, the medications prescribed were dispensed by the surgeon's mate assisted by an enlisted helper or two who were called loblolly boys.[2] They usually fed the patients who could not feed themselves, handled the bedpans and urinals, and gave "nursing" care. In cases of serious illnesses or wounds, the surgeon treated the patients himself, assisted by his mate. He was kept informed of the condition of patients while he was away from the sick bay, and in serious cases he paid periodic visits. At other times he tried to maintain his records and pursue his own interests. Speaking of his environment in the *Constellation,* Surgeon George Balfour complained of "the impossibility of obtaining even a moment's privacy, on board a ship built as this is.—Our Gun Room is too confined & dark to write in—, and what little I can make shift to do is on the open Deck, amid a crowd of persons, a great obstacle this to medical enquiry or correct observation."[3]

Early in a cruise ailments or disabilities that had escaped the eye of the recruiting officer or examining physician showed up. Also, men who had claimed at the time of recruitment to have certain experience were sometimes found to be wanting in that skill. Among the inexperienced hands were some who could make the transition to sea life easily and some who could not. Breaking in a crew frequently involved resorting to the cat-o'-nine-tails to instill discipline and promptness in executing commands. Stopping the bleeding caused by flogging and treating lacerated backs became one of the routine tasks that naval medical officers performed. During the Quasi-War sailors were enlisted for only one year. This brief term of service proved to be an impediment to extended operations, but short cruises and stays in various locales minimized the risk of exposure to some diseases. The captain needed to get the maximum use of his men during their term of enlistment, so that if a man was seriously ill or had an ailment that could not be cured in a few weeks at most, it was better to get rid of him and enlist a healthy replacement. Thus as early as July 26, 1798, we find Captain Barry discharging a marine and an ordinary seaman as unfit for duty and his master-at-arms for "his lingering illness." Likewise, when the *Constellation* reached Hampton Roads that same month and Captain Truxtun found that a good supply of men was available in the area, he seized the opportunity to discharge "a Number of Rotten and inanimate Animals that found their Way into the Ship, by imposing on the recruiting Officers and Surgeon's Vigilance."[4] While such men were no longer the concern of Truxtun, they were still the responsibility of the navy, as we shall see.

Much attention was paid to keeping the ship clean as a means of pre-

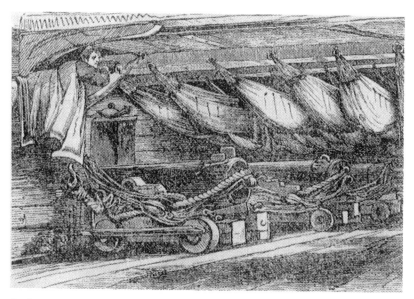

Sailors in Hammocks on the Gun Deck of a Warship. Smithsonian Institution, Washington, D.C.

venting disease. Decks were scrubbed, fumigated, sprinkled with vinegar, and ventilated as much as possible by rigging a sail to divert wind down the hatchways. The cockpit was never washed but rubbed dry and cleaned with sand. Frequently water would be let into the hold and then pumped out to keep the dirt and probably the rats under control.

One of the problems associated with the frequent washing of the decks was that spaces below the main deck had insufficient light or heat to dry them fully before the next scrubbing. The result was a damp and often dank environment that could have been conducive to colds and made respiratory problems more difficult to resolve. One remedy was to heat the lower decks by means of stoves, specially constructed metal pots filled with sand and hung overhead, into which heated shot or burning sulphur were placed to produce warmth. These stoves were especially important during the winter months when men would go below with wet clothes, yet under the best of circumstances they were probably not very effective. One officer who appreciated the need for heat and dryness was Truxtun. In late July 1798 he established a regular schedule: large fires were to be made in the stoves below decks every Monday, Thursday, and Saturday. On the other days the crew's quarters were to be washed with vinegar and brimstone was to be burned in the hanging pots.[5]

Poor ventilation below decks was also a recurring problem as gun ports and hatches had to be closed during bad weather. Men slept in their hammocks with only 17 inches between them and condensation from wet clothes, and the sweating of unseasoned timber combined with the constant washing of decks created a fetid condition that required a great deal of ventilation. Also, butter and cheese stored in the hold became rancid. Carbolic acid and firedamp, an explosive mixture of methane gas and air, developed down below. In the Royal Navy a man would hold a candle to determine whether there was sufficient air in the hold, another method was to see how many minutes it took for a silver spoon to tarnish.[6] It is not known if the U.S. Navy had a similar test. Nor can the effects of poor ventilation on health be calculated at this late date.

Most of what is known about matters of sickness and death comes from records prepared by line officers, where a death would often be recorded without any indication as to cause, much less what might have been done to save a man's life. From existing records it is possible to piece together some of the medical aspects of the war in terms of the officers and crews of specific ships.

Sickness, Injuries, and Death in the *Constellation*

The *Constellation* is of special interest because it was active for most of the war and because its first commander, Captain Thomas Truxtun, had a well-deserved reputation for organization and conscious effort to instill pride and establish traditions in the naval service. He was also much interested in matters of health.

The muster roll of the *Constellation* for August 16, 1798–July 16, 1799, shows that out of the 507 officers and men who entered service there were 12 confirmed deaths. The first to die was an ordinary seaman whom Truxtun described as having "an old sore Leg, and a Complication of Disorders." He was buried at sea on July 23, 1798, the day he died. Another ordinary seaman died at St. Kitt's Island of a fever of some kind in May 1799, and a marine private died at sea the same month of the flux, or dysentery. Two other seamen died of wounds during the battle with the French frigate *L'Insurgente* in February 1799. Still another is listed as having died at Staten Island on July 16, 1799, but no cause is stated. Of the remaining 6, 1 seaman, missing at sea, was presumed drowned, 4 are listed as having drowned, and one boy was killed when he fell from a mast in March 1799. Thus of the dozen deaths, half were the result of accidents. Two others are listed as having either deserted or drowned.

In a 10-month period, 23 men in the *Constellation* were regarded as too

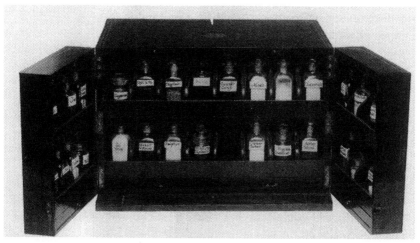

Eighteenth-Century Medical Chest of the Type Used in the U.S. Navy. The Francis A. Countway Library of Medicine, Harvard University. Photographed at the USS *Constitution* Museum, Boston, Mass.

sick to remain on board. Eight of these were sent to sick quarters at Norfolk on May 22, 1798. Seven other sick men were discharged at their own request in August 1798, and another on December 29 of the same year. It is interesting that 5 seamen were discharged at their own request by supplying substitutes. Another seaman suffered from dropsy and was discharged at Norfolk in August 1798.[7] One who suffered from the flux was sent ashore at St. Kitt's and was subsequently returned to the United States in a prize schooner. Still another was sent ashore because of a rupture (hernia) on June 1, 1799. Perhaps the most poignant case was that of Ordinary Seaman John Hilsberry, who became mentally deranged as a result of a fall in the ship and was sent to Norfolk in August 1798. Other injuries were the result of the battle with *L'Insurgente.* Midshipman James McDonough lost a foot and was sent ashore at St. Christopher's to recuperate. With him went Ordinary Seaman John Andrews, who was shot through both legs. Both recovered and were sent home in a prize schooner. As was noted earlier, two other wounded men later died.

It subsequently developed that there were more casualties than Truxtun knew about. William Brown, a black powder monkey, was struck in the left foot by a French bullet. He was taken to the cockpit, where the wound was dressed. When it was partly healed he returned to his duties. Brown continued to serve in the ship for some months, but his wound never healed completely. Later he applied for a pension on the basis of his injury. William Palms claimed he was wounded in the head, neck, legs, and ·

stomach and was later transferred to a hospital at Norfolk, where he remained for a year or so.[8]

On the French side the casualties in this battle were 29 killed and 41 wounded. When the battle was over, the U.S. medical men assisted the French doctors in treating the wounded. The French wounded were kept on their ship until they reached St. Christopher's, where they were transferred to a hospital ashore. After the battle, Lieutenant John Rodgers was placed in command of *L'Insurgente,* and Surgeon's Mate Isaac Henry was temporarily transferred to it. After undergoing repairs and adjudication by a prize court, it entered the U.S. service.[9]

When the *Constellation* again saw action on the night of February 1, 1800, it was with the French frigate *La Vengeance.* During the two-hour fight the French ship struck her colors, but this was not seen in the darkness. At 1:00 A.M. it ceased firing and struck again. Before the Americans could take their prize, the main mast of the *Constellation* collapsed. As they struggled to clear the wreckage, the two ships drifted apart, and *La Vengeance* escaped and put in at Curaçao. Here it was officially reported that it had sustained 28 dead and 40 wounded, but an American seaman on the ship, who did not participate in the fight, later reported 100 killed and 60 wounded. In the *Constellation,* Isaac Henry, now the surgeon, had his hands full. Captain Truxtun's report of February 2 gives the casualties as 14 killed and 25 wounded. On Surgeon Henry's list 11 men are recorded as having slight wounds and 5 others as having fractured legs or thighs. But in a letter to his father on February 3, Henry put the cost of the battle to the *Constellation* at 15 killed and 25 wounded, "all badly."[10] One of those who was badly wounded was John Hoxse, a carpenter. He recorded his recollections nearly forty years later.

> Towards the close of the action, as I was standing near the pumps, with a top maul in my right hand, with the arm extended, a shot from the enemy's ship entered the port near by, and took the arm off just above the elbow, leaving it hanging by my side by a small piece of skin; also wounding me very severely in the side, leaving my entrails all bare. I then took my arm in my left hand, and went below, into the cock-pit, and requested the surgeon to stop [the bleeding in] my arm [as it] was already off. He accordingly stopped the effusion of blood, and I was laid aside among the dead and wounded, until my turn came to have my wounds dressed. The cock-pit at this time was full of the dead and dying, but I was so exhausted that I fell asleep, and was not sensible that any thing had happened, until I was called up to have my wounds examined and dressed. I was then taken up, laid on a table, my wounds washed clean, and my arm amputated and thrown overboard.[11]

Truxtun brought his damaged ship to Jamaica to transfer the wounded to a hospital ashore and to be repaired. Henry again wrote to his father about the battle. "I have had I can assure you a most disagreeable time with the wounded—Six Amputations of Limbs with a number of very severe flesh wounds—some of them have died since we got in with Lock Jaw. All my amputations are doing as well as I could wish—and I am extremely anxious to get them to the Hospital, but we want the permission of the Admiral."[12] The admiral in question was Vice Admiral Sir Hyde Parker of the Royal Navy, who was in command at Jamaica.

The British naval hospital at Port Royal, Jamaica, had a poor reputation. The U.S. wounded who were transferred to it soon had their own problems there. John Hoxse notes that Surgeon Henry thought it prudent not to move the men until their wounds were healed. By the time the *Constellation* left Jamaica, only four of the wounded were still alive. They were transferred to the hospital, where they faced further ordeals. Hoxse had bitter recollections of his time on the island.

> All the attendance we received was from the black women, and they were insolent, lazy, filthy, and abused their patients in every manner of way they could devise. If we asked for a drink of water, we seldom got it, unless we crawled after it ourselves. Our wounds were not half dressed, nor the bandages kept clean, otherwise we should have got clear of this lazarhouse, weeks before we did. But what could be expected from such heartless wretches? They had no feelings or sentiments that could be wrought upon by suffering humanity! Their own condition was that of slaves; and their owners, the Doctors of the Hospital; who were so penurious that they would allow only one slave to wash and attend upon twenty patients. The four of us, however, recovered, and wrote to our agent, at Port Royal, to procure us a passage to the United States.[13]

Hoxse's situation once he got back will be noted later in this narrative. But for the moment it should be pointed out that on the basis of the testimony of Surgeon Henry and Hoxse, the final tally of U.S. casualties in the battle with *La Vengeance* was 36 dead and 4 who recovered from their wounds.

Casualties in Other Ships

Records from the Quasi-War provide other glimpses into the toll of battle. For example, when the former enemy frigate, now in the U.S. service under the name *Insurgente*, captured the French schooner *Aurora* on January 25, 1800, Midshipman Richard Bland Randolph boarded the prize and was attacked by a Frenchman wielding a cutlass. Randolph lost a finger on his left hand. A second Frenchman fired a pistol at him, and the ball struck him in the right ankle. He was later reported to have suffered a severe rupture. Randolph was presumably treated by the surgeon or mate of his ship. He died later when the *Insurgente* sank.[14]

In another instance, off St. Christopher's in February 1800, the *Baltimore* exchanged fire with a French privateer, and one marine was killed by a musket shot. The schooner *Experiment,* while convoying merchant ships, was becalmed off the island of Gonaive in January 1800 and attacked by 400 or 500 pirates in armed barges. Two barges were sunk, many pirates were killed or wounded, and two the merchant ships were lost to the attackers. But in the *Experiment* no one was killed and only one man was slightly wounded.[15]

On the general question of shipboard health, a picture somewhat similar to that experienced in the *Constellation* emerges from the records of Captain Silas Talbot in the *Constitution*. From November 1798 to November 1799 17 deaths were recorded. In five instances no cause is given. Accidents, such as falling overboard and a shooting, accounted for 7 other deaths. Diseases are mentioned as the cause of death in only five instances. One of these deaths was from "Bilious Fever" (a fever probably associated with jaundice), 1 from scurvy, 1 from a cramp in the stomach, and 2 from "a complication of diseases." On the other hand, the record of deaths compiled by Captain Tyrone Martin, USN (Ret.), from the log of the *Constitution* shows 3 deaths in 1798 including those of Surgeon Read, a midshipman who succumbed to yellow fever, and a marine who died of fever or scurvy. Sixteen deaths were recorded in 1799, including those of two marines, with the following attributions: bilious fever, 4; consumption, 3; several disorders, 3; gout, 2; and 1 case each of fever and stomach cramp. During 1800 only 4 deaths were recorded, including those of two marines, one of whom died of a fever and the other of "complication of the lungs." One seamen died of a fever and another of bilious fever.[16]

A marine lieutenant, reporting to his commandant the arrival of the brig *Richmond* in the Chesapeake in October 1799, announced the recent death of Lieutenant Jeremiah Rose. The marine noted that Rose died as the result of an inflammation of the liver accompanied by a bilious complaint.[17] In the case of yellow fever, records tend to be more precise. For example, in 1800 the *Ganges*, whose normal complement was 220 men, recorded 19 dead of that disease, and the *Warren* lost 39 out of a complement of 160. The atmosphere in the *Warren* when the fever was at its worst was described by Surgeon John Park as "horrid, beyond description."[18]

The fear that a fever-ridden ship could bring to a community can be seen in the case of the frigate *General Greene*. After his ship was damaged in a gale in the West Indies, Captain Christopher Perry put into Havana for repairs. While there he lost 20 men to yellow fever out of a complement of 220. The ship then sailed for home, and en route 2 more men died of the fever; 5 others were stricken but recovered. When the ship reached Newport, Rhode Island, on July 21, 1800, it became a source of serious concern to local officials. The frigate was quarantined and a local physician went on board to inspect the men. He reported that there were no patients on board with any malignant or contagious diseases; the small number of sick were convalescing. Before the town council would lift the quarantine, however, it wanted the sick transferred to another vessel in the harbor or to some remote place on shore that would serve as a hospital. In reporting these things to Secretary Stoddert, the local navy agents used the occasion to point out the need for a marine hospital at Newport. They said that the frequency with which the sick from ships were landed and placed within the limits of the town was causing anxiety to the inhabitants. Through the navy agents, Stoddert ordered Perry to discharge his crew, which he did, but this caused an uproar when new deaths were reported among them.[19]

To calm the public, Surgeon William Turner wrote a letter to the local newspaper setting forth the facts. Three men had died while the ship was in port, but one of these deaths was due to intemperance. Two others who died of the fever were predisposed to it by their intemperance. After most of the crew had been discharged, one of them, a boy in Providence, and three men in Newport died of the fever. But there were no signs of the fever among the nurses who attended the patients. Only one person on board had a slight complaint about fever, but a day later he was well and walking about the town. Furthermore, the ballast had been removed, and the ship had been washed, scrubbed, and fumigated, whitewash had been applied to the decks and hold, and the ship was now "in a state of the most healthy cleanliness."[20] These explanations and assurances presumably allayed the anxiety of the citizenry of Newport.

The *Congress* and the *Essex*

When Secretary Stoddert ordered the frigates *Congress* and *Essex* to the Dutch East Indies for convoy duty, he set in motion a series of events that had a great influence on the health and morale of the officers and men of both ships. The convoy sailed from Newport on January 6, 1800. Five days later it encountered a severe storm at sea. During the second day the fore and main masts of the *Congress* were torn off, as well as the top of its mizzen mast. In this battered condition the ship made for the nearest port, Hampton Roads, Virginia. The crew was wet, seasick, and tired but otherwise in good condition. Surgeon Larkin Thorndike and his assistant, Edward Field, survived the storm in reasonably good shape.

While the ship was being repaired, there was criticism of the conduct of Captain James Sever, and a court of inquiry was ordered. Stoddert insisted that the investigation not delay the repairs on the ship or interfere with Sever's command functions. As Stoddert told Sever, "The Men of the Congress have too long to serve to be discharged, and the expense of keeping them idle in port is not the worst consequence which will accrue— ill humor & insubordination must arise out of such a state of things."[21] These words proved to be prophetic.

Before the court of inquiry could take place, Sever was confronted with a mutiny. He nipped it in the bud by arresting eight men and holding them for trial. This incident again drew the attention of Stoddert to the state of affairs in the *Congress*. From a navy lieutenant in the ship, the Secretary learned that "the whole officers of the Ship are at variance with the Captain—No wonder the men are disorderly."[22] According to Captain Alexander Murray, the problem was that Sever had little practical knowledge of seamanship and did not appreciate opinions different from his own. He was aloof and distant from his officers and men. This allegation of discontent among the officers would seem to include the medical men as well as the line officers, but there is no way of knowing for certain. It seems likely that the medical men would have stayed in the background during the arguments, charges, and countercharges about the functions of command. Yet living and working in such a close and tension-filled environment must have created its own share of worry for Surgeon Thorndike and Surgeon's Mate Field. Many years later, after Field's death, it was claimed that he was injured during the mutiny: his right wrist and tendons were damaged in circumstances that were not explained. Presumably he received attention from his colleague, but apparently he had to function for some time with a disability. This injury later became the basis for a pension when Field left the service at the end of the Quasi-War. The unfortunate Dr. Field thus became the first medical officer of the U.S. Navy to be pensioned for a service-connected disability.[23]

Meanwhile his senior colleague, Larkin Thorndike, had his own share of problems, and it is intriguing to speculate about his mental state. Whether Captain Sever, the mutiny, or other deep seated personal problems—or all three—were troubling Thorndike cannot be ascertained, but something drove him to suicide. On May 24, 1800, he cut his throat.[24] This must have come as a great shock to Dr. Field. The small area of the ship reserved for medical activities could not help but make each man aware of his colleague's personal habits and idiosyncracies.

Two days after Thorndike's death, Field was made the acting surgeon of the *Congress*. He continued in this capacity until July 3, when Dr. William Turner assumed the duties of senior medical officer. While Field was in charge, most of the crew was transferred to the *Chesapeake* and a new crew was recruited and reported on board. Of the old crew, eight were tried for mutiny and two of the ring leaders were found guilty and sentenced to be hanged. Commodore Truxtun, who reviewed the record of the trial, considered the sentence too harsh. Instead he ordered that each of the ringleaders receive 100 lashes with a cat-o'-nine-tails on the bare back and be discharged from the service. Four other mutineers found guilty received 72 lashes each. One man was acquitted.[25] A new lieutenant was sent to Sever as his second in command. With these changes it was hoped that the ship would again be well disciplined and able to carry out its mission. About mid-July the *Congress* was ordered to relieve the *Constellation* off the coast of Santo Domingo.[26]

Meanwhile the *Essex* with its compliment of 300 continued on alone to the East Indies. From the Cape of Good Hope, Captain Preble reported to Secretary Stoddert that his surgeon, Dr. Hector Orr, "is ever attentive to the health of the ship's company, they are all now in perfect health except for one man sick with a cold."[27] The log of the *Essex* shows that three weeks before this, one man had died, but the cause of death was not recorded; nevertheless, the health of those on board remained good. While at Cape Town, Preble acquired a copy of *Instructions for Navy Surgeons*, distributed by the British commissioners for taking care of sick and wounded seamen.[28] It is quite possible that Preble bought the pamphlet at the request of Dr. Orr; if not, he no doubt shared the insights gained from it with Orr either directly or indirectly.

Preble sailed from Cape Town on March 27, and the *Essex* anchored in the harbor of Batavia, Java, on May 15. Here Preble waited four days for the arrival of the *Congress*. With no sign of that ship, he notified the captains of the U.S. merchant ships about the departure time of the convoy. While he waited, 7 men were reported sick on June 5, probably with malaria or dengue fever. The next day an able seaman died and the number of sick remained the same. On June 19, the convoy sailed for the United States. The sick list grew: three days later it had reached 12.[29] Four days later, Surgeon Orr reported to Preble that the unhealthy climate and the size of the sick list made it necessary to have another surgeon's mate. He suggested Midshipman Thomas Marshall, "who has been regularly educated [as] a Surgeon & Physician, and appears upon examination to be well acquainted with the theory of both Surgery & physics."[30] Marshall seems to have been given an acting appointment. After the return of the

Essex, he was not commissioned but given a warrant dated December 13, 1800.[31]

In the meantime, when the *Essex* left the East Indian seas, the health of the crew began to improve. By early July the number on the sick list had dropped to 8. In September it rose again to 13, and 1 seaman died of unrecorded causes. Preble's journal contains the notation, "The Scurvy appears among the people."[32] But from St. Helena on September 15, Preble reported to Stoddert that the ship's company was "in general good health."[33] That situation continued for the rest of the trip, which ended in New York on November 28. The long voyage to the East Indies and back had cost only seven lives. But in the course of the mission, Preble's own health was undermined, and that was destined to cut short his promising naval career.[34]

Medical Cases of Interest

Above and beyond the cases recorded in the logs and letters of the line officers, there were some health situations that were of special interest to the surgeons and their professional colleagues in the civilian world. Early in the Quasi-War, Surgeon George Balfour of the *Constellation* wrote to Benjamin Rush about some cases he had treated.

While the ship was at Hampton Roads in June 1798, Balfour was faced with several cases of fever. Midshipman Samuel Henry, aged 20, had been walking around, apparently in perfect health, before lying in his hammock on the berth deck. While there he was seized with great pain in his legs and arms and suffered a headache. Dr. Balfour was called and observed that Henry's face was flushed, his eyes were red, and he was unable to get out of his hammock. Balfour had him moved to the gun deck, where the air was better, and began to bleed him. After 14 ounces of blood had been taken, the headache disappeared and Henry was able to sit up. The midshipman was then given a purge of calomel and jalap. Six hours later he had a good pulse, but headache and pain in the limbs returned, although not as intense as they had been previously. Henry was bled again and afterwards he felt no pain anywhere.

During July 1798 several sailors were stricken with fever and were bled. Balfour's usual practice was to take 8 ounces of blood first, and later 24 or 30 ounces. He had great success in overcoming fever by this method. Balfour also noted that, contrary to popular belief, sailors did not object to being bled.

On the morning of July 9, Balfour was called to examine Seaman Thomas Foss, who had a high fever. The doctor found him suffering from pains in the front part of his head, and he observed that Foss had a flushed face, a tense pulse, a "great degree of Coma," and an inability to stand. Balfour removed 8 ounces of blood. The patient was very dirty, so he was washed with vinegar and water and given 15 grains of jalap and 14 grains of calomel. Foss said that these measures gave him much relief. But that afternoon, Balfour found that his patient's pulse was still tense and that he was in a kind of coma. He bled Foss again, this time taking 12 ounces, and then gave him an ounce of castor oil to make up for the inaction of the calomel and jalap. Next came the application of a large blister to his chest, which made him feel uneasy. To deal with this problem the doctor gave him 25 drops each of tincture of opium and antimonial wine. Later in the day, seeing that the coma persisted and that Foss's pulse was high, Balfour took another 14 ounces of blood. The patient reported that his head pains were considerably relieved. That evening the doctor removed another 14 ounces of blood.

On July 11, Foss complained of pains in his head, so Balfour took a further 8 ounces of blood. The patient experienced considerable relief. Foss had not been able to take anything but lime juice and water since he became ill. By the evening of the 11th, his stomach was so irritated that he could not keep down any food. His pulse was still tense. Another 8 ounces of blood were taken.

When Balfour came by on July 12, he found Foss vomiting frequently, but his head felt better. Balfour attributed this improvement to the bleeding. The patient's pulse was very active. There appeared to be no break in his fever except after the previous day's bleeding, so Balfour decided to bleed again, this time taking 16 ounces. The doctor was surprised to see the blood flow more freely than at any previous time. During the night Foss complained of pains in his breast. A new blister was applied on July 13. Balfour noticed that the patient's eyes and skin were now yellow. He vomited whenever he tried to drink, and he showed signs of debility, restlessness, and anxiety. His pulse was about 100 per minute. Again Balfour bled him, this time taking 16 ounces. Foss was removed from the gun deck to the spar deck, where the sea air refreshed him. He had no appetite for food and his stomach could not hold any. Lime juice and water continued to be his only nourishment. That evening, finding that his pulse was still hard and throbbing, Balfour took another 10 ounces of blood. Foss received five grams of calomel, which Balfour hoped would increase his salivation and slow his pulse rate. Half an ounce of mercurial ointment was rubbed on him.

By July 14 Foss was much relieved of pain in his head and chest. His fever was down and his bowels were open. His pulse was still a bit tense.

For the first time in days he was able to eat a little food and keep it down. The next day his pulse was softer but there was no other change. A day later he still had a touch of fever and a slight amount of salivation. The fever was completely gone by July 17, and Foss was no longer vomiting; he was salivating to a considerable degree because of the calomel. Balfour described Foss's skin as yellow as a pumpkin. The patient remained free of fever, coma, and pain the following day and was asking for broth made from fresh meat. That night, Foss was stricken with diarrhea, for which Balfour gave him a few drops of laudanum the next day. Foss was now very weak.

The seaman was much better on July 20. His diarrhea had been checked, and he was allowed a little wine. Foss continued to improve despite a little diarrhea, and by July 23 he was placed on a convalescent status. He had survived his various ordeals. Reflecting on the case, Balfour told Rush that if he had taken 24–30 ounces of blood at the beginning, he probably would have cured Foss sooner. Since then Balfour had had several other cases of yellow fever, which he treated by immediately bleeding the patients, taking 24–40 ounces of blood, and administering a powerful cathartic. The results were so successful that it was frequently not necessary to repeat the bleeding. In those few cases where additional treatment was required, only one additional bleeding was necessary before the patient was cured. Only one man with the fever had died since the ship had sailed, and his death was due to an accident and not to his ailment. The Foss case suggests how much drama may have been lost if the only account of a death is a brief entry in a log or a muster roll or payroll which does not give a cause.

Balfour went on to recount to Rush that he resorted to bleeding patients in cases not only of fever but also of injuries from falls, and in one instance of dysentery. He was convinced that bleeding prevented "the most violent local inflammations."

There was also the case of James Morgan, a gunner, who on July 23, 1798, complained of a pain in his breast and difficulty in breathing. His face was flushed and he had an incessant cough and "an oppressed pulse." Balfour's response was to take 76 ounces of blood during the first 12 hours after the injury, and another 30 ounces the following night and again the next day. The continuance of violent symptoms led him to take another 40 ounces. This meant that in a 36-hour period, some 146 ounces of blood were removed. After the last bleeding the violent symptoms disappeared. The patient recovered.

Despite his belief that the lancet was "worth all other remedies on shore" and that it was especially valuable on ships, Balfour did not bleed all his fever patients. When men were not vomiting but had generally languid dispositions and complained of pains in the forehead, he believed that these symptoms preceded the onset of fever. To ward it off, he gave a dose of tartarized antimony, which not only prevented the fever but also relieved the head pains. Sometimes blisters were applied to such patients, as the Royal Navy's Surgeon James Lind had suggested, but Balfour had not found them to be very effective.

Surgeon Balfour was also sure that Rush would be interested in a case involving a crew member who had a liver complaint that he had concealed for several days. When Balfour saw him, he complained of acute pain in his right side extending up to his shoulder, and he had some fever. He was bled repeatedly, his bowels were kept open, and mercurial ointment was rubbed on his side. He discharged a small stool and quantity of "pure Pus." Balfour believed that the man's liver was infected, but since there was no sign of pus in subsequent evacuations, he deduced that abscesses were forming in the liver. Over the next five days, the patient's pain was not so acute but he was steadily growing worse. His pulse was down to 40. Rubbing him with mercurial ointment was not helping, and it seemed likely that he would die. So, as a last resort, Balfour took three ounces of nitric acid and diluted it with water, followed by as much water as the patient desired in the course of the day. After three days of this treatment the patient's mouth began to show the effects of the mercury, but his pain was gradually diminishing. Believing that the nitric acid was affecting the patient's mouth, Balfour cut the dosage in half and continued the treatment. Eleven days later, the pain was entirely gone and the man was completely recovered.[35] What Rush thought about this case is not recorded, but the modern reader should be aware that the patient's recovery had nothing to do with the medication he received.

Another unusual case involved Surgeon John Rush and his colleague Surgeon's Mate John Parker. While the *Ganges* and the *Retaliation* were lying off Marcus Hook in the Delaware River in August 1798, the crews were stricken with yellow fever. Each time a man came down with it, the patient was transferred from the ship to one of the tents set up on an elevated and healthy spot on shore. Eventually 60 men, suffering from various stages of the fever, were sent to the tents, where the surgeons treated them under the supervision of the captain. Four of the 60 men died. One of the cases from the *Ganges* that made a vivid impression on the doctors was that of Ordinary Seaman James Clark, aged about 19. Clark showed the symptoms of yellow fever, and his pulse was low. Twenty-four ounces of blood were taken from his arm and he was purged with strong doses of calomel. His pulse then became full and strong. On the second day the bleeding and purging were omitted in favor of small doses of calomel, and he was rubbed with mercury. About noon he was pronounced dead and his body was placed in a coffin. Later, at about four o'clock that afternoon, Surgeon Rush examined the body. He noticed that Clark's complexion, which had been a pale yellow, was now orangelike with purplish spots. There was no evidence of a pulse or warmth in the body, and a mirror held before the mouth showed no signs of breathing. Despite this, Rush noted, the lower jaw was still flexible and there was no sign of decay. The surgeon felt or thought he felt a slight trace of warmth in the epigastric region. It was enough to make him try an experiment. Rush ordered that the body be covered with warm ashes from the cook's fire and that every half hour a gill of very strong brandy be poured down Clark's throat. Rush had to leave before the effects could be observed, but he asked Surgeon's Mate Parker to keep up the treatments. When Rush returned at sunrise the following morning, he found Clark propped up and eating soup. From Parker he learned that at about eight o'clock the previous evening, and after a quart of brandy had been poured down Clark's throat in the course of the treatment, the seaman began to breathe. The brandy treatment continued until eleven o'clock that night, when the patient complained about the heat of the ashes. He was then taken out of the coffin and laid upon some straw on the ground. Port wine sangree was now substituted for the brandy and was administered every half hour until daylight. At that time Clark refused to take any more wine and asked for food. Soup was given to him and it was shortly after this that Rush arrived and was able to rejoice in the success of his experiment. Clark probably returned to duty. It would be interesting to know the details of his subsequent life and whether his narrow escape from being buried alive had any long-range effect on him.

The whole story of Clark's revival would have been lost had it not been for Rush, because Parker took his daily journals with him when he left the navy at the end of the Quasi-War, and nothing is known of his or their subsequent history. Rush published his account of this case in 1804 in the interest of encouraging efforts at resuscitation in cases of doubtful death .by fever and to prevent premature burials.[36]

Another account of the treatment of an outbreak of yellow fever in the ship *Delaware* was recorded by Surgeon's Mate Samuel Anderson for the benefit of Dr. Benjamin Rush. The *Delaware*, with a complement of 180, was off the island of Curaçao on December 16, 1799, when the men began to show symptoms of the disease. Within three days 50 men were affected. By Christmas the situation had become alarming, and a hospital was established on shore to which all the sick were removed. Presumably this hospital was of the tent variety similar to that used off Marcus Hook for the men of the *Constellation*. Within a few hours after being moved to the shore, the great majority of the sick began to show milder symptoms, and many recovered with very little medical assistance. Anderson attributed the rapid change to the salubrious air. He added that the air between the decks of the ship was so bad that he frequently vomited while administering medicines. On the matter of symptoms, he noted that in many cases the beat of pulse was quite different. "In a word[,] so various was the state of the pulse that frequently I was at a loss to know how to act."

The experience gave Anderson the opportunity to witness a number of different states of fever as well as the methods of treatment used by Surgeon George Wright, his senior colleague. Wright used emetics and sometimes other medicines, followed by a cathartic, and then nitre and paregoric. After the fever had subsided, he gave Peruvian bark and wine to complete the cure. Anderson had studied under Dr. Philip Syng Physick, from whom he learned Rush's ideas about bleeding. He had also attended a public lecture by Rush and was familiar with his writings. Anderson told Rush that it was through the study of his works that he recognized the symptoms of yellow fever. Convinced that the course of treatment he observed on the ship was wrong and that the medicines prescribed had a tendency to aggravate the disease, he tried to change Wright's mind about them. "Many arguments did I use to convince Dr. Wright that the principles impress'd on his mind, were false; and that a practice founded upon them would not only be inefficacious, but highly injurious; but in vain did I argue; for firmly were those Ideas impress'd on his mind, that no reasoning, nor even facts would have eradicated them."

It was only after the hospital was established ashore that things began to change. Anderson came down with the fever himself, and the captain engaged a local physician, Dr. Forbes, formerly of New York, to help in the hospital. Also assigned to the hospital was Surgeon's Mate Richard C. Shannon of the *Scammel*. These two physicians shared Anderson's views about bleeding, and even though Wright believed that it was an improper procedure, he was induced to try it. Wright observed that bleeding was very successful in arresting yellow fever. Anderson was proud to report to Rush that out of the 140 cases they had had, only nine men died. It seemed as though bleeding had proved itself an effective treatment. At any rate, Anderson became even more convinced that victory over yellow fever was due to the lancet.[37]

Anderson was also involved at Curaçao when Captain Thomas Baker of the *Delaware* became affected by what was described as a violent inflammation of the brain which caused him to become deranged. He remained this way for some weeks, after which he had no memory. Being incapable of command, he was relieved of it in July 1800. Before that, however, his appearance and conduct were observed by several line officers who made their own judgments as to Barker's fitness to command. Anderson seems to have been the only medical officer who examined Captain Baker, who was discharged from the service in April 1801 and pensioned the following August. Such was the way a case diagnosed as insanity was dealt with.[38]

Some useful thoughts on the practice of medicine during the Quasi-War were also recorded by Surgeon's Mate Benjamin G. Harris of the frigate *Philadelphia,* presumably for his own reference. While the ship was attempting to cross the bar below Ft. Mifflin on Delaware Bay, it went aground on April 9, 1800. All hands were put to work unloading the ship's guns and provisions, a task made more difficult when nearly all the officers and crew came down with cholera morbus (diarrhea). This was not Asiatic cholera but diarrhea and cramps. It was noninfectious and rarely fatal. Harris believed that this was caused or aggravated by windy weather in temperatures from 60 to 65 degrees and by low river water. The hard work made the men thirsty, and they drank water from the river. Harris treated the men with "evacuarts, succeeded by astringents with opium." Later the water rose and the ship moved to Bombay Hook. Three days after the crew began drinking the ship's water, there was little cholera morbus among them. Later in April some of the men complained of irritation of the mouth. Harris thought this might be due to the potash that some bakers put in their bread or to the lime that was put into the water casks to sweeten them. He does not indicate what he did to help the men.

The month of May saw many members of the inexperienced crew become victims of accidents. While ramming home a cartridge in one of the cannon, a sailor exploded it and had his arm shot away. Surgeon Benjamin Champney immediately performed an amputation. Since the temperature in the cockpit that day was between 75 and 80 degrees and that on the gun deck between 70 and 75, the operation took place in the space above the cockpit. Before Champney had finished with this patient, another sailor was injured by an exploding powder horn. His hands were lacerated and he lost one of his little fingers. Both men recovered within six weeks. Later that month a sailor fell from the main topmast and suffered a fracture of his right humerus and a severe concussion. He was bleeding from his right ear and his senses were greatly deranged. Harris does not indicate how that case turned out.

Harris was quite busy in late September when there were nearly 30 on the sick list with scurvy or pulmonary complaints or sometimes both. He noted that the pulmonary complaints were very obstinate and required copious bleedings. On the matter of scurvy, he was careful to record a method of preserving lime juice that was recommended by Captain Stephen Decatur Sr. This involved boiling the juice in an earthen vessel and removing the sediment with a wooden ladle. When one-fourth of the juice had evaporated, it was removed from the heat and strained through a piece of flannel cloth. Half a pint of brandy per gallon of the acid was added and the mixture sealed in a bottle. Decatur told Harris that the sealed mixture could be preserved for several years without being impaired. Harris thought that if the oil of olives was added, it would help to exclude air, and if the acid was more concentrated, it would be better preserved and more convenient for travelers. Harris's generation did not know that heating destroyed most of the antiscorbutic value of the fruit, but he was correct in his observation that the concentrated acid was better.

While the *Philadelphia* was en route to St. Pierre in November 1800, Harris had a few cases of scurvy, one of which was serious. At St. Pierre all but the serious case recovered quickly. This astonished Harris because these men had fresh provisions only one day, except for any that they bought themselves from the local populace. The one serious case was that of a marine who died from a combination of scurvy and a lung infection.

In December 1800, Harris tallied the death statistics for the ship. Only three had died. One landsman, or inexperienced seaman, died of "Pulmonary inflammation." He had a very troublesome cough, and at the time of his death was hemorrhaging by the rectum. A second death was attributed to "violent Remittant Bilious Fever" and deranged senses. The third was the case of scurvy and lung infection mentioned above.

In addition to these ailments, Harris had to deal with cases of venereal disease. He was careful to note details that did not fit the generally accepted view of how things were supposed to look. Also, he records reports of cures as a result of various remedies.[39] Since venereal disease was not the result of official duties, there seems to have been discussion about how and if such cases should be treated. In the Royal Navy physicians were allowed to charge patients a fee for venereal treatment; was a similar fee to be allowed in the U.S. Navy? In response to this inquiry, Stoddert set forth a fee schedule by rank: marines paid $3; seamen, ordinary seamen, and petty officers $5; and warrant officers $10. These fees were not for each visit but for treatment until a "cure" or a remission took place. After circulating the fee schedule, Stoddert undermined it to a degree by stating that officers and men were not to be charged the fee unless they consented to it.[40] It is not known to what extent they did consent, but since their options at sea were limited, it is believed that most agreed to pay. Thus another practice began which in a few years would become a problem.

Sometimes a physician was so busy taking care of others that he forgot about himself. Hanson Catlett, the surgeon of the *Ganges*, suffered from heart complaints, coughing, and the frequent spitting of blood. He assumed that his condition was due to the use of salted provisions and the consumption of more spirituous liquor than he was accustomed to in civilian life, as well as to less exercise. He wrote to Benjamin Rush, who recommended regular habits and the use of tar pills. Catlett said he found these helpful. But when the Quasi-War ended and he was discharged in April 1801, he was still suffering from his complaints. Catlett went to Tennessee to start a new life.[41]

While in the *Ganges* many of Catlett's shipmates were surely aware of at least some aspects of his health. In his case and especially those of Lieutenant Samuel Angus and Surgeon's Mate Edward Field, we have glimpses of the long-range effect of illnesses or injuries in the naval service. But for many others there no way of knowing how many serious injuries there were which might have resulted in death or disability later. A systematic examination of all the pension records would doubtless shed some light on these questions. Some indications of the outcome of battle casualties has already been noted.

Let us now consider the case of Seaman Daniel Hawthorne, who somehow got information to Secretary Stoddert about the beatings he had received from Captain Mullowny in the *Montezuma*. Stoddert rescued Hawthorne from a jail in New Castle, Delaware, and had him brought to Philadelphia, where he was presumably examined and treated. Hawthorne expected to go to sea again during the winter of 1800–1801, but he was worried that he might never regain his health. "My Skull is much hurt, and I fear I shall lose my sight; The blows I received from him [Mullowny] were disgraceful to humanity; they forced the blood from [my] Mouth, Eyes, Ears & Nose." Hawthorne said he had heard from his former shipmates that Mullowny's conduct toward the men had improved, and he expected that this was due to the action of the secretary.[42] We do not know the subsequent history of this case, but Mullowny was not among the officers selected for retention at the end of the war. It would be interesting to know what Hawthorne's subsequent life was like. Nowhere in his letter does he indicate whether or what type of medical treatment he received for his injuries, but there must have been some. Were there other cases similar to Hawthorne's? We will probably never know. But it seems clear that what he suffered was never considered part of the cost of the war.

Health Care for Navy Men on Shore

The shortage of navy doctors in some areas made it necessary to employ civilian medical men for some services, most commonly to examine recruits for the navy or marines. Such duties were of short duration. A more serious problem was the care of invalid officers and seamen by civilian practitioners. For example, when Lieutenant Wilson Jacobs of the frigate *George Washington* became ill, he was allowed to return to his home in Providence to be with his family during his recuperation. There he was treated by two civilian doctors at intervals between November 1798 and April 1800. The total cost of this care, including consultations between the doctors, came to $137.31. Lieutenant Jacobs was most anxious to have the bills paid by the government before he went to sea.[43] Presumably they were.

Another claim against the government, and one that provides information on the transportation practices of Philadelphia physicians, was that filed by Dr. Joseph C. Strong. He was hired to attend the marines in the city from August 2 to November 30, 1798, when a new outbreak of yellow fever struck. Strong was asked to examine navy recruits during the same period. Since the distance between the navy and the marine corps installations was two miles, he hired a horse to get around the city, dividing the cost between the navy and the marines. This method of accounting, as well as his bill for $555.00 for his services and the horse rental, raised some questions in the mind of the navy's accountant. At this point, Dr. Benjamin Rush wrote a letter to the accountant justifying the charge for the horse. All the other physicians in the public service visited their patients in sedan chairs that were rented for $3.00 a day, and if Strong had done the same, their charge would have been higher than the horse rental. As it was, Strong was out in all kinds of weather and was exposed to danger. It was Rush's view that Strong could have charged four times more than he did, for individuals had paid Rush that much. An additional justification of the charge, said Rush, was that Strong had sacrificed his private practice at a time when it was very profitable.[44] The accountant was apparently convinced, and the Treasury paid the full sum requested.

There was also the case of Midshipman Daniel Eldridge of the frigate *United States*, who, while off Marcus Hook in November 1800, fell off the gunwale of the ship and received a dangerous wound. Gangrene set in, and Lieutenant Cyrus Talbot ordered him to be placed under the care of a Dr. May of Chester, Pennsylvania, because when the ship moved down river it would not be possible for the surgeon or his mate to attend to Eldridge. Dr. May was willing to take the case but first wanted to know how he was to be paid for his attendance and for nursing care. Presumably satisfactory arrangements were worked out, for Eldridge recovered and went on to serve in the *Constellation*.[45]

Another midshipman, Jesse N. Lewis of the *Ganges*, became sick while on the Havana station in 1800. He was given a furlough to recover his health and he went to Boston. Having no funds for housing or food, he applied to the navy agent for two months' pay, producing, as proof of his character and connections, a letter from Secretary of State John Marshall and one from Congressman Josiah Parker of Virginia. Lewis told the agent, Stephen Higginson, that if he had any doubt about the bill, Marshall, who was a relative, would pay it. Higginson advanced the money and informed the accountant of the guarantee. Lewis was discharged from the navy in January 1801 and disappeared from sight soon afterward. Higginson subsequently learned that he had been taken advantage of, and the money he advanced was never repaid.[46]

A somewhat different environment prevailed in the cases involving enlisted men. When Captain Truxtun discharged five invalids at their request at Norfolk in August 1798, he promised them that the navy agent would furnish living quarters until they could shift for themselves or receive instructions from the secretary of the navy. Truxtun so advised the agent, William Pennock, and added that no public money should be spent on them that could be avoided, for they were not worth the rations that they drew.[47]

Other captains followed similar practices. In September 1798, Stoddert wrote to the secretary of war that sick sailors had been left at Norfolk and Newport, and others would probably be left in New York, Philadelphia, and Boston. Those left at Norfolk and Newport were boarded and doctors were paid to attend them. This was costing quite a bit, and there was no guarantee that once a man recovered, he would not be lost to the service. Stoddert therefore wondered if the War Department had troops and surgeons stationed at any of these ports whose services could be used for sick sailors.[48]

Apparently nothing came of this novel suggestion of cost sharing by the armed forces. As a consequence, the navy continued to pay for the care of its invalids on shore. For example, Francis Higgins, a steward at the Pennsylvania Hospital in Philadelphia, was paid $36.57 for the board of one Robert Smith, an invalid sailor from the schooner *Retaliation*. Unfortunately we do not know the length of the convalescence, but it may well have been two months. In another case the navy paid William Allen, the health officer at Staten Island, $18.66 for the board of an invalid marine named Peter Kelly. Another account shows that one Dwight Foster was paid $17.90 for taking care of an invalid marine at Brookfield from April 13 to May 1, 1799.[49]

How much was to be allotted for the treatment of the sick sometimes became a matter of dispute. For example, Captain Barry had a sick sailor from the *United States* who was left in the care of Lewis Albertus of

Philadelphia. Dr. Strong attended the man from June 25 through mid-July 1800, but he did not submit any evidence that the sailor needed a longer convalescence. Nevertheless, Albertus billed the navy for nursing care from June 25 to November 25. Thomas Turner, the navy's accountant, refused to pay unless Albertus could justify the long-term care.[50] The outcome is not known.

Hospital and medical costs were on Stoddert's mind when he wrote to Captain Henry Geddes of the *Patapsco* about a wounded man. Stoddert suggested that instead of sending the man to the hospital, the captain should give him an extra month's pay and discharge him. Other wounded men of the *Enterprise,* who were left in the hospital by Captain John Shaw, should be discharged unless they were well enough to be taken on board the *Patapsco.* If they remained in the hospital, it must be at public expense for as long as necessary.[51]

Meanwhile the New York navy agents faced additional problems. Two men who were wounded in the battle between the *Constellation* and *La Vengeance* went to New York to await the arrival of the ship's purser, who would pay them off. One was disabled, and under the act of Congress of March 2, 1799, he was entitled to half pay for life, and if he married, for his wife's lifetime as well. The disabled man wanted to learn a trade, and the New York agents felt that they could probably get him a place to acquire a skill. But first the agents needed to hear from the government how the man was to get his half pay. Presumably the accounts of his naval service would first have to be settled. While awaiting the arrival of the purser from their ship, both men applied to the agents for funds, soon exhausted the sums earmarked for their use, and ran into debt. The agents asked that the navy accountant send them a copy of the purser's records so that the matter could be resolved.[52] There is no record known to the writer of the outcome of this case.

There was also the case of John Hoxse, a seaman from the *Constellation* who had lost his right arm and been wounded in the side during the battle with *La Vengeance.* Hoxse and others had been left in a British hospital in Jamaica, where some of his shipmates died. He got out of Jamaica and went to Rhode Island, where he was treated until his wounds healed. When they looked into the matter of half pay, the New York agents told him that he had been discharged from the service as of May 22. Hoxse wrote to the accountant stating that his date of discharge should be when he was cured at the hospital, and not earlier; he also asked for his pay during that interval. Hoxse won his appeal. Not only did he get his back pay, but the navy agents were sent a copy of the regulations governing the payment of his pension.[53]

Medical care for the French prisoners and the marines who guarded them was also an issue that was brought to Stoddert's attention. French prisoners were sent from the West Indies to New Castle, Delaware, in the fall of 1798 where they were turned over to the U.S. marshal and lodged in a barracks. They were guarded by a marine corporal and nine men. The discipline and cleanliness of the marines had improved since they were first assigned to this duty, but they were inadequately clothed. By October they were suffering from the want of socks and watch coats. Lieutenant Anthony Gale urged his superiors to send these items quickly. The clothing did not arrive, and between October 30 and November 24, three men had died. One was reported killed, but no details survive about the circumstances. Two other marines had been sick and died of unspecified diseases. The rest of the marines were "in a dreadful way," probably for want of adequate clothing.[54] We do not know how well this group survived the winter or when or if they got their clothing.

Meanwhile some French prisoners were sent to Philadelphia, where they were confined in a jail and became ill. Stoddert wrote to the managers of the Pennsylvania Hospital asking that they be admitted and promising that the Navy Department would be responsible for the costs incurred.[55] The final cost is not known.

In attempting to assess the health record of the Quasi-War years, a researcher is hampered by a lack of data from many ships and installations and the knowledge from other sources that not all injuries and illnesses were reported. Furthermore, some of the injured were discharged from the navy within a short time, and the final outcome of various cases will probably never be known. For example, Truxtun discharged at Norfolk a man who had a brain injury as the result of a fall on shipboard.[56] This was clearly what later generations would call a service-connected injury. Yet leaving him at Norfolk was but a short step away from having him discharged by navy agents, who were conscious of the need to keep costs down. In fairness to them, and to the state of medical science at the time, there was little that could be done for such unfortunate men. Midshipman Samuel Angus suffered a similar fate when he was struck on the head by a block or splinter during the battle between the *Constellation* and *La Vengeance* on February 1, 1800. The impact knocked him flat. The ship's surgeon examined him but did not consider the wound serious enough to be reported as a battle casualty. From subsequent events it seems likely that Angus suffered a fractured skull or a severe concussion. He had a scar on his head for the rest of his life. In the months that followed the battle, his fellow officers often heard Angus complain about pains in his head. It proved to be only the first of several wounds that Angus suffered in the course of his career which eventually led to mental disturbances.[57]

If there are many unanswered questions about naval medicine during the Quasi-War, there are also some facts from which tentative conclusions can be drawn. The vast majority of deaths were due to accidents, high on the list of which is the sinking of the revenue cutter *Pickering* and the frigate *Insurgente* in a gale in September 1800. The loss of these two ships with all hands meant that over 400 men died.

On other ships in more tranquil settings, missing men were assumed to have fallen overboard and drowned at night. If the ship was in a harbor, the man might be listed as having deserted and/or drowned. Death in battle was a comparatively rare fate. Wounds of various types were common, but when the injured were transferred to hospitals ashore, it is impossible to know with any certainty how many recovered and how many died at a later time from the effects of their wounds. Apparently only a very small number of those who were permanently injured were pensioned.

It is known that 99 men died of yellow fever. How many others died of this disease in ships for which no reliable sources survive cannot be known. But it is assumed that if there had been any large number, some record of it would have survived, at least in correspondence. In addition, many of the deaths due to unspecified diseases or simply to fever may or may not be related to yellow fever. It is known that 9 marine officers and 194 enlisted men died during the Quasi-War years. The 9 officer fatalities included 1 lost in the *Insurgente* and 1 killed in a duel. Of the 194 enlisted men, 31 were lost in the *Insurgente* and 11 in the *Pickering*, 4 were killed in action, 2 died of wounds, and 1 was accidentally killed. Six enlisted men are recorded as having drowned. This leaves a total of 139 with no known cause of death, but many of these may have been due to diseases. When all causes of death are considered and estimates made for the unknown, it seems likely that service in the navy during the Quasi-War led to the demise of at least 600 men out of a total force variously estimated at between 2,559 and 7600.[58] Perhaps another 50–100 suffered lasting effects from injuries received during their service. The general good health was due in part to one-year enlistments for sailors in contrast to three years for marines, to keeping ships at sea as much as possible and away from Caribbean ports where the men would be exposed to disease, and to discharging as soon as possible any sailor or marine who seemed to have any long-term health problem.

Chapter 4

The Barbary Wars

One of the men who played an important role in the medical story of the navy in the early nineteenth century was Surgeon Edward Cutbush, and he was very nearly lost to the service. By the end of the Quasi-War, he had grown tired of life at sea. His rations were inadequate and he was contemplating leaving the navy and establishing a civilian practice. But when he received word that he was among those selected for retention in peacetime, he felt honored: he had not asked to stay on but had been selected. It seemed he had been favored by the government, and if this was true, then his prospects looked bright. Even so, there were doubts in his mind during the months that followed his selection. While waiting for orders for active duty, he looked into the possibility of setting up a practice near Monticello, Virginia. If he chose to do this, he knew that there would be expenses related to moving his family and getting established. He weighed the advantages and disadvantages. Finally he decided to remain in the navy, and soon he received orders assigning him to the *Constellation*, then being prepared for war service in the Mediterranean. Cutbush did not realize it, but he was about to participate in an enterprise that would do much for his career and for the navy.[1]

Between 1801 and 1807 the U.S. Navy was active in the Mediterranean as a result of threats to U.S. commerce in that region. The wars between Napoleonic France and the allied powers of Europe focused the attention of those governments largely on affairs on the Continent. This encouraged the Barbary pirates in North Africa to seize ships involved in trade in the Mediterranean and demand tribute. Small powers were especially vulnerable to such harassment. U.S. merchant ships tried to use their nation's status as a neutral to trade with both France and the allied powers, especially Great Britain. U.S. ships were easy targets, and the pirates had little to fear from the naval force that had been largely dismantled at the end of the Quasi-War. Tripoli declared war on the United States, and from time to time there were concerns that Algiers and Morocco might join in the conflict. For a brief period, Morocco was technically at war, until new understandings were worked out. From the point of view of the Jefferson administration, the problem was whether it was wiser to pay tribute or wage war. Congress was divided. Jefferson was concerned about reducing national expenditures and was therefore initially averse to becoming involved in extensive and expensive naval operations. There were also differences between Secretary of the Treasury Albert Gallatin and Secretary of the Navy Robert Smith over the course of action to be followed. As a result, when it was decided to resort to force, the war had to be waged on a peacetime budget.[2]

From a naval point of view, the Barbary Wars were important for helping to preserve the sea service, for giving its young officers a sense of pride and professionalism, for developing leadership, and for affording experience in such areas as maintaining blockades, the use of gunboats, support for operations on land, overcoming problems of supply, and diplomatic negotiations. For medical men the war provided new opportunities to observe the effects of climate and food, as well as additional experience in the treatment of wounds, injuries, and diseases. It also meant expanding the number of doctors in the navy only a few years after it had been reduced. Once again several medical men had to adjust to a naval environment in the midst of war, with the additional complication this time that waging war on a peacetime budget meant something had to be sacrificed. The indications are that the enlisted men of the navy bore the brunt and that some of the resulting strain may have contributed to their health problems.

To give a better appreciation of some of the naval operations and the health questions that arose during them a few words about geography may be helpful. The Barbary coast of North Africa was more than 3,000 miles long. On the western end was Morocco. Tangier, its principal seaport was nearly opposite to the British base at Gibraltar. East of Morocco was Algiers, whose capital city bore the same name as the country. From Tangier to Algiers was 500 miles. The next state to the east was Tunis, whose capital city bore the same name. From Algiers to Tunis was 550 miles. To the east was Tripoli, whose capital city was also named Tripoli. The distance from Tunis to Tripoli was 370 miles. The two most powerful of the four Barbary states were Algiers and Tunis. Algiers had a navy of

15 large ships, 60 gunboats, and 150 galleys. Tunis had 94 large vessels and 30 gunboats. By contrast, Morocco's navy had only 5 vessels and Tripoliti's 8 large ships and a fleet of gunboats. If these four powers combined forces in a struggle with the United States, the peacetime navy would have its hands full. Therefore the economy-minded Jefferson administration first attempted to deal with its Mediterranean problem by a small show of force.

A squadron of four vessels under Commodore Richard Dale in the frigate *President* was sent to the Mediterranean in May 1801 to ascertain the situation there and punish the seizures of U.S. vessels. When Dale reached the Mediterranean, he learned that Tripoli had declared war on the United States. He tried to bring Tripoli to terms by a show of force and a blockade, but his squadron was too small and the port of Tripoli was too well protected. His effectiveness was further limited by the need to convoy U.S. merchant ships from port to port and the need for ships to leave the blockade to chase and try to capture Tripolitan vessels. While this sort of activity resulted in little sickness and death, the replenishing of water, food, and supplies was a constant problem.[3]

The British allowed the Americans to purchase supplies and refit at Gibraltar, but fresh food and water were hard to get. Dale was hopeful that supply ships from the United States would soon bring staples to Gibraltar. Meanwhile he sent the schooner *Enterprise* to the island of Malta for water. En route the *Enterprise* captured a Tripolitan cruiser without the loss of a single man wounded or killed. But the Tripolitans lost 20 killed and 30 wounded. At Malta the Americans had to wait their turn while the British filled their casks and as a result had to leave the island and return to their duty station before all the casks had been filled. The *Enterprise* brought back so little water that there was none to share with the other ships. Dale was obliged to take the *President* off blockade duty and to go to Malta himself for water. Despite hardships the crew was still healthy. While he was at Malta, Dale sent the *Enterprise* to Sicily to investigate the water supplies at Sargossa. By August 25, 1801, Dale was back on blockade duty before Tripoli, but an outbreak of influenza and a shortage of food soon forced him to go to Gibraltar. Early in September, Dale reported to William Eaton, the U.S. consul at Tunis, then living in Leghorn, Italy, that out of a crew of 409, he had 152 men on the sick list and that the number was growing every day. He did not indicate the nature of the illnesses; perhaps influenza was one. By the time he reached Gibraltar, the sick list had been reduced to 37, but 3 men had died. One was an old marine who had fallen from a gun to the berth deck. Despite a week of ministrations by the medical men, he expired. The causes of the other two deaths are not

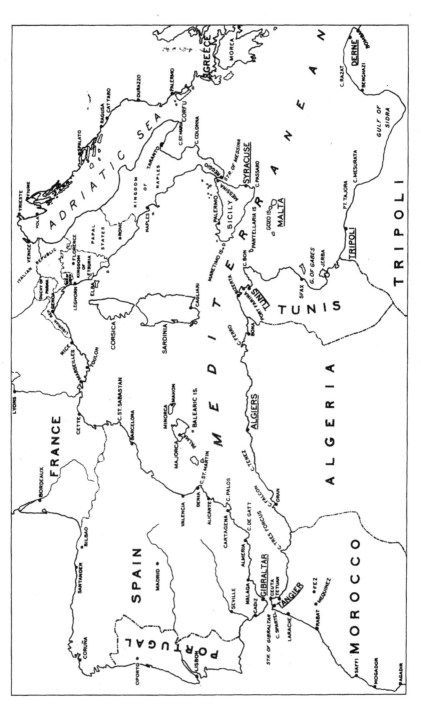

Map of the Mediterranean Region during the Barbary Wars. U.S. Navy Department, *Naval Documents Related to the United States Wars with the Barbary Powers*, 1:140.

recorded. One marine, suffering from cramps, was transferred to a British hospital at Gibraltar.

When Dale reached that British base, he was disappointed to find no U.S. store ships waiting for him. Hearing that the Spaniards had detained U.S. merchant ships at Algeciras, he went there and got his provisions. He was surprised that no butter, cheese, molasses, rum, or candles had been sent, and he found that the bread was full of weevils. Dale was also shocked that the supply ship was carrying rice and flour for private merchants. He wrote to the secretary of the navy, about these matters. His diplomatic words to his civilian superior were presumably designed to make President Jefferson ponder why the naval force that he sent to the Mediterranean was not being fed and supplied adequately fashion.[4]

Dale's search for supplies continued with the frigates *Philadelphia* and *Essex* sailing to Malaga, Spain. the The U.S. consul there supplied bread and fresh meat but no salted provisions. Captain William Bainbridge of the *Essex* had to content himself with the purchase of only four barrels of pork. Both ships watered at Malaga and were on duty off Tripoli by September 29. While cruising off the coast, the *Essex* lost two men to accidents. One was a 16-year-old boy who fell from a yard, fractured his skull, and died half an hour later. Were these accidents attributable in any way to the lack of an adequate diet? We will never know. Certainly men who were presumably adequately fed in the years both before and after the Barbary Wars had similar accidents. Yet a shortage of food and water must have had some effect on the ability of the sailors to do their jobs. Three days after the boy died, a lieutenant died of a lingering illness, the nature of which has not been preserved.[5]

Continuing to search for the additional supplies that he needed, Dale returned to Gibraltar. Here a seaman deserted, was apprehended, and deserted again. Two midshipmen captured him once more. While one went for a guard, the second got into an altercation and stabbed the deserter twice in the chest with a dirk when he attempted to escape. A British doctor who examined the wounds said they were dangerous. The man was then brought on board the *President* and examined by its surgeon, who told Dale that the wounds were slight and not dangerous. The deserter now claimed to be a British subject, and a naval officer from that service came on board the *President* and demanded his release. Dale refused but offered to let a British naval surgeon examine him. This was done, and the surgeon reported to Dale that the wounds were of no consequence. On October 20, 16 days after he had been stabbed, the deserter died. It seems the appearance of the wound belied an infection that took the man's life.[6]

Two days after this there was a serious accident. On the way back to the *President,* a cutter overturned and all but one of its occupants were drowned. This probably represented the loss of six to eight men.[7]

November 19 found the *President* at Port Mahon on the island of Minorca, where it was placed in a quarantine despite Dale's objections. The authorities at Mahon noted that approximately 100 men in the squadron were on the sick list, but none had contagious diseases. The actual situation was somewhat worse: there were 70 sick men in the *Philadelphia* and 80 in the *Essex.* Complicating the situation in the *Philadelphia* was the fact that Surgeon William Turner had become ill and had been put ashore at Tunis to stay with William Eaton, the U.S. consul. By the end of November, the squadron's sick list had been reduced to 50, and Dale set sail.

While leaving Port Mahon, the pilot ran the ship on a rock and caused some damage to the hull. Dale headed for the French port of Toulon in search of repairs. The French also insisted that the ship be placed in quarantine and returned the men who had been sent ashore. Dale protested that he had no contagious diseases on board, only men with slight colds. There were "no more sick on Board, than is common on Board of ships of this description." The quarantine continued, but the ship was allowed to take on the supplies it needed. A preliminary examination of the bottom revealed an obstruction, and Dale was unwilling to take his ship to the United States until he was confident about the state of its hull. He also told the secretary of the navy that an Atlantic passage in midwinter would be long and exposed to severe gales. The ship's company was feeble, "many of them down with the Scurvy and other diseases, also [sic] a number without shoes or stockings, and badly clothed otherwise." Consequently the *President* did not sail from Toulon until February 11, 1802, and it reached Gibraltar on February 26. From there it proceeded to the United States in March.[8] As far as can be ascertained from surviving records, the loss of life in Dale's squadron was small. The *President,* with a crew of about 400, lost 8 or 9 to accidents and 3 to disease; the *Essex,* with an authorized complement of 228, lost 2 men to accidents and 1 officer to an unknown illness.[9]

By this time it had become apparent to the administration that Dale's force was too small to accomplish much, and plans were underway to replace it with a larger force. Congress enacted a law on February 6, 1802, which was the equivalent of a declaration of war against Tripoli. Originally, Commodore Thomas Truxtun was to head the new squadron, but a disagreement arose between him and the Navy Department over its failure to send him a captain to command the ship so that he could devote himself to the duties of commodore. Truxtun resigned and Richard V. Morris was named to replace him as commodore. The new squadron consisted of the frigate *Chesapeake*, which was the flagship, and the frigates *Constellation, John Adams, New York,* and *Adams,* and the schooner *Enterprise.* Men for these ships were enlisted for two years instead of one. In addition, Morris was authorized to purchase gunboats from European powers which could be used for blockade duty and the protection of U.S. commerce in the Gibraltar Strait. Ships of the squadron sailed at different times from February to October 1802, their captains carrying with them a new set of navy regulations issued by the president in January 1802.[10]

These regulations set forth the duties of officers and petty officers, as well as instructions about convoys, clothing, provisions, courts martial, and the keeping of logbooks and journals. The surgeon should "inspect and take care of the necessaries sent on board for the use of the sick men; if not good, he must acquaint the captain; and he must see that they are duly served out for the relief of the sick." He must also visit the sick men under his care twice a day, or oftener if necessary. He was also obliged to see that his mates did their duty, "so that none want due attendance and relief." It was the duty of the surgeon to inform the captain daily of the state of his patients. In difficult cases, he was to consult with the other surgeons in the squadron. No men were to be sent to sick quarters ashore unless their illnesses or numbers were such that the surgeon could not care for them on shipboard, and the surgeon must certify such before the patients were moved. When sick men were transferred to hospitals, the ship's doctor was to send to the surgeon there an account of the time and manner in which each man was taken ill and the treatment he had received. If the surgeon at the hospital found that a patient who was transferred there might have been cured in a few days on his own ship, the doctor who recommended the transfer would be fined $10.

In a combat situation the surgeon and his mates and assistants were to be ready before the battle was joined. They were to have at hand all the things "necessary for [the] stopping of blood and dressing of wounds." At all times the surgeon was obliged to keep a daybook of his practice containing the names of his patients, the date and nature of their illnesses, the method of treatment, prescriptions used, and the disposition of individual cases. Using this daybook as a source, the surgeon was to prepare two other journals: one containing a record of his "physical" practice and one for his surgical work. These two journals were to be sent to the Navy Department at the end of every voyage. He was also to keep a regular account of his receipts and expenditures for all stores furnished to the medical department on his requisition. The surgeon was to be held accountable for all such expenditures, of which he was to transmit a report to the accountant of the navy at the end of every cruise.[11] The regulations of 1802 made no mention of the duties of surgeon's mates. We can thus assume that they did everything that the surgeon ordered them to do, which on some ships and in some conditions could be a considerable amount. There were also instances where a mate had to act as surgeon, or a surgeon had to function without a mate. Both situations could involve a great deal of time and energy, especially with a big patient load. During the Barbary Wars some surgeons and mates were placed in situations that tested them greatly.

The *Constellation*, with Surgeon Cutbush on board, was the first frigate of the new force under Commodore Morris to reach Tripoli, and it began hostile operations by attacking some gunboats that had been driven ashore. In April the ship lost one marine to a severe respiratory infection and another seaman and marine to smallpox. Six weeks later, Captain Alexander Murray reported that he had a healthy crew that was in fine condition. On August 16 he lost an ordinary seaman, but no cause of death is stated. Three days later the *Constellation* had a battle with eight gunboats. Eight of the Tripolitans were killed, but no Americans were reported injured.[12]

Meanwhile when Morris reached Gibraltar in the *Chesapeake* on May 25, he found the *Essex* blockading a Tripolitan ship in that harbor. At that time there was a danger that Morocco would join in the war against the United States. To guard against that possibility, Morris kept his squadron near the Strait of Gibraltar. It was not until August 16 that he learned that the dispute with Morocco had been resolved peacefully. Morris was now free to deal with Tripoli. His orders were to send the *Enterprise* to Leghorn to pick up James L. Cathcart, the former U.S. consul at Tripoli, who was to negotiate a new treaty with that state. The rest of the squadron, with the exception of the *Adams*, which relieved the *Essex* off Gibraltar, were to proceed to Tripoli. Morris heard that there were Tripolitan cruisers near the Spanish coast, so he decided to use the *Chesapeake* to convoy a group of Swedish and U.S. merchant ships around the northern coasts of the Mediterranean and go for Cathcart himself. When he reached Leghorn on October 12, he found the *Constellation* there under Captain Alexander Murray. Arriving off Tripoli on June 7, Murray had cruised in those waters until early September, when he convoyed Swedish and U.S. ships to Gibraltar. From there he proceeded to Leghorn, where he met his commander.[13]

At his meeting with the commodore, Murray gained the impression that Morris intended to sail for Tripoli at once and open negotiations with the pasha of that country. Instead Morris remained in Leghorn until November 3. There a duel took place between a marine and a naval officer of the

Constellation which resulted in the death of the marine. A midshipman from the *Constellation* and three seamen from the *Enterprise* were drowned in a boating accident while returning to their ships. Meanwhile Morris ordered Murray to take his ship to the French naval base at Toulon for repairs and then pick up supplies at Gibraltar and take them to Malta. After leaving Toulon, Murray ran into heavy weather and sprang a foremast yard. He ran out of bread and had to put his crew on half rations until he reached Malaga on November 26.[14]

Shortly before the arrival of the *Constellation,* the U.S. consul at Malaga received instructions from the Department of State concerning how he should deal with distressed seamen. He replied that the 12¢ a day allowed by the government would "procure a very scanty fare" for anyone in Malaga. Earlier the *New York* had been denied water there and had had to proceed to Algiers. Fortunately, Murray was allowed to make his repairs. While this work was being done, a marine died of unstated causes. To bury him at sea, it was necessary to use one of the frigate's boats to carry the body out of the harbor to an unrestricted area, where the commitment service took place.[15]

Both Murray and the consul were relieved when the frigate *John Adams,* the last of the Morris squadron to sail from the United States, arrived in Malaga the day after the *Constellation.* Before leaving, it had picked up supplies of food, gunpowder, and other items at Hampton Roads and delivered them to Gibraltar before moving on to Malaga. Murray took most of the supplies that were still on the *John Adams* and gave some to the *Enterprise,* which arrived a few days later. The *Enterprise* then returned to Morris. Since the *John Adams* needed some caulking, Murray sent it back to Gibraltar to have the work done, as well as to pick up more supplies and a foreyard for the *Constellation.* Among the items Rodgers was to acquire were medicines and clothing for the marines.

Originally it was Murray's intention that when both ships had been repaired and supplied, they would join Morris at Malta. But in December, Murray received an unsealed letter from the secretary of the navy to Morris directing that the *Chesapeake* and the *Constellation* return home without delay. Murray assumed that the letter had been left unsealed so that whoever saw it first would act on it. Knowing that the period of enlistment of his crew would soon expire and that Morris was 1,200 miles away and not easily consulted, Murray decided to return to the United States without waiting for orders from his commander. He wrote to Morris of his decision and gave the letter to Rodgers to deliver. While the *John Adams,* with a complement of 220 men, was at Malaga in November and December 1802, one marine died of a fever. The rest of the marines were so sickly that their commander could rarely muster 15 men for duty. We do not know the cause of this illness. Despite this problem, Rodgers carried out his orders.[16]

Meanwhile Morris reached Malta on November 20, where the *Chesapeake's* bowsprit had to be repaired. Before the ship could get underway again, an outbreak of influenza immobilized the crew. By Christmas Day the disease had abated sufficiently for Morris to sail for Syracuse in search of provisions cheaper than those at Malta. He returned to Malta on January 4, 1803, to find the *New York* and the *John Adams* waiting for him and to learn of Secretary Smith's order and Murray's departure. The provisions brought by the *John Adams* were distributed to the squadron. Morris and Cathcart finally sailed for Tripoli on January 30 in company with the *New York* and the *John Adams*.[17]

When the squadron arrived off Tripoli on February 3, it was buffeted by strong winds and currents, which made Morris decide that he could not operate against Tripoli in the winter. The squadron returned to Malta, then went to Tunis for a meeting with William Eaton, the U.S. consul there. The pasha of Tunis was preparing for war with the United States. Eaton told Morris that he must meet with the pasha, who wanted to discuss the return of some of the cargo of a Tunisian-owned ship that had been seized by the *Enterprise*. During the interview the commodore and the consul lost patience with the demands of the pasha and departed without taking formal leave of him. En route to the ship, Morris was arrested by agents of the pasha, who refused to release him until the seized cargo was paid for. At length Morris agreed to pay $22,000, or about two-thirds of the claim. This was acceptable to the pasha and Morris was released.[18]

By this time the Eaton's feelings against the pasha were so strong that he could no longer function effectively as consul, and he was replaced by Dr. George Davis, who had been serving as the ranking surgeon of the squadron. At their first meeting the doctor and the pasha discussed the differences between yellow fever in America and the plague in the eastern Mediterranean. Davis became the U.S. chargé d'affaires at Tunis and served from March 1803 to August 1805. Later, in July 1806, he was appointed U.S. consul at Tripoli. While this change of careers was good for Davis in financial terms and prestige, it meant that another experienced surgeon was lost to the navy.[19]

On March 19, Morris's squadron arrived off Algiers, where he learned from James Leander Cathcart that the dey was angry because Jefferson had sent him money instead of the naval stores he expected. The dey showed his displeasure by refusing to receive Cathcart as the consul and successor to Richard O'Brien. Morris did not go ashore but took his force to Gibraltar, where he made some changes in the squadron. The *Chesapeake* was sent home, and Morris transferred his flag to the *New York*. The ships received a new supply of provisions, then headed for Malta and some repairs. By early May only the *John Adams* was ready for service, and Captain John Rodgers was ordered to take it to Tripoli. He was to cruise off that port for three weeks or until the pasha made a peace overture.[20]

In the midst of chasing and boarding various neutral ships, Rodgers captured the Tripolitan cruiser that had been blockaded at Gibraltar for two years. It had gotten out of that predicament when the emperor of Morocco laid claim to it, and Morris accepted the argument. Rodgers took his prize to Malta, where he found the *New York* and the *Enterprise* now ready for sea. The squadron returned to Tripoli and engaged in hostile action. This resulted in the death of several men and the wounding of others, which will be noted below. It soon became clear that the pasha was not easily frightened and was not ready for peace. Turning the blockading squadron over to Rodgers on May 10, Morris returned to Malta. Rodgers attacked enemy gunboats, and the threatened capture of an enemy cruiser led to its being blown up.

These were small gains that did not change the overall picture of the war much. Morris now decided that he would abandon operations against Tripoli and return to Gibraltar by way of Messina, Naples, and Leghorn. The squadron sailed from Malta on July 11. When Morris reached Gibraltar on September 14, 1803, he found Commodore Edward Preble, the head of a new squadron, waiting to relieve him. Morris returned to the United States in the *Adams*. A court of inquiry censured him for his lack of activity, and President Jefferson dismissed him from the service.[21]

Before considering Preble's operations, we should note that our knowledge of the medical record of the Barbary Wars has been greatly enhanced by the discovery of a hitherto unknown log kept by Surgeon Peter St. Medard of the frigate *New York.* This log has been analyzed by J. Worth Estes, M.D., and the results of his study have been published. From September 1, 1802, to December 9, 1803, St. Medard kept records on the 237 men and one woman who came under his care. About two-thirds of the crew needed some medical attention at least once, and half the complement required more than one visit. This meant that 488 new cases, or an average of 1.1 a day, were added to the sick log. There were 30 deaths in the course of the voyage.

The most common complaint was disorders of the respiratory tract, or catarrahs, in the language of the surgeon. These accounted for 214 cases, or 60 percent, of all new admissions and one-third of the lost work days. St. Medard initially treated his catarrah patients with diaphoretics 40 percent of the time, with emetics, another 40 percent, and with cathartics about 17 percent. After a few days these gave way to the use of various mixtures of tonics and other drugs.[22] Next came disorders of the gastrointestinal tract, which amounted to 20 percent of the total admissions, and which were most often fatal. Recovery took two to four weeks and was responsible for almost one-fourth of the lost work days. They were also the cause of most of the medical discharges. Of all the gastrointestinal problems, dysentery and bilious disorders were the most frequent at the beginning of the voyage and recurred from time to time. Patients were treated with emetics or cathartics and absorbents in cases of dysentery and, less frequently, diarrhea. In the case of bilious disorders, the treatment began with emetics and cathartics, followed by diaphoretics and bleeding if there was a fever. Treatment continued with Peruvian bark, which was a source of quinine, and febrifuges, or something to reduce fever, as well as opiates for pain. The next most common problems were the critical fevers: typhus, slow, and nervous. Available evidence is insufficient to tell us whether some of these were the same as modern typhus or typhoid fever, but that is possible. Almost one-fifth of those who died suffered from one of these fevers. St. Medard had 32 patients with rheumatism, 56 percent of whom were treated with liniments, 21 percent with gum guaiac given orally, 12 percent with diaphoretics, and 5 percent with cathartics. Next in frequency was lues, or syphilis, which affected 12 men, or 1.2 percent of the ship's compliment. These cases were treated with mercury.

The voyage to the United States in the fall of 1803 took 50 days, during which 8 percent of the crew became ill with scurvy. Five men died of it. Treating the sick was particularly difficult for St. Medard because he was shorthanded. His mate, Nathaniel T. Weems, had been transferred to the *Constitution,* which continued to be a part of Preble's squadron. St. Medard's situation might have been much worse had the voyage lasted any longer. At Norfolk most of the crew were discharged. Enough hands were retained to take the ship to Washington, D.C., where it was to be decommissioned. When the *New York* reached Washington in early December 1803, most of the sick (6.1 percent of the original complement) who were transferred to the hospital ashore were suffering from scurvy. Some of St. Medard's problems on the homeward voyage were the result of the eight invalids transferred to the ship before its departure.

In the course of his Mediterranean assignment in the *New York,* St. Medard had only 29 patients with surgical problems, or 6 percent of the total admissions. For the most part this involved immobilizing fractures and dressing wounds.

Part of St. Medard's caseload was the result of an explosion on April 25,

1803. A ship's gunner directed his mate to return some signal lanterns to the storeroom. Later, when the gunner went down to see that this had been done and that things were in their proper place, he found that the mate had left a candle lit in a lantern. The gunner blew it out, returned to the deck to reprimand the mate, then returned to the storeroom, where he discovered while moving some sheepskins that sparks had fallen from the lantern and ignited the skins. Some sparks had also gone into a bucket containing damaged powder, and flames had moved from the floor to some powder horns. Both the horns and the bucket of powder exploded, damaging one of the bulkheads in the adjacent marine storage room and exploding 37 blank cartridges that had been left there. Nine men were injured and three of these died within eight hours. The dead included the gunner, the commodore's secretary, the captain's clerk, and the loblolly boy. Among the wounded was Surgeon's Mate Nathaniel Weems, two midshipmen, the purser's steward, and a marine sentinel, who were under treatment for burns from 8 to 28 days. They were purged on the fifth and sixth days. One man had to be transferred to the British hospital at Malta, where he died.[23]

Surgeon St. Medard got three new burn cases a month later, when a powder horn exploded in one of the ship's boats. One of these men had to have two of his fingers amputated. On another occasion a man suffered a concussion and was burned. His wounds were dressed and he was bled three times in two days, and he recovered after three weeks.

There were three cases of gunshot wounds, two of which were the result of efforts to prevent the Tripolitans from unloading boats that had run the U.S. blockade. St. Medard saw both men as soon as they returned from the raid, and both were bled. For the next two days they were treated with cathartics. One of died on the seventh day, probably from an infection, and the other recovered after nine days of treatment. The third gunshot case resulted from a duel. Young naval and marine officers had a highly developed sense of personal honor, which often led them to fatal encounters. In this case a young naval lieutenant was struck by a ball fired by a marine officer on the ship. It passed through both thighs and the perineum. Treatment involved bleeding the lieutenant on the first two days, then prescribing several doses of cathartics, and an epispastic to try to control his fever. The ball was removed. After seventeen days of treatment, the lieutenant died.

Among the lesser problems with which St. Medard dealt was one case of an unspecified leg injury. The man was bled on the first day and had his wound dressed for three days. In another case, an ankle injury involved the application of dressings over a three-week period. One man who was flogged had his back treated for 12 days. Still another man who was beaten, evidently during a fight with a shipmate, had his superficial injuries treated and was given an emetic on the second day and Peruvian bark on the third and fifth days. Peruvian bark also figured in the first 8 days of treatment for nonscorbutic leg ulcers in one man, followed by occasional cathartics during the 11 days he was under medical care. There were two cases of abscesses in unidentified locations which were treated by applying dressings. One man recovered after 9 days, the other after 37. Another sailor was described as suffering from "Testicular trauma," probably incurred while working aloft. He was bled on the first day and had dressings applied to his injury for a week.

The most unusual case in St. Medard's records involved a 19-year-old woman, most likely the wife of one of the seamen. Wives were in naval vessels of the early nineteenth century but rarely appear in the surviving records. She came to the surgeon's attention as a result of an abortion, probably self-induced. St. Medard prescribed warm baths, emmenagogues, or medicine to stimulate the menstrual flow, elixir vitrol and an antiemetic during the first five days of treatment. He seems to have decided that her case was hopeless and for the next six days he gave her only bark and sedatives to make her as comfortable as possible. On the 12th day she died.[24]

Supplementing this complete record are fragmentary bits of information from other ships in the squadron during the same period. In July 1802, two men fell overboard from the *Essex* in a storm and were drowned. While the *Boston* was en route to Malta in July 1802, the purser came down with "a violent fever" that lasted 16 days. He recovered. The ship's surgeon, John Goddard, also became ill, but his condition was not considered dangerous. Then he died suddenly, after two years and three months of service. In August 1802 the *Constellation* lost an ordinary seaman to an unrecorded cause. A fall from a mast was responsible for the death of a marine in the *New York* in September 1802.[25]

The payroll of the frigate *Constitution* for the period from May 1, 1803, to November 8, 1804, contains information on the 425 officers and men assigned to it. There were 18 deaths: 9 due to illness, 7 to combat, and 2 to accidents. In addition, seven of the sick seamen were transferred to other ships, and one sick midshipman was sent home with despatches. Eleven other sick men were transferred to hospitals ashore, seven to the marine hospital at Ft. Independence, near Boston, Massachusetts, and four to facilities at Malta. When the ship was preparing to go to sea, four men were discharged as unfit for duty, and one petty officer was let go for intemperance. One midshipman resigned. Of the 47 supernumeraries who were carried to the Mediterranean, only 1 had serious health problems. A seaman became insane and was sent ashore at Malta for care.[26]

When Preble took command, there was more action, resulting in more casualties. Upon reaching Malta on November 27, 1803, he heard that the *Philadelphia* had run aground and been captured while chasing a Tripolitan ship. Preble offered the pasha $40,000 for the release of Bainbridge and his men, but this was refused. The capture of the frigate made the Tripolitans more stubborn and resistant to negotiation. Commodore Preble now decided that the *Philadelphia* would be destroyed, and Lieutenant Stephen Decatur of the schooner *Enterprise* was given that responsibility. A Tripolitan ketch was captured, renamed the *Intrepid,* and fitted up for the task of destroying the *Philadelphia.* While this was taking place, Decatur informed Surgeon's Mate Lewis Heermann of the plan and asked him to report any officers and men in the *Enterprise* who were physically unfit for the undertaking. The *Intrepid* could hold only 75 men, and every one of them had to be dependable. The brig *Siren* was to follow the *Intrepid* into the harbor, recover the attackers, and cover the retreat. Decatur intended to have Dr. Heermann accompany him but to transfer him to the *Siren* just before the *Intrepid* entered the harbor. Heermann said that he would do as ordered but that he wished to accompany the volunteers in the attack, for he thought his professional services might be in demand. Decatur tried to discourage him by pointing out that he might be killed or wounded, in which case it might reflect badly on him. Heermann was said to have replied as follows:

> My life, Sir, is not more valuable than that of any of the other brave officers and men who are to accompany you; and should I be killed or wounded, the officers and crew would be as well provided for after their achievement by Dr. Marshall alone, as by him and myself united. Again, Sir, allow me to observe, with all due deference to your better judgement, and with a perfect consciousness of the bravery of your officers and men who have volunteered to accompany you on this expedition, that the presence of a professional man to assist the wounded, might save many valuable lives, which may be sacrificed from loss of blood, for the want of a surgeon, conversant with the most effectual means of staunching it, and will not sailors more regardlessly expose themselves, when they know that professional aid is near at hand? Should you have many wounded, would not some confusion arise, to impair your effective force?

To this Decatur replied, "Well then, Doctor, you may go with me; but be sure that you get into a place of safety on board the vessel in the moment of danger." Heermann thanked Decatur and said that he regarded the permission to go as an order. A day or two before the expedition was to depart, Decatur told Heermann that he could not not spare an officer to stay with him in the *Intrepid* when they boarded the *Philadelphia,* so he would be left in charge of seven men. Once the attackers had subdued those in the *Philadelphia,* Heermann and his men were to see that the combustible material on board was transferred to the frigate as quickly as possible. Arms and ammunition were left with the doctor and his men in case the *Intrepid* was attacked. If this happened, he was to get word to Decatur as quickly as possible. Heermann and the men under him would be expected to defend the *Intrepid* to the last man.

All arrangements having been completed, on the night of February 3, 1804, Lieutenant Stephen Decatur led a party of 75 volunteers into the harbor and destroyed the frigate without the loss of a man and with only one wounded. The Tripolitans lost about 20 killed, and 1 wounded man was taken prisoner. During the attack a Tripolitan crewman jumped from the frigate onto the *Intrepid.* He was found to be severely wounded, and there being no need to refrain from taking prisoners, Heermann treated him and saved his life, earning Decatur's praise. The courage and daring of those who destroyed the *Philadelphia* was widely recognized at home and abroad, and they received the thanks of the president, the secretary of the navy, and Congress.[27]

From his base at Syracuse, Preble launched five attacks against Tripoli in August and September 1804. The first resulted in the loss of Lieutenant James Decatur, the brother of Stephen, and the wounding of 13 men. A second attack killed a lieutenant, a midshipman, and 6 other men, and several were wounded. The third was a failure because cannon balls fell short or did not explode. In the fourth attack, carried out at night, 30 of the crew of the *John Adams* were lost. A fifth attack was carried out on September 3, but no Americans were killed or wounded. Afterward the bomb ketch *Intrepid* was filled with powder and combustibles and sent into the harbor. For some reason, perhaps because it was boarded by the Tripolitans, it blew up prematurely and killed three officers and 10 men. This brought the total casualties of Preble's operations to 54 killed and 24 wounded.[28]

Events in the Mediterranean had been closely followed by the administration. Jefferson had become thoroughly aroused by the loss of the *Philadelphia* and the imprisonment of its officers and men. He decided to increase the naval force being sent out under Commodore Samuel Barron. This consisted of five frigates: the *President,* which became Barron's flagship, the *Congress,* the *Essex,* the *Constellation,* and the *John Adams.* A corresponding increase was made in the number of medical men sent to the Mediterranean. For some reason, Secretary Smith expected Preble to serve in a subordinate capacity to Barron, but this was not Preble's intention. John Rodgers already outranked Preble but worked under him. The new arrangement would make Preble third in command, which would be intolerable. Preble did confer with Barron about the latter's discretionary authority to help Hamet Caramanli, the deposed brother of the pasha of Tripoli, regain power and thereby make a treaty favorable to the United States. The idea had long been advanced by Consuls William Eaton and James L. Cathcart. For a time, Preble had considered the project and later dropped it. He now recommended it to his successor.

At Barron's request, Preble traveled to Naples in the *John Adams* to ask the Neapolitan government for the loan of bomb ketches and gunboats in the 1805 campaign against Tripoli. The Neapolitan government was friendly but in the end decided that it needed the vessels for its own defense. The best Preble could do was to suggest that Barron might rent or buy suitable vessels at Malta and convert them to gunboats. Otherwise he would bring Barron's needs to the attention of the government. Preble then sailed for home and reached New York on February 25. He found himself a national hero, and on Jefferson's second inauguration day, Secretary Smith took him to meet the president. Work with the secretary followed on plans for reenforcing Barron.[29]

While Barron continued the blockade of Tripoli, plans for aiding Hamet Caramanli were implemented. An army was assembled in Egypt which was made up of 25 artillerymen of various nationalities, 38 Greek mercenaries, about 400 Arabs, who served as cavalrymen, camel drivers, and footmen, and 10 Americans. The 10 consisted of 7 enlisted U.S. marines under Lieutenant Presley N. O'Bannon, Navy Lieutenant John H. Dent, and General William Eaton. This force marched 520 miles across the North African desert to the city of Derne, on the eastern edge of Tripoli. Aided by bombardments from the schooner *Nautilus,* the sloop *Hornet,* and the brig *Argus,* Eaton and Hamet's force attacked and captured the city on April 24. Casualties among the attackers were highest for the Greeks. The Americans had 1 marine killed and 2 wounded, 1 of whom subsequently died. Eaton was also wounded. As soon as the battle was over, Isaac Hull, the captain of the *Argus,* ordered the ship's boats ashore to pick up the wounded.[30]

It was originally believed that the capture of Derne would help to put pressure on the pasha to make peace. If this failed, there would be an attack on Tripoli itself. Bainbridge and Dr. Cowdery were fearful that if it came to that, they and the other *Philadelphia* prisoners would be killed before the pasha capitulated. Barron was unaware that Preble's work in Washington was about to bring him the reinforcements he needed, and hence he saw no prospect of ending the war soon. There was also the matter of his health. Because of his liver complaint, he designated Rodgers acting commander of the squadron in November 1804. By the following spring he had not recovered his health and as a result was not interested in offensive operations. On April 21, 1805, a peace overture from the pasha arrived through the Spaniards and was studied by Tobias Lear, the consul general of the United States at Algiers. The pasha demanded a ransom for his prisoners, but Lear was convinced there was hope for a settlement. After discussing the matter with Barron, Lear decided that the pasha would settle for less and therefore set out for Tripoli in the *Essex* to see what might be done. Barron relinquished the command of the squadron to John Rodgers on May 22.[31]

Lear's gamble was successful, and preliminary articles of peace were agreed upon on June 3, 1805. Under the terms the United States agreed to evacuate Derne and the pasha's territory, to cease giving supplies to those hostile to him, and to try to persuade the brother of the pasha to withdraw from the ruler's domain. Both sides were to release the prisoners they held, but since the United States had about 100 fewer Tripolitans than the number of Americans held by the pasha, it paid the pasha $60,000 for the difference in the totals. Also to be released from the custody of the pasha were the wife and children of his brother. Although the Senate ratified Lear's treaty on April 17, 1806, it was not a popular one. Citizens, editors, naval officers, and historians have discussed whether it was the best resolution in long-and-short range terms of the problems with Tripoli and its neighbors.[32]

Peace brought the release of Bainbridge and the other men of the *Philadelphia* on June 3, 1805. It was a source of surprise that during their 19 months and 2 days of captivity, only 6 men died out of 300. The enlisted men were kept separate from the officers, put to forced labor, and beaten. Much of what we know about the captivity comes from a journal kept by Surgeon Jonathan Cowdery. From March 28 to April 13, 1804, Cowdery was too ill to write anything. At the end of July, the pasha moved him from the prison to the castle and told him that henceforth he would be the pasha's family physician as well as being responsible for caring for the U.S. prisoners.

Cowdery's environment improved, but he was afraid he might become so valuable to the pasha that he would not be exchanged, so he pretended to lack skill. When called upon to treat an Arab patient whose hand had been injured by the bursting of his blunderbuss, Cowdery amputated all but ne of the man's fingers with a dull knife. He then dressed the wound in a bungling manner, "in hopes of losing my credit as a surgeon." The surgeon saw firsthand some of the effects of Preble's bombardment of

Tripoli, and he expected to have his hands full with wounded Arabs. Despite his efforts to minimize his skill, the pasha thought highly of Cowdery and told him that he would not take $20,000 for him. Later, Cowdery was taken to a palace in the country, where he bled the oldest son of the pasha. In the end, Cowdery was redeemed along with the other captives.[33]

One of the Americans who was a prisoner of the Tripolitans at this time was a marine named William Ray. When Cowdery's journal was later published in the newspapers, Ray was a critical reader. Subsequently he accused the doctor of being more interested in the health of the officers and the pasha and his family than that of the enlisted men. Ray also marveled that so few men died in captivity, and he attributed their good health to their habit of mixing vegetable oil with all the food they received. But it was not just the captives who were concerned about matters of health; the subject was in the mind of the secretary and many of the officers.[34]

Hospitals in the Mediterranean

Believing that the lazarettos in the Mediterranean were the cause of death of all who were forced to enter them, Secretary of the Navy Smith tried to provide an alternative. He instructed Captain Morris that if possible he should "establish a temporary hospital in some of the most healthy ports in the Mediterranean." Smith thought that Syracuse, on the island of Sicily, might be an excellent place since it was healthy and close to Tripoli. But the choice was left to Morris. Once the hospital was established, Morris was to assign a surgeon and allow him to take a surgeon's mate with him; Smith was inclined to think that Surgeon Davis might be the best choice. The secretary promised enough funds to provide for all the hospital stores needed. If there were enough patients to justify it, Smith believed that both humanity and economy argued in favor of a hospital. He urged Morris not to lose sight of these considerations.[35]

Anticipating an early decision by Morris on the site of the hospital, Smith ordered Surgeon Bullus to prepare an assortment of medicines and instruments suitable for 1,000 men for one year. The medicines were assembled and packed in black bottles and the other items wrapped. When everything was ready, Bullus was to send the items to Norfolk for shipment on a vessel bound for Gibraltar.[36]

A site for the hospital had not been selected by the time the decision was made to entrust Captain Edward Preble with the command of the squadron. In his instructions, Smith told Preble that the hospital had been authorized and the choice was now up to him. The secretary thought that

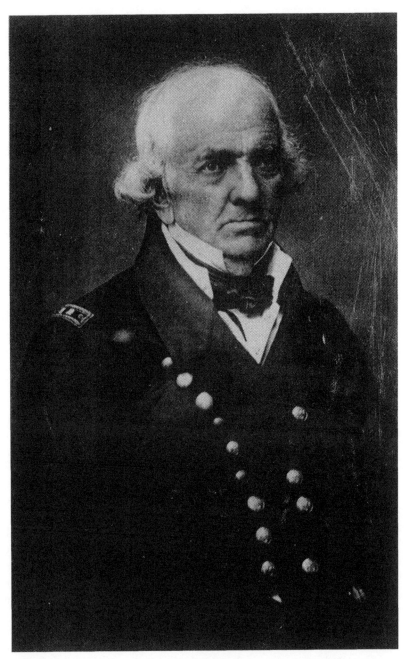

Surgeon Jonathan Cowdery in His Later Years. Naval Historical Center, Washington, D.C.

Malta might be a good spot if permission could be obtained; if not, Preble was to find some other suitable location. "Care must be taken of our seamen," wrote Smith, and "great advantages will result from their being made sensible that we regard them as an useful class of citizens in all respects deserving of our care and attention."[37]

When Preble reached the Mediterranean, he found himself trying to cope with the number of desertions from his force. Gibraltar and Malta were especially good spots for sailors to leave the U.S. service for the British. When U.S. officers tried to recover their deserters from the British, they were frequently rebuffed. The same was true of British officers seeking their men who had deserted to the Americans. This state of affairs had a bearing on where the hospital would be located, for there was always a danger that men would desert from the hospital. John Gavino, the U.S. consul at Gibraltar, suggested to Preble that Syracuse would be a better place for depositing supplies. Ideally the spot chosen for the storage of supplies would also be a good location for a hospital. By October 1803, Preble had come to the conclusion that, to minimize the desertion problem, stores shipped to Gibraltar should be transshipped to a store ship that could also function as a hospital ship, and he asked the secretary for authority to arrange this. Meanwhile Preble sent home his invalids from the *Philadelphia*, the *New York* and the *John Adams*. The invalids, 2 petty officers dismissed for incompetence, the deserters, and the 10 men and a boy Preble supplied to man the ship going home had left Preble 49 men short of his prescribed complement. This threw extra work on the remaining men, yet four days after these shortages became apparent, Preble recorded in his diary, "Our Ship's Company [is] remarkably healthy."[38]

To maintain this good luck as well as the morale of crews, there would have to be adequate provisions. When a supply ship arrived from Baltimore in early November, Preble was disappointed to discover that its cargo did not include cheese, butter, molasses, or candles, all articles that were expensive in the Mediterranean. He also found that the captain of the supply ship would not carry the cargo to Syracuse without the payment of $30,000, or a total of $800 more than the British vessels normally charged. Preble advised the U.S. consul at Gibraltar to pay. Clearly, if Preble was to use a store ship for that as well as for a hospital, it would have to be one owned by the U.S. government. He therefore advised the secretary that the next supply ship sent out should carry slop clothing in addition to its other cargo and that it should go directly to Syracuse. Fortunately another U.S. ship soon arrived in the Mediterranean with a cargo of the needed items, as well as fish, salt, and dry goods. By this time, Preble was convinced that he must travel to Syracuse and make the necessary arrangements to use that port for future supplies. The hospital question remained pending, and new health problems brought it to mind.[39]

The early days of November 1803 brought sickness to the *Constitution*, but the exact nature of it is not known. The number of men who were ill went from 12 sick and 10 convalescent on November 10 to 30 sick, 13 convalescent, and 1 discharged as of January 21, 1804. By January 30 the figures had dropped to 13 sick, 4 convalescent, and 1 additional man discharged.[40]

The spring of 1804 brought serious health problems to the schooner *Enterprise*. One man died and one-third of the crew were sick with fever. The term of enlistment of most of the crew had expired, and Preble decided to grant discharges to the 12 who demanded it and asked others to wait a few weeks longer for the expected replacements. To care for the sick he had the ketch *Intrepid* fitted up as a hospital ship and transferred the sick of the *Enterprise* to it. In June 2 men sent from the *Constitution* to the hospital ship died. That September the *Intrepid* went back to war. Loaded with explosives and manned by volunteers under Lieutenant Richard Somers, it was sent into the harbor of Tripoli. It exploded prematurely, killing all on board. Another vessel was used as a hospital ship but its identity is unclear. By November 1804 a surgeon's mate was necessary on the ship, and John H. Beall was transferred from the *Congress* to perform that duty. Apparently this was only a brief assignment for the hospital ship appears to have been replaced by a facility ashore.[41]

While Barron was preparing to go to the Mediterranean to relieve Preble, the secretary informed him that a hospital had been authorized, but thus far a site had not been chosen. Barron was given discretionary authority to establish a hospital at Syracuse or any other healthy port near Tripoli. Meanwhile Preble, in anticipation of Barron's arrival, set up a temporary hospital "in an excellent house" at Syracuse in September 1804 and placed Surgeon's Mate John W. Dorsey in charge. Any hospital stores that were needed should be ordered through the navy agent at that port. Preble informed Barron that the sick were being comfortably accommodated there.[42]

When Barron arrived in Syracuse, he presumably visited the hospital. For reasons that are not clear, he asked George Dyson, the navy agent there, to find another house to rent for a hospital, one big enough to accommodate 100 men. When a house was found, Barron placed Surgeon Edward Cutbush in charge of it in November 1804. Cutbush had originally gone to the Mediterranean in the *Constellation* as a part of Commodore Morris's squadron, but that assignment was short. After a brief period at the Philadelphia navy yard, he returned to the war zone in the *President*.

Shortly afterward he was ordered to establish a hospital that would accommodate 75 patients. He was to draw on the navy agent for any articles necessary being as economical as the comfort and convenience of his patients would admit. Cutbush was given the title of hospital surgeon and the authority to hire nurses and other employees and draw up the internal rules governing the establishment. Any person who violated these rules was to be reported to the senior officer of the port, and if in Cutbush's opinion could be sent back to his ship, it would be done. No officer of the squadron who was not on the books of the hospital would be permitted to lodge there.[43]

Armed with this authority, Cutbush set up a hospital to which the sick of the squadron were transferred. The hospital of course needed surgical instruments, and Barron asked Rodgers to try to get them in Lisbon. These would probably be items of British manufacture that were for sale in that city. If they were not obtainable, the order was to be left with the consul at Lisbon, who was to send to London for them and then forward them to Malta for transshipment to Syracuse. As things turned out, the order did have to be sent to London. It is not known how long it was before Cutbush received the instruments, but apparently he did not have the benefit of them for long.[44]

At the peak of its operation, the naval hospital at Syracuse seems to have cared for about 100 patients. Most were casualties from Derne who were evacuated by the *Argus*. Cutbush later wrote that he "received all the sick and wounded of Genl. Eaton's forces, consisting of Greeks, Turks and renegades of all nations, the Hospital was filled, and I had no medical assistant for a great part of the time." Surgeon's Mate Joseph J. Schoolfield was ordered to assist Cutbush at the hospital, but he did not arrive in the Mediterranean until July 1805, and he returned to the United States in December.[45]

One of the patients at the hospital was marine Private David Thomas, who was wounded in the right leg in the attack at Derne. In the hospital at Syracuse, he came to the attention of Surgeon Cutbush, who certified in September 1805 that Thomas, a tanner in civilian life, would not be able to maintain himself in his trade because of his leg injury. Thomas was later given a pension of $3 a month. Most of the U.S. patients seem to have been men suffering from an array of ailments that could not be treated or cured within a limited time on their own ships. We know that the sick and wounded of the *Nautilus* were ordered there, as were some sick marines from the *Constitution*. There is no record of any deaths in the hospital, but there must have been at least one. In a discussion of the accounts of the local navy agent, there is a mention of funeral expenses. It is possible that this may have been one of Eaton's international army.

The signing of a new treaty with Tripoli in 1805 meant that there would be no further need for a hospital at Syracuse. In August 1805, Rodgers ordered Master Commandant John Shaw to pick up all the invalids under the care of Cutbush and carry them back to the United States. The following March, Cutbush was ordered to transfer to the *Siren* and the *Enterprise* all of his patients who were able to make a voyage. In April 1806, Rodgers ordered Cutbush to close the hospital and transfer the furniture, stores, and other items times to the navy agent. When this was done, Cutbush was ordered back to the United States in the frigate *Essex*. So ended a unique experiment in the care of the sick of the navy overseas.[46]

Cutbush was wise to leave the payment of all bills to the navy agent. That individual was unfaithful to his trust and resigned after the war ended, leaving others to untangle his accounts. This process took many years. When Cutbush returned from the Mediterranean, he learned that because he had no vouchers, he could not get credit for the money he advanced for boat hire to bring supplies to the hospital.[47]

If the return of peace meant that there was no longer a need for a large hospital facility, there were still the day-to-day matters of health on every ship to consider. In June 1805 the *Essex*, which had an authorized strength of 228 men, had between 50 and 70 men on the sick list suffering mostly from fever. For a time Surgeon's Mate John Butler had trouble keeping up with his caseload. By early July the fever was abating.[48]

While Rodgers was in command of the squadron, there was a special emphasis on cleanliness, which no doubt helped prevent disease. Surgeon James Dodge of the *Constitution* was so impressed with what had been accomplished that he told Rodgers that his internal regulations had made surgery unnecessary and medicine almost superfluous. There was no complaint of a serious nature in the ship. To illustrate this point, he gave Rodgers a rundown of his daily report, which that day showed 20 patients: 4 had intermittent fever and syphilis; 2 had a sore leg; 2 had a pain in the breast; and there was only a single case each of rheumatism, pneumonia, cramp, bilious fever, debility, boils, and diarrhea.[49]

Rodgers also made sure that the men in the gunboats had adequate care. Surgeon Thomas Marshall was given this duty and was to live in one of the boats. While they were in port he was to visit all of them once a day and minister to the sick. A boat was provided for his use in making his rounds, and no one else could use it without his permission. Any gunboat needing a surgeon was to hoist a black ball about the size of a bushel basket (presumably a flag with a black circle on it) on the main-topmast. This signal was to be answered by any gunboat that had the doctor on board by raising the U.S. flag on the main-topmast.[50]

The gunboats were also the scene of an interesting development in the history of inoculation in the U.S. Navy. When a man on gunboat 8 came down with smallpox in October 1805, it was believed that five or six others had been exposed to the disease. Therefore Surgeon's Mate Thomas Marshall requested permission from his commanding officer, Lieutenant David Porter of the *Enterprise*, to inoculate those who had been in contact with the infected man. Porter turned the question over to Surgeon Cutbush at the naval hospital. He, in turn, consulted with the other surgeons in the squadron. They all agreed that the men who had been the most exposed on the gunboat should be inoculated. Given the unanimous approval of the medical men, Porter allowed Marshall to do as he proposed. The record is silent on whether the men were polled for their opinions; most likely they were not. Since the proposal was for the good of all the crew, it is probable that once the decision was made, more than just the five or six high-risk cases were inoculated. A few days later, Midshipman Daniel McNeill complained to Porter that the inoculation had made it necessary to postpone his plans to get the gunboat ready for sea: only four sailors and the marine contingent were able for duty. Sailing Master Alexander Harrison reported that since the corporal and one of the marines were inoculated, he had only three men who could stand sentry duty.[51]

While the frigate *John Adams* was cruising off Sardinia in December 1804, a seaman was found to have smallpox, which he apparently picked up in Naples. Captain Isaac Chauncey mustered the ship's company, read the Articles of War, and had all the men examined. He found 24 who had not had smallpox and ordered his surgeon to inoculate them. In the *Constitution* 27 men were inoculated, presumably on the order of Commodore Edward Preble.[52]

With the ending of the war and the withdrawal of most of the ships from the Mediterranean, new health problems arose. In 1807, Captain Hugh Campbell of the *Constitution* complained to the secretary of the navy that the squadron was suffering from a want of medical assistance. Patrick Sim, the surgeon's mate of the ship, had died of consumption in Lisbon the previous October, and for 10 months prior to that, his illness had made him of little use to the squadron. A second surgeon's mate, Thomas G. McAllister, was suffering from rheumatism, unable to use his right arm, and "incapable of exerting himself." At that time he was worse than at any time earlier. The result was that the ship was "without any person capable of performing any Surgical operation where the least judgement is required." Nearly 30 of the crew were ill with various diseases, but there was no one to care for them except the loblolly boy. He had acquired some skill and judgment in pulling teeth and "applying the Lancet to a well filled vein."

In addition, Surgeon Samuel D. Heap of the schooner *Enterprise* was dangerously ill at Messina. This situation made it necessary to provide the *Enterprise* with a surgeon from the *Hornet*. Until the wishes of the Navy Department were known, it would be necessary to employ local medical help temporarily. It is not known just what was done in regard to local doctors; it may be assumed that British physicians in Malta or Gibraltar were hired.[53]

Medical Personalities

The war with the Barbary pirates offered a second chance for a naval career to Surgeon's Mate Gershom R. Jacques. He wanted to remain in the service, but he was discharged at the end of the Quasi-War. When he appealed this decision and asked Secretary Smith for reinstatement, he was told that it was impossible. Smith did tell him that his name would be kept in mind when other appointments became available, and he was as good as his word. A vacancy occurred when Surgeon's Mate Daniel Mc-Cormick resigned unexpectedly in January 1802. The Secretary asked Captain Alexander Murray of the *Constellation* to make inquiries about the competence of Jacques. The answers apparently satisfied the captain and the secretary, for Jacques was given a new commission and assigned to the *Constellation*. He was promoted to surgeon in November 1804 and saw additional wartime service in the *Nautilus*. At the end of the war, he was given leave to make a cruise in the merchant service.[54]

Service during the years of the Barbary Wars made it possible for some of the surgeon's mates retained in the peacetime navy to become surgeons. This was the case with Starling Archer and James Boyd, who were promoted in 1803, and Jonathan Cowdery, Lewis Heermann, and Larkin Griffin in 1804.[55]

The demands of war also brought out the shortcomings of some officers. When the brig *Argus* was at Boston preparing for duty off Tripoli in 1803, Surgeon's Mate Nathan Tisdale wrote to Captain Stephen Decatur that he would not report on board unless he were promoted. Decatur immediately wrote to the secretary of the navy to advise him of a potentially dangerous situation. A detachment of recruits was expected soon from New York, of whom some had died from an undiagnosed contagious disease. In the circumstances, Decatur could not put to sea without a surgeon and a surgeon's mate. Tisdale was dismissed from the navy in April 1804. Meanwhile, John W. Dorsey was commissioned as a surgeon's mate in July 1803 and ordered to the *Argus* in early August. On August 21, Decatur told the secretary that Dorsey had not yet reported. With the sailing date fast approaching, Decatur was concerned that he might have to leave without any medical officer on board. Again the secretary sent orders to Dorsey saying that if he had not departed yet he must go at once to Boston. Dorsey made it in time to sail with his ship.[56]

Orders for sea duty posed a special problem for Surgeon George Balfour, a veteran of the Quasi-War. He was married, with a large family dependent on him. Most of his income came from his position in a civilian hospital in Norfolk. So he resigned his commission in April 1804.[57]

Another experienced surgeon was lost to the navy when John K. Read Jr. was furloughed in 1803 to make a sea voyage for his health and died in 1805. Surgeon William Turner died en route to the Mediterranean in 1802. Two other Quasi-War veterans, Surgeons George Davis and James Dodge, accepted diplomatic appointments in North Africa. Thus by 1805 all the surgeons who entered the navy in 1798 were gone. Of those who were commissioned in 1799 and were retained under the peace establishment act, only Cutbush, St. Medard, and James Wells were still in service at the end of the Barbary War. Wells died in 1807. Also, of the eight surgeon's mates promoted to surgeon in 1799, only one, John Bullus, was retained for peacetime service, and he left medicine for the more profitable position as navy agent at New York in 1808. That same year, Thomas Marshall died. He had entered in 1799 as a surgeon's mate and saw extensive service during the Barbary War. With his death only one of those who had entered the navy as a surgeon's mate in 1799 still remained in service.[58]

Between 1802 and 1807 the names of 45 medical officers were added to the rolls of the Navy Department, including three who acted for brief periods. The largest number of the new appointees, 15, came from Maryland. Next came New York with 6; Pennsylvania with 5; the District of Columbia with 6; Virginia with 4; Massachusetts with 3; and Georgia with 2, one of whom saw no active service. The states from which two other surgeon's mates came are not known to the author. One surgeon, two surgeon's mates, and one acting mate resigned during this period, including three who had been retained at the end of the Quasi-War. Two surgeons and one surgeon's mate who had been discharged in 1801 came back into the service during the Barbary War years. Three surgeons became inactive as the result of diplomatic appointments. Three surgeons and two surgeon's mates were dismissed, and the fate of one other surgeon's mate is unknown to the author. One of those who resigned was subsequently reappointed and later dismissed and is counted in the dismissed category. Another of those dismissed was Isaac Kipp, who was involved in a duel in the Mediterranean. He was court-martialed, but the details of his case are not known. When he advised the secretary that he was sending the doctor home, Commodore John Rodgers said he was "a poor simple creature and deserves to be pitied." One of the mates who was promoted to surgeon later died of an illness. John Ridgely, one of the surgeons commissioned in 1803, was lost to the navy when he became the charge d'affaires of the United States at Tripoli.[59]

Casualties

In his analysis of the costs in men of various wars, Louis H. Roddis stated that 31 navy and 2 marine corps officers and men were killed and 54 navy men and 4 marines were wounded. These figures are for 1800–1804 and cover the engagements of the gunboats off Tripoli in July and August 1804, the loss of the crew of the *Intrepid* in September 1804, and the boarding and burning of the *Philadelphia* in February 1804. Although Roddis's findings appeared after the documentary volumes on the Barbary Wars had been published, he does not seem to have consulted them. Based on these volumes, the work of Dr. Estes, and manuscript sources, the known totals for 1801–7 are 101 officers and men dead. Included in this total are 43 combat related deaths, 19 deaths from diseases, 12 from unknown causes and 27 from accidents. Of these totals, 7 of the dead were marines. If we include the deaths from duels during the same period, another 3 navy and 1 marine officers must be added to the totals for the war years. Those known to have been wounded in duels were 3 navy and 2 marine officers. During the Barbary War years, 7 surgeons and 1 surgeon's mate died, 2 as the result of duels.

Marine Corps records for the years 1802–7 show the deaths of 4 officers: 1 the lieutenant colonel commandant, 1 a captain who died in a duel in 1802, and 2 lieutenants who died of unknown causes. In the case of enlisted men, Marine Corps deaths during the same period total 187, of which 2 were killed in action, 2 died of wounds, 3 were lost in gunboats, 1 committed suicide, and 11 drowned. If we deduct these 19 from the above total, we have 169 unexplained deaths of enlisted men, some of which must have been due to illness. In light of these figures, it would seem that the Barbary War years saw the deaths of at least 181 men including officers and men of the navy and Marine Corps.[60]

Chapter 5

New Orleans

In the years that followed the American Revolution, the state of affairs at New Orleans became a matter of concern to the settlers west of the Appalachian Mountains, as well as to the central government of the United States. For the western settlers the only practical outlet for their crops was via flatboat down the Ohio and Mississippi rivers to New Orleans, then in Spanish hands.

Arrangements had been made with the Spanish authorities to warehouse the goods until they could be picked up by U.S. ships and carried to distant markets. From time to time, Spanish authorities had threatened to cut off this access to New Orleans, a move that would ruin western farmers. From the point of view of the Spaniards, it was desirable to win the allegiance of the western settlers from the weak United States to Spain. This would protect the frontiers of Louisiana from the steady increase in U.S. settlers. The only leverage the Spaniards had was the need for access to New Orleans. On the other hand, the central government of the United States under both the Articles of Confederation and the Constitution needed to protect the economic future of its citizens and keep their political loyalty. For the fledgling United States it was a matter of great importance that their southern neighbor continue to be a weak Spain rather than a powerful France or Great Britain. This situation changed on October 1, 1800, when, under the terms of the Second Treaty of San Idefonso, France secured the Louisiana territory from Spain in return for a promise to enlarge the area of the state of Parma in Italy. But, as things turned out, the French did not take formal possession of Louisiana until 1803.[1]

Given the importance of New Orleans, it is not surprising that conditions there were of interest to a number of Americans. Just how healthy was the city? One of those who tried to find out was John Watkins, who had studied medicine at Edinburgh and the University of Pennsylvania. In June 1800 he wrote to Benjamin Rush about his experiences. He said, in part: "The people of New Orleans last summer persuaded themselves and wished to make the world believe that the yellow fever was imported from Kentucky in tobacco and flour—from Kentucky the healthiest climate upon earth, where no contagious disease ever existed except the small pox and measles; and in consequence of this belief many poor fellows were shut out of Doors and lost their lives—How absurd was the Idea and how cruel and inhuman was that conduct."[2] Yet this was only one part of the clash of cultures and medical philosophies. Another and more significant comment came in August 1801 when a U.S. citizen named Evan Jones, who was residing in New Orleans, wrote to Secretary of State James Madison about the plight of his countrymen. When seamen and boatmen became sick in the city, he reported, they usually turned to the charity hospital for help. This institution did what it could, but the number of sick Americans was too great for its capacity. Local hotels and boardinghouses would not take sick men, who had to treat themselves in ships and boats or in miserable cabins on the shore. Jones estimated that during the past year over 3,000 sailors had arrived in the city and suggested a tax on them to provide a fund that could be used to care for those who became ill. Jones asked if this was not a subject worthy of the attention of the government. Madison thought so and sent the letter to Jefferson.[3]

The president considered the matter important enough to include in his message to Congress in February 1802. He asked that Congress give New Orleans priority over other foreign ports in the matter of providing hospital care. Jefferson said that since a number of Americans had dealings with New Orleans, Jones had probably underestimated the number of unfortunate people who needed help. The House of Representatives referred the president's proposal to its Committee of Commerce and Manufactures.[4]

News of Jefferson's recommendations reached Governor William C. C. Claiborne of Mississippi Territory, and he wrote to Madison to express his approval. Claiborne said that a marine hospital was needed for humane and economic reasons: the bare necessities it would furnish would mean the difference between life and death to those who traveled on the river, and it would encourage both rivermen and merchants to make more trips.[5]

Meanwhile on April 6, 1802, the House committee reported a bill to amend the act of 1798, which was read twice and then postponed until it could be considered by the whole House. Six days later, when the matter was taken up, there was some opposition to the proposal to place all the money deducted from the pay of the seamen in a general fund to be applied as the president saw fit, rather than using the funds in the ports where they were collected. Efforts to amend this provision were narrowly defeated. The next day, Representative Phanuel Bishop of Massachusetts introduced an amendment to appropriate $20,000 to build a marine hospital in his state. Congressman Samuel Smith of Maryland, who was the sponsor of the original bill, agreed that Massachusetts had a right to a hospital, but he asked that the sum requested be reduced to $15,000. Bishop accepted this and the House agreed to the amendment. Then John Milledge of Georgia tried to get $5,000 for a hospital at Savannah, but the House did not accept this proposal. The final bill was approved by a vote of 39 to 29.[6] In the Senate, the bill was read twice and referred to a special committee. Fifteen days later it was again taken up and this time approved with two amendments, probably on matters of wording, and the House subsequently accepted these changes. Final approval took place on May 3, 1802, by a vote of 15 to 5. Jefferson signed it into law on that same day.[7]

Part of the law dealt with marine hospitals in general. Directors of these were given a commission of 1 percent on the funds expended. Eligibility was enlarged by permitting the admission of foreign sailors who became ill in the United States. The sick man's captain had to request that the sailor be admitted to the hospital and pay 25¢ a day to the collector of the port. Hospitals were to receive such foreign seamen as long as it did not inconvenience them. Most of the law dealt specifically with New Orleans. The president was authorized to spend up to $3,000 to furnish the city with a hospital, a director, and the necessary supplies provided that it could be done with the consent of the government having jurisdiction over the port. The costs of running the hospital would be met by taxing the U.S. crews of each barge, flatboat, or other craft traveling down the Mississippi the sum of 20¢ per man, to be collected at Fort Adams, located south of Natchez.[8]

With the necessary legislation in place, Jefferson turned his attention to the task of finding a suitable director for the marine hospital. Writing to his friend Dr. Caspar Wistar of Philadelphia, he asked for a confidential report on Dr. William Barnwell of that city. The president had seen a book by Barnwell which impressed him, but he wanted the opinion of one of the doctor's colleagues. Wistar gave Barnwell an excellent recommendation, but before it could be acted on, there was a new complication. Dr. William Bache, a grandson of Benjamin Franklin, had earlier asked Jefferson for a government job, and the president now learned that he was planning to move to Mississippi Territory. For Jefferson this was an opportunity to do a favor for a friend as well as getting a qualified director for the hospital, and so Bache got the job. Before he could take up his position, however, arrangements had to be made with the Spanish authorities in New Orleans.

Upon learning that Daniel Clark, the U.S. consul at New Orleans, was then in New York, Jefferson requested Treasury Secretary Gallatin to get in touch with him so that he could advise Bache on his forthcoming assignment. As it happened, Gallatin had already written to Clark for information. In his reply, Clark expressed pleasure about the news of the hospital and his certainty that the Spanish authorities would consent to the project. He suggested that the medical supplies be ordered in the United States and shipped to New Orleans. Surgical instruments might not be available there, so the doctor should take these with him. Food, drink, and other staples could be obtained cheaply in the city.

One thing that disturbed Clark, however, was that the amount of money allocated for establishing the hospital was inadequate. He suggested that to keep the costs down, a structure might be rented instead of built. He recommended spending the entire appropriation during the city's unhealthy months and charging for medical care the rest of the year. The consul also felt that he and the director should consult frequently in order to conserve money. Finally, he wanted to know whether the doctor's salary and medical supplies were to come from the appropriation. Clark's suggestions were passed on to Dr. Bache before he set out for his new assignment.[9]

Arriving in New Orleans on March 27, 1803, Bache called on William Hulings, the U.S. vice consul. Hulings knew of Bache's appointment, but he could not account for Clark's optimism about getting permission from the Spanish authorities for a hospital. No such permission had been granted. Bache wrote to Jefferson that he intended to take the matter up with the Spanish governor of Louisiana, but this matter could not be decided until the much larger question of the ownership of the area was resolved.[10]

While waiting, Bache began treating the sick Americans in the city. Within three weeks of his arrival, 18 men had come to him, and arrangements were made with the charity hospital to provide space for those who were ill. The doctor soon discovered that the sum allotted to him was inadequate, and he, Clark, and Hulings consulted on how to deal with the money problems. Within a few months of his arrival, Bache asked for a salary increase, which Jefferson, on Gallatin's advice, denied. Bache left, and Jefferson appointed Dr. William Barnwell to replace him.[11]

Meanwhile events had taken place that would change the whole future of Louisiana. On October 16, 1802, the authorities at New Orleans withdrew from the Americans the right to deposit their goods in the city while awaiting shipment. This was a violation of Pinckney's Treaty of 1795, and it led to a U.S. effort to buy New Orleans and other territory in east and west

Florida. Napoleon Bonaparte, the ruler of France, had earlier induced Spain to cede Louisiana to his country. As part of his desire to recreate some of the old French empire in America, Napoleon intended to reestablish French control over the island of Santo Domingo. But the troops he sent there were virtually destroyed by yellow fever, a disaster that, coupled with the anticipated renewal of war in Europe, probably made Napoleon change his plans. The U.S. minister at Paris was astounded when the French offered to sell not just New Orleans but all of Louisiana. He quickly seized the opportunity. The Louisiana treaty was signed on May 2, 1803, and the U.S. Senate gave its approval on October 20. On December 20, 1803, Louisiana was formally transferred to the United States.[12]

The cession of Louisiana to the United States led to some administrative problems in regard to sick seamen, for Clark's position as consul no longer existed, and he stopped collecting funds for their care. William Claiborne, the new territorial governor, wanted Clark to continue. Also, the charity hospital could not handle all the sick sailors, and the governor's home was constantly being visited by men seeking treatment. At that point, Hore Brown Trist, the collector of the port of New Orleans, assumed the responsibility. He made arrangements with the charity hospital to accept sick sailors and hired Dr. John Watkins, the physician of the port, to care for them until a new director of the marine hospital was appointed. Gallatin wrote to Trist informing him that Dr. Barnwell had been appointed to succeed Bache, and he also sent to the collector a long letter clarifying procedures in regard to the directorship of the hospital and the rules governing the admission of American and foreign seamen. Gallatin suggested the expediency of operating a separate hospital rather than continuing to use the charity hospital. The appropriation for New Orleans was increased to $5,000 a year, but Trist was told to keep down expenses, and only the most urgent cases were to be treated. Now that the area was part of the United States, it was anticipated that there would be an increase in commerce. So, early in 1804, Congress extended to Louisiana Territory the laws concerning sick and disabled seamen.[13]

When Dr. Barnwell reached New Orleans in August 1804, he was too sick to take up his duties. Soon after this, Trist became ill and died of yellow fever. William Brown took over the duties of the collector, and he continued to employ Dr. Watkins. Brown recommended to Gallatin that Watkins be retained as an assistant. Barnwell had also indicated to Brown that he wanted a separate marine hospital because he could speak neither French nor Spanish, the languages used in the charity hospital. Brown said that he did not believe that there were sufficient funds for a separate hospital. When Barnwell recovered his health he found himself with a large number of patients. He also found that he greatly missed the society, the institutions, and the intellectual stimulation of his native Philadelphia. Although a man of learning himself, Barnwell was not welcome in local society, and he began to spend his free time exploring the local country-side. As a result he asked Jefferson for the position of surveyor general of Orleans Territory, but the president denied this request, and Barnwell remained at his post until 1812.[14]

As soon as the Louisiana transfer arrangements had been completed, there was a concern in Washington that a U.S. military presence be established in the territory as quickly as possible. Army troops were stationed there, but New Orleans was a port in a strategically important part of the United States, and a naval presence was also deemed necessary. Until a naval force could be established there a marine detachment would have to be sent at the earliest possible date.[15]

At the Navy Department, the chief clerk, Charles W. Goldsborough was busy with the arrangements for sending the marine detachment under Captain Daniel Carmick to the territory. Goldsborough had been told by Surgeon John Bullus that a doctor would have to be sent with the troops, and he was looking for a suitable person. He talked to William Rogers, who had served briefly as a surgeon's mate in the Mediterranean in 1802–3 and had since resigned. Goldsborough said that the assignment would last only a few months until the army arrived, and he probably also offered Rogers a surgeon's commission. The doctor was noncommittal. Later, while at dinner, Rogers was approached by Bullus, who again pointed out the need for a doctor to go with the marines. Rogers agreed to go. On March 13, 1804, he received orders to depart from Washington with Carmick and his troops.[16]

Carmick, along with two other marine officers, Surgeon Rogers, and 102 enlisted men, reached New Orleans on May 4. One part of the detachment was stationed in the city, and the other nine miles away at Camp Claiborne. No sooner had they settled in when yellow fever made its appearance in the area. Surgeon Rogers found himself obliged to commute between the two camps to care for the sick and rented a carriage, the expenses for which Carmick allowed in the doctor's accounts.[17]

Rogers was also having trouble providing suitable food for his patients. In May he wrote to the secretary of the navy to see if something could be done to provide for more flexibility in the issuing of food for the sick. Under the existing arrangements, a surgeon had to draw rations for four days at a time. One day he might have 10 men on the sick list, but the next day the number might have doubled, in which case rations had to be stretched until a new issue was available. There was an even greater problem in trying to preserve fresh meat in the intense heat of Louisiana:

within 24 hours it would begin to decay and would only make patients sicker.[18]

There was also the more general problem of the daily allowance of food. The ration of each marine consisted of three-quarters of a pound of pork or one-half a pound of beef, one gill of liquor, about one-half tablespoon of salt, and one tablespoon of vinegar. It was Rogers's opinion that the consumption of meat in a hot climate tended to make the men warmer and hence more uncomfortable. Men were also issued bread or flour. When they received flour to make their own bread, they tended to eat it when it was only half-baked. This made the surgeon apprehensive that the men would be susceptible to scurvy, dysentery, or yellow fever, which would kill them. It was then the most healthy season in the area, but nearly one-quarter of the force was on sick report that day. Marines were allowed to exchange their rations for locally grown vegetables but had to do so at an exorbitant discount. This trade was troublesome also because it was the source of liquor introduced into the garrison.[19]

Rogers was also concerned about his status. Although he had been appointed as a surgeon, he had yet to receive his commission. Suppose there was a war and he was captured—would he be treated as an officer? He wrote to his friend Judge William Kilty and asked him to take up the matter with the secretary. Kilty did so.[20] The government had not forgotten Rogers; it was just that things moved slowly. On January 2, 1805, the Senate confirmed his appointment as a surgeon effective March 13, 1804, the day he was ordered to leave Washington. Rogers felt relieved, but he was now faced with a series of queries from the secretary.[21]

Smith asked if instruments and medicines sent to Rogers had been received. They had, but Rogers replied that some of the medicines had spoiled. Bullus had included alkaline salt and a bundle of orange peelings; both were unnecessary, since the salt was of little use against the effect of the climate on northern constitutions and since orange trees flourished locally. It had become necessary to purchase additional medicines, and Carmick had approved these requests. As of late March 1805, all the marine officers were in good health and the enlisted men "nearly so," but a fresh outbreak of yellow fever was expected at any time.[22]

When the expense accounts from New Orleans reached the Navy Department, they set off new requests for justifications. The navy accountant inquired about the $280.00 for quarters for Dr. Rogers for three months. Carmick furnished a statement that there were no quarters in the garrison that were fit for the doctor, and that $20 a month was considered "a moderate charge, considering the rates of house rent in New Orleans."[23] The accountant also challenged the expense of renting a carriage to attend the sick at Camp Claiborne. Rogers pointed out that he was under the impression that he was entitled to $10 a month for forage in addition to his pay, and this might be applied. Also, since Carmick had approved this expense, the doctor had not kept vouchers on his actual expenditures. After much perseverance and taking of oaths, Rogers was allowed $2 a day in additional pay for every day that the marines were at Camp Claiborne.[24]

Another troublesome question related to the arrangement whereby marines were compensated for acting as nurses in addition to their regular pay. Rogers pointed out that he had read an advertisement in a New Orleans newspaper offering $30 a month for nurses to attend the sailors in the section of charity hospital that functioned as a marine hospital. Later, Rogers saw two blacks acting as nurses there. One was a slave belonging to the collector of the port, who told Rogers that $30 a month was paid to him for the black's services. Furthermore, the army paid its men extra for such nursing activities. As an additional justification, Rogers noted that the local military surgeon, Dr. Oliver H. Spencer, did not stop the rations of sick soldiers, as was customary. Instead he drew them and sold them to raise funds to buy items he needed, such as bowls.[25]

The secretary of the navy referred this troublesome matter to Thomas Turner, the accountant, for further study. Turner reported that under the law of May 30, 1796, fixing the military establishment, nurses were allowed $8 a month. But the law of March 16, 1802, on the military peace establishment, allowed the matrons and nurses one ration each. The War Department was interpreting the new law as prohibiting any other allowance, but the navy accountant was not sure whether that part of the earlier law allowing pay was not still in force. Still, he doubted that either law applied to the marines. Nevertheless, the general principles governing contingent expenses "would authorize any allowance that may appear to you to be just and equitable to the Marines who have been employed in attending on the Sick at the Hospital at New Orleans, in addition to their pay as Marines." Turner also felt that the secretary could allow Rogers to incur any extra expenses as long as they were properly recorded on vouchers. The matter was eventually settled equitably, but new complications marred the relationship between Rogers and the department.[26]

When Rogers arrived in New Orleans, he found opportunities for private practice outside his official duties. He was also impressed by the country in the Opelousas region of Louisiana, and he had a friend purchase a farm for him there. Rogers sent for his family and located them on the farm. Recalling that the chief clerk of the Navy Department had originally spoken to him about a short-term assignment at New Orleans, he made plans to resign his commission. Before he could do so, however, the marine contingent was ordered to abandon the post because of the unhealthy climate. In August 1805 the marines returned to Washington and Rogers went with them. Secretary Smith was out of town when he arrived, so he did not report to him. He did have a conversation with Thomas Turner about his accounts. At the Navy Department he found that the news of his intended resignation had preceded him. Goldsborough, the chief clerk, told him that a naval establishment was going to be built at New Orleans and that Rogers should not resign until he had had an interview with the secretary.

Following this advice, Rogers traveled to Baltimore, where Secretary Smith was visiting his father. Smith asked Rogers why he wanted to resign. The surgeon replied that he had a family for whom he must provide, and that going to sea would be a great inconvenience. Then, according to Rogers, Smith replied that he saw no necessity for him to go to sea, and from this Rogers assumed that when a hospital was established at New Orleans, he would be in charge of it. Accordingly, Rogers put aside thoughts of resigning from the navy. He returned to New Orleans in October 1805 and went to his farm to await the call from the Navy Department for new responsibilities. Meanwhile he tried to be helpful.[27]

In November 1805 the secretary of the Navy ordered the reestablishment of the marine post at New Orleans. To start the process, 19 marines under First Lieutenant Samuel Baldwin were sent to the city, in the expectation that they would augment their strength through local recruiting. Meanwhile Rogers had looked into possible sites for a naval hospital and wrote to Smith about them. He suggested a building then being used as a magazine which could be made comfortable at little cost. He also suggested that the marine and naval hospitals be combined, so that one surgeon and one mate would be sufficient to care for the sick. The pay of the present marine and naval surgeons should be combined, so that surgeons at the hospital could live comfortably and not have to supplement their income by private practice.[28]

Nothing came of this suggestion, and in the meantime there were developments that Rogers did not anticipate. He learned that another medical officer, Surgeon James Wells, a veteran of the Quasi-War and the Barbary War, had been assigned to New Orleans. With him came Master Commandant John Shaw, who was to take charge of the newly arrived gunboats in the area. Stunned by this turn of events, Rogers first contemplated resigning his commission but on further reflection decided to go to New Orleans and see what he could find out about how he was regarded in naval circles. Some unnamed informants suggested that since the surgeon had bought a farm, or perhaps because the secretary had inferred from his letters that

Rogers was no longer interested in a naval career, Smith had turned to another doctor. Additional questioning and theorizing failed to resolve the problem, so Rogers wrote to Smith asking if there were any unfavorable reports about him and if he was still in the navy. Smith replied that no unfavorable reports had been received, that Rogers was still considered a naval surgeon until he resigned or had his commission revoked, and that he presumed Rogers knew that until he was ordered to active service, he was on half pay.[29]

When Surgeon Wells left New Orleans for service on the gunboats stationed below the city, he was accompanied by marines in the area under the command of Lieutenant Baldwin. The lieutenant was concerned about the sick marines he had to leave behind, and he asked Master Commandant Shaw if he knew of a doctor to whom he could entrust their care. Shaw said that the only surgeon he knew of was Dr. Rogers, and he was on furlough. Shaw did not feel authorized to call him back into service for this purpose, and therefore Baldwin hired him as a private physician. For Rogers this arrangement raised questions of how he would be paid, whether the Navy Department would consider him as being on full pay, and whether he would be entitled to an allowance for rent and hiring servants to attend the sick, questions he put to Secretary Smith in a letter. Before Smith had time to reply, Surgeon's Mate George C. Quackenbos arrived on the scene to help with the sick on the gunboats and bomb ketches, and he arranged to pay Rogers as a private physician.[30]

Suddenly there was a new demand for the medical talents of Dr. Rogers. Keith Spence, the navy agent at New Orleans, was diagnosed as suffering from insanity. As Rogers described it, Spence went to bed on the evening of November 27 feeling perfectly normal. The next day, Rogers found him "with wild staring eyes and gritting his teeth like one who was recovering from an apoplectic fit." Spence made no complaints but was found to have defective sight and hearing. He answered yes or no without regard to the question being asked. As Spence later told his wife, when he awoke, he found that he could not speak. When he tried to write, he could not control the pen: characters and figures different from what he intended appeared on the paper and looked like hieroglyphics. He could not read, but he still had the use of his senses. A modern diagnosis might be either a small cerebrovascular accident, or a transient ischemic accident from an arterial spasm with residual sequelae. Surgeon Rogers bled Spence copiously three times in the course of two days. In a few days he began to show signs of improvement. He began to speak in sentences and ask questions. The agent could not recall things that he had read before he became ill, and he began to show some concern about the state of his affairs. After seven days he recovered his health but not his reason. He had only a partial understanding of words and sometimes seemed to want to start a conversation but could not express the words. According to Rogers, at times Spence wore "an idiotic grin" and told jokes. He seemed unaware of the effect he had on people.

Three or four weeks passed without any change in Spence's condition. Then Surgeon Wells saw him and instantly recognized the problem. Wells's father had suffered from the same affliction and he knew what to do: he began to treat Spence with mercury pills and the patient began to improve. By January 1, he could dictate a short letter to his wife, and on January 30 he wrote a single-page letter in his own hand. Two weeks later he wrote his wife about his ordeal. He was then back at work, but he found that he sometimes got a pain in his head which would confuse him, and he would occasionally get lost in long calculations. But he was getting better every day, and by the end of February he told his wife that he had recovered.[31]

While Keith Spence was struggling to regain his health, Louisiana experienced a major scare. In 1806 former Vice President Aaron Burr had been talking to various people in the West about a scheme to raise a body of armed men and send them to New Orleans. From there they would be used to detach from the Union the states west of the Allegheny Mountains, where a new nation under Burr's leadership would be established. Others understood that there would be an attack on Spanish-held territory in Mexico. Some believed that both projects were contemplated. Burr told different versions of his plans to different people, so that there is no definitive evidence of just what he intended to do. In late October 1806, Secretary Smith directed the commandant of the marines to organize a detachment of 74 enlisted men and four officers "to reinforce or take the place of the garrison at New Orleans with a view of Spanish operations." On December 11 the detachment, under Captain Daniel Carmick, set out for New Orleans in the U.S. brig *Franklin*. Meanwhile, in early December, Governor Claiborne of Louisiana and Major General James Wilkinson, the commander of the army troops in the region, met with New Orleans merchants to determine the best method of raising a sufficient number of seamen to man the gunboats in order to meet a "premeditated attack on the Territory, by a formidable body of men assembling on the Ohio." Earlier, Wilkinson had told the chamber of commerce that Burr had 7,000 men and that 2,000 of these would reach Natchez on December 20.[32]

A few days before this meeting, Master Commandant John Shaw told Surgeon Rogers that circumstances made it necessary for him to use every available officer in the area. Shaw therefore ordered Rogers to establish a hospital for the reception of sick seamen and marines. If possible he was to secure a public building, but if that could not be done, then he must choose a suitable house. Rogers was also to look over the stock of public medicines available and give Shaw a list of what he needed. The doctor replied that the number of men on the sick list was increasing daily and there was no place to put them; he had no bedding or fireplaces to provide some comfort; and the present environment made it impossible for him to give his venereal patients the usual course of mercury treatments. One remedy for overcrowding was to acquire a large house across the Mississippi River then occupied by General Wilkinson, which could be transformed into a hospital at little expense. Rogers had made a similar suggestion to the secretary of the navy, adding that since the proposed hospital was in a good location, merchant ships could discharge their sick there before proceeding to New Orleans. The location would present some difficulties for the surgeon, however, for he could not live in the city and work at the hospital, and therefore Rogers asked what arrangements should be made.[33]

Before these problems could be resolved, events took a new and more ominous turn for Rogers. Surgeon's Mate Quackenbos delivered an order to him from Shaw to join the bomb ketch *Etna* immediately and place himself under the command of Lieutenant Jacob Jones. This was a part of the process of placing the naval force in the river to resist an attack by Burr's forces. There was nothing in the order that said what the doctor was to do with the patients now under his care or about the plans to move them to new and larger quarters. What should he do? Rogers wrote to Shaw that he could not comply with the order. Unfortunately he did not say that his patients needed him but based his refusal on other grounds:

> I have long since resolved never to act again as Surgeon on shipboard—
> this resolution was personally communicated to the Secretary of the
> Navy—it must at least have been acquiesced in by him, or I should not
> have been continued on the Navy list—had I known that you harbored
> the idea of sending me on Shipboard, when I received your letter of the
> 1st Inst. [concerning the establishment of the hospital] I should have
> done as I now do, & rested on the Secretary's furlough, from which
> State, in my opinion, none but the Secretary can remove me.[34]

Shaw was stunned when he received this note. He showed it to General Wilkinson and asked his advice. The general apparently agreed with Shaw on what needed to be done, and Shaw informed Rogers that he was placing him under arrest on two charges: unofficerlike conduct and disobedience of orders. Copies of these charges and pertinent letters were being sent to the secretary. For his part, Rogers wrote to the secretary that at the request of Shaw, he had taken charge of the sick men of the navy and the medicines and was preparing Wilkinson's former quarters as a hospital.[35]

Meanwhile in letters to the secretary, Shaw detailed the steps that had been taken to stop any attack by Burr's forces. Smith approved of what had been done. On the matter of Dr. Rogers, he ordered Shaw to convene a court-martial as soon as circumstances would permit it. He added: "I am astonished at his [Rogers's] observation, that his resolution not to act as Surgeon on ship board was personally communicated to me. Had I understood this before, the course to be pursued with respect to him was obvious—He could not have continued in the service."[36] Smith ordered Rogers to report to Master Commandant John Shaw, and the doctor did so on January 29, 1807. Shaw said that the services of Rogers would be required until the wishes of the secretary were known. The secretary had other matters on his mind.

As things turned out, Burr's boats were seized, and he surrendered to the authorities in Mississippi Territory in February 1807. Brought to trial in Richmond on a charge of treason, he was acquitted. Once Burr was in custody, the navy could turn its attention to the situation with Dr. Rogers.[37] A court-martial was held on the bomb ketch *Etna* on June 8. The court consisted of six line lieutenants and Lieutenant James Leonard as prosecutor. Shaw testified that during the previous summer he had often heard Rogers say that he would never do duty on shipboard again. On one of these occasions, Shaw told the surgeon that he should resign his commission. He also warned Rogers that if he disobeyed an order from him he would be arrested. Shaw quoted Rogers as saying that he did not give a damn for the government of the United States. Rogers was found guilty of the charges of unofficerlike conduct and disobedience of orders and dismissed from the navy in August 1807.[38]

In an effort to meet the medical needs at New Orleans, the secretary ordered Surgeon's Mate Thomas Marshall to the city, and he set out from Clarksville, Tennessee, in May 1808. No sooner had he become a part of the force than he died of unknown causes in November 1808. Because of confusion or a lack of system in Washington, Marshall's friends in Farmingham, Massachusetts, did not learn of his death until 13 months later.[39] Others had already taken over his duties.

Fate was much kinder to newly appointed Surgeon's Mate Amos A. Evans, who reached New Orleans safely by sea. Writing to his father about his assignment, he was very pleased to be in a beautiful and settled environment. Speaking of the house then being used as a hospital, he wrote:

It is large & nearly square, 2 stories high with a wide porch all around it, on the second story. The rooms are large & full of doors & windows: from one room you can pass to all the others in the same story. There is no communication between the stories on the inside of the house. There are steps on the outside leading to the porch from there you may enter the house by doors on every square. The doors & windows are double— the outside one, wood & the inside glass—& both open like window shutters. The panes of glass are very large, some of them 18 by 24 inches. The glass of the upper story of this house cost $200. The rooms are handsomely papered, & have a picture of some kind & a large square looking glass set in the chimney place, above the fireplace in every room. The U.S. pay $100 per month for the rent of this house—It is a receptacle for the sick men & officers of the Navy on this station. I have a good advantage of practice here—as the house is generally full—and having them all together can attend them with less trouble. I have a room to myself and a servant to attend for me. The Surgeon—Dr. S. D. Heap, has a good library which I have the liberty of using.[40]

Here we see a young surgeon's mate able to keep up with his intellectual and clinical education in a hospital that was generally full of patients in normal times. But later in that same year, additional strains were placed on the system. The number of marines and the size of the naval force in the New Orleans area increased, placing new demands on the medical personnel. During the summer of 1809, there was an outbreak of sickness, presumably yellow fever, which killed a number of persons. Until then it had been customary to keep distinct the duties of the hospital and fleet surgeons, but when Dr. Wells was ordered to join the marine detachment at Natchez, the hospital he ran in the house rented by Dr. Rogers came under the direction of Surgeon Samuel D. Heap. Heap also attended the marines in the area and the sick in the arsenal as well. When he needed supplies or medicines, Heap requested them from the principal line officer in charge of each of these departments. They examined and signed the requisitions and passed them on to the navy agent, who then scrutinized them and supplied only what he considered to be proper. At least one officer was concerned about the fact that the agent was not responsible to the naval commander of the station.[41]

The medical situation in New Orleans was a matter of concern to Master Commandant Shaw. Weak and ill from a violent "bilious attack" and awaiting permission to depart for Ohio for his health, he wrote to the secretary and suggested that Surgeon Lewis Heermann be assigned to the hospital. Heermann, then on duty in Norfolk, also requested the assignment. To Heermann the responsibility for the naval hospital at New Orleans offered a greater field for an important medical practice than he had in his present

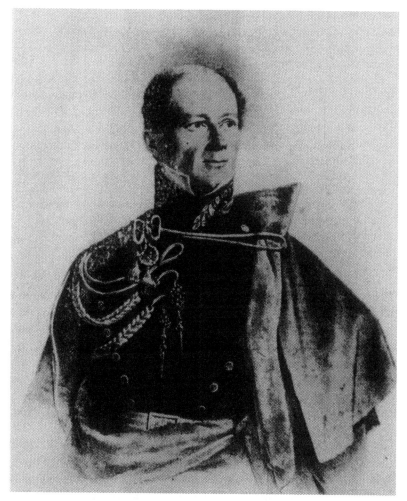

Surgeon Lewis Heermann. National Library of Medicine, Bethesda, Md.

post. Also, with the title of hospital surgeon, he would make more money. One obstacle in the way of such an assignment was that Surgeon Samuel Heap was already there and wanted to stay. His wishes were not fully honored. He served briefly at Norfolk before being sent back to New Orleans in 1811.[42]

One of those who wanted to leave New Orleans, at least briefly, was Surgeon John A. Brereton. He had scarcely completed his medical education in Philadelphia when he entered the navy in 1808 and subsequently had seen a good deal of sea duty. He had been promoted to surgeon in

March 1811, and he now wanted to go home to put his affairs in order. At that time he pointed out that there were six surgeons, two acting surgeons and one surgeon's mate attached to the New Orleans station, so he would not be missed. The secretary granted him permission.[43]

If there were enough doctors to handle the caseload, the hospital facilities still left much to be desired. Shaw called the secretary's attention to the problem.

> The rented house at present occupied as a Naval Hospital, is a tolerably good one, and sufficiently spacious for the accommodation of a considerable number of officers at the same time; but by no means calculated, from its elligant [sic] and costly structure, and its want of apartments sufficiently distinct, for the reception of the common seamen and other ordinary hands, such of these as require the benefits of the hospital are necessarily placed together in a mere shed, situate[d] at a small distance in the rear of the principal building; where they are much less comfortably situated than ought to be wished, as indeed expected.

Shaw believed that instead of paying $1,500 a year plus damages to rent the building, the government would be better off in the long run building its own hospital. Heermann, who was now in charge of the facility, could prepare estimates of the cost.[44]

After Heermann took over the supervision of the naval hospital, he tried to apply his European concepts of order to it. He considered the hospital one of the most important in the United States and therefore felt that he was entitled to more pay. He pointed out to the secretary that a hospital surgeon in the army made $123 a month plus an allowance for rent and fuel. This was in keeping with what a professional man deserved. Heermann's income as a naval surgeon was not commensurate with his responsibilities and inadequate considering the cost of living. At Captain Shaw's request he had not engaged in private practice on his own time. To Shaw he indicated his feelings that his duties were as important as those of Surgeon Samuel R. Marshall in New York, who had the title of hospital surgeon. Certainly the cost of living in New Orleans, which exceeded that of all other naval station, was an argument for higher pay.[45]

If his own status and income were much in his mind, they did not prevent Heermann from doing what he could to improve the hospital accommodations. In May 1811 the navy agent advertised in the local newspaper for a "commodious House in an airy situation, with suitable out house, for the Navy Hospital." Apparently this led to the renting of another house in an area known as Faubourg Marigny, and the hospital was moved there sometime during the summer. As for Shaw's argument that it was

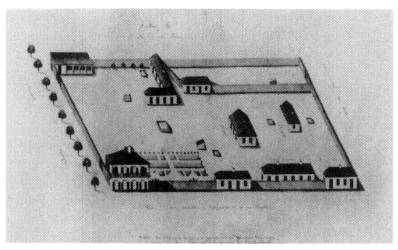

Surgeon Lewis Heermann's Naval Hospital at New Orleans. National Library of Medicine, Bethesda, Md.

better to build than rent, Heermann was convinced that it was impossible to get a good location with adequate accommodations for a hospital on the local scene.[46]

The new hospital had been functioning only a short time when its staff was faced with a major crisis: a "malignant bilious fever" struck the marines in August. Two officers and 16 men died. Many others became sick, including Surgeon Heap and the surgeons of the U.S. brig *Syren*. This threw additional work on Heermann and Surgeon Amos A. Evans. After 24 days, Heap was able to resume his duties. Six weeks after the outbreak, all his patients were convalescing. It was a source of some surprise to Heap that despite four years of "seasoning" in New Orleans, he was still prone to an attack of the fever. Yet he was happy to tell the secretary that the city was becoming more healthy.[47]

When the health crisis was nearly over, Heermann again wrote to the secretary about his need for more money, saying that he made less than the most menial journeyman mechanic in that region. He was not the only one who was discontented about his compensation: Surgeon's Mate Julius R. Shumate wrote to the secretary about the laborious duty he had had at New Orleans and saying he felt he should be promoted. Frustrated by his inability to advance himself in rank, Shumate resigned from the navy in July 1812. By that time the nation was at war and new challenges and opportunities awaited medical men.[48]

Chapter 6

Medical Care Ashore: Boston

When the act of 1798 relating to the care of sick sailors was passed, no action was taken in Boston for another eight or nine months, apparently in the belief that the fund needed to be built up first. At that time, Boston had an almshouse for paupers with various kinds of physical and mental illnesses. There was also a quarantine hospital on Rainsford Island where persons with contagious diseases who arrived in ships could be held. If someone came down with a contagious disease in the city, a public hospital would place that individual in isolation while care was administered. At the public hospital people could be inoculated against smallpox and remain there while they recovered from the virus. So a marine hospital near Boston would be an important advance in health care. Where would it be built?

One suggestion came from the secretary of the Treasury. In May 1799, Oliver Wolcott wrote to Benjamin Lincoln, the collector at the port of Boston, suggesting that Castle Island (later known as Castle William and as Ft. Independence) would be a suitable location. It had been fortified since 1634, and in 1798 there were 20 buildings on the site. An army contingent took over the post in October 1798. Dr. Thomas Welsh was appointed acting surgeon and took up his residence at the fort. Welsh had graduated from Harvard College with honors in 1772 and had studied medicine under Dr. Isaac Foster of Charlestown. He was also a member of a group that organized the Massachusetts Medical Society in 1781, and a decade later he was elected a member of the Boston Marine Society. When asked if he would be willing to care for sailors as well as soldiers, Dr. Welsh said yes. Though Castle William would be suitable for a temporary hospital, it would be necessary to repair a barracks then being used and to construct one or more additional buildings. The secretary of war, James McHenry, had assured Welsh that when a suitable place for a hospital was chosen at Castle William, Major General Alexander Hamilton, who was then serving as inspector general of the army, would be advised. In addition to the buildings, it would be necessary to provide beds, bedding, utensils, and the services of a steward and a nurse. Dr. Welsh suggested to the collector the expediency of having Secretary Wolcott take up the needs of Castle William with McHenry.[1]

The matters were broached to Wolcott, who took them up with his colleague the secretary of war. McHenry wrote to the collector on June 25, 1799, to inform him that orders had been issued to one Jonathan Jackson to make the repairs and to build the barracks in accordance with the directions of the collector. In order that the new barracks not create any obstruction that would hinder the defense of the island, McHenry advised that it be built a distance from the quarters occupied by the garrison. Presumably the work was done during that summer, and Dr. Welsh probably moved his patients into new quarters when temperatures became cooler in the fall.

In February, Welsh sent the collector a list of proposed regulations for the hospital, and Lincoln forwarded them to the secretary of the Treasury, who approved them a month later. These rules provide a glimpse of the operations of this early hospital. All officers and men of the navy and marine corps, as well as all officers and seamen of the merchant service, could be admitted whenever wounds, sickness, or infirmity made it necessary. If they suffered from a contagious or malignant disease, they would be subject to the orders and regulations relating to such afflictions. No gambling of any kind was allowed in the hospital, and no one could leave it without permission. The steward was charged with the responsibility of procuring, issuing, and keeping safe all supplies not otherwise furnished by the hospital. It was also his job to preserve order. The principal nurse had responsibility for keeping the wards, beds, bedding, patients' clothing, and utensils in neat order and exercising the most exacting economy in her department. For every 10 sick or wounded patients under her care, an additional nurse would be allowed to assist her. Convalescent patients might be required to perform reasonable services, as the surgeon might direct.

The daily issue of food was regulated by the steward according to diet. For a full diet, the issue consisted of one pound of fresh meat, two gills of rice or four gills of Indian meal, one gill of molasses or eight gills of milk, and one pound of bread. Those on a half-diet got no meat and only three-fourths of a pound of bread, but the same amounts of rice or Indian meal and molasses or milk as in the full diet. The low diet consisted of one gill of rice or two gills of Indian meal, one half-gill of molasses, one gill of milk, one half-ounce of coffee or chocolate or one quarter-ounce of tea, two ounces of sugar, and one pound of bread. The milk diet contained two gills of rice or four gills of Indian meal, three pints of milk, and one half-pound of bread. Those patients on the fever diet got water gruel, panada (bread boiled to a pulp and served with sugar, currants, and nutmeg or other spices), and herb tea according to the surgeon's orders in the particular circumstances. The surgeon also determined what amounts of soap, salt, candles, vinegar, spirits, wine, vegetables, and wood a patient was to receive.

In 1802, while discussing the need for a marine hospital at New Orleans, Congress adopted an amendment providing $15,000 "for the erection of a hospital in the district of Massachusetts."[2] Three days after this law was passed, the secretary of the Treasury advised the collector at Boston of it and suggested that that city was the best place for the hospital. The collector was requested to report the best location and the probable expense of the ground and buildings, and it soon became apparent that the best site was one of interest to the navy.

In 1799, during the Quasi-War, Congress had appropriated funds for timber and timberlands, ship construction, and dry docks. Accordingly, Secretary Stoddert acquired land for navy yards at Portsmouth, New Hampshire, Boston, New York, Philadelphia, Washington, D.C., and Norfolk. In Boston the navy had scarcely acquired the land when it became necessary to sell up to five acres of it to the Treasury Department for a marine hospital. The secretary of the navy directed Samuel Brown, the navy agent at Boston, to select the ground to be transferred.[3] The area staked out came from the north or lower end of the yard. Brown was also to advertise in local newspapers offering a prize of $50 for the best plan for a hospital. The specifications were that the structure would occupy an area of 4,000 square feet, have two stories of 10 and 8 feet high, and have cellars below. The rooms for the sick were to be well aired and vary in size from 12 to 20 square feet. Economy of space and in construction, as well as convenient distribution of rooms, would be important factors in the final selection. Entries were to be sent to the secretary of the Treasury by August 15, 1802.

Asher Benjamin submitted an entry, the only one received, so he won the prize. With some alterations it became the basis for the new hospital. Before construction began, Professor Benjamin Waterhouse of the Harvard Medical School, wrote to the collector on February 9, 1803, to express his views on what should be done at the hospital. He had long felt the need for a hospital where medical students, especially those in his courses in physic and surgery, might observe the treatment of patients. The new marine hospital would offer such an opportunity, and Waterhouse was therefore contemplating applying for the post of physician there. If appointed, he would try to see that all requirements for the care of the sick and wounded be fulfilled.

The rules of the hospital would supersede all others. He would introduce students studying physic and surgery to the patients in the hospital, to all important operations, and to the rules in established hospitals in Europe. In addition he would give clinical lectures on the "extemporaneous practice of physic and surgery" and "a short course of lectures on the most approved mode of preserving the health of seamen," as well as on matters that might arise out of unforeseen circumstances. Waterhouse went on to say that he had communicated these ideas to Representative Samuel Latham Mitchell of New York, who had studied medicine at the University of Edinburgh before taking up the law and had, between 1797 and 1813, served as editor of the *Medical Repository,* an early medical quarterly published in New York. Mitchell expressed his approval of Waterhouse's plans and urged him to apply for the position in Boston.[4]

Despite this endorsement, the position of physician in charge of the marine hospital went to Charles Jarvis. He was a graduate of Harvard College, class of 1766, and had studied physic and surgery in Boston and England. Like his predecessor, he was one of the founders of the Massachusetts Medical Society, and he was also a member of the American Academy of Arts and Sciences. At the Boston Marine Hospital, his salary was $1,000 a year.[5] When the hospital was completed, Jarvis moved his patients from Castle Island to the new building in January 1804.

Meanwhile Surgeon Peter St. Medard had returned from Mediterranean service and was attached to the navy yard at Boston. "It will be your duty to attend to all the officers, Seamen and Marines, who may belong to the yard, or who may be in Boston or in its vicinity and under the control of this department," wrote Secretary Smith. The navy agent would supply him with any medicines he needed.[6] Within a matter of weeks a jurisdictional question arose. There were marines being treated by Dr. Jarvis at the marine hospital, adjacent to the yard. Did these men fall within St. Medard's responsibility? No, said the secretary. St. Medard was in no way connected with the hospital. "You are considered as attending the marines at the Navy Yard."[7]

Six days later, St. Medard was ordered to report to Washington, but he did not leave Boston, apparently because of illness. The order was repeated, and again he did not go. As a result, the secretary apparently decided that St. Medard was not well enough to attend to his duties at the yard. So, in May 1804, Smith arranged with Jarvis to attend to the marines at the temporary hospital in the navy yard and those in the neighborhood of Charlestown and Boston for $506 a year. St. Medard was informed of the decision and placed on furlough. When he was ordered to sea in March 1805, he wrote to the secretary that he had had a long and active service but had now reached an advanced age and was suffering from diminished vision, sciatica pains, a weakness in his limbs, a broken constitution, and a rupture dating from the Revolutionary War. He asked the secretary to take note of his faithful service and give him the post of superintendent of a marine or naval hospital. If the secretary wished, he would resign his commission. Instead Smith placed him on furlough, where he remained for most of the rest of his life.[8]

A few months after this problem had been resolved, Smith received a complaint from Lieutenant Colonel Franklin Wharton, the commandant of the marine corps, about the arrangements in Boston for his sick men. When marines went on sick call, they were sent to the marine hospital, which was used mainly by the men in the merchant marine at the lower end of the yard. Here they were beyond the vigilance of their officers, and if so disposed, they could desert while convalescing. To guard against this, Wharton wanted a room added to the present barracks where the sick marines could be kept. Smith forwarded his letter to the navy agent at Boston and asked for ideas and estimates on the proposal. The agent met with First Lieutenant Newton Keene of the marines, and they decided that it would be most convenient to construct a building 30" × 16" near the barracks. The estimated cost was $700. Smith approved but had no funds available for construction, so the project languished.[9]

If funds had been available, a more urgent case could have been made for their use in repairing the marine barracks, where the troops suffered from exposure to the weather. It was not until the fall of 1810 that contracts were signed to build a brick barracks with marines supplying most of the unskilled labor. A month later it was determined that a second story was needed on the wings of the building. Difficulties in funding followed, and it was not until February 1811 that the men could move into the still unfinished barracks. Work was completed in August of that year largely through the efforts of the marines.[10]

Meanwhile problems has arisen in regard to medical direction of the marine hospital. Jarvis was stricken with "lung fever" and after an illness of about 60 hours, died at the hospital on November 23, 1807.[11] He was succeeded by Dr. Benjamin Waterhouse, who now proceeded to carry out the suggestions he had made two years earlier about using the hospital in connection with his teaching at Harvard. Waterhouse assumed that his appointment included all the duties and emoluments of Jarvis, views endorsed by Commodore Samuel Nicholson, superintendent of the Boston Navy Yard, as well as by the commander of the marine detachment. But when Waterhouse called on the navy agent, he was informed that he would not be recognized as the successor to Jarvis without a letter from the secretary of the navy. Until it was received, the doctor was to submit no accounts for payment. Waterhouse took up the matter with the secretary of the navy.

Waterhouse pointed out to the agent that the navy and marine corps patients were almost as numerous as those from the merchant service and that no other physician could come into the marine hospital and prescribe for the patients regardless of his organizational affiliation. In addition, Waterhouse noted that he spent a portion of every day examining recruits for the navy. These arguments failed to sway the agent, and it took a letter from Smith to resolve the dispute.[12] In requesting the intervention of the secretary, Waterhouse mentioned that some of the opposition to his appointment came from local medical men who, in turn, had influenced the members of the Boston Marine Society. This may have been related to his plans to use the marine hospital to educate surgeons for the merchant marine. His local medical colleagues knew of his plan, and they apparently saw that this would take pupils from them. But when writing to General Henry Dearborn, the newly appointed collector of customs at Boston, one of the local doctors, William Eustis, advanced other arguments. Eustis said that Waterhouse had never pretended to practice surgery and that in politics he was a Federalist, belonging to the party opposed to that of Jefferson. Eustis had been acting as the physician at the marine hospital since the death of Jarvis, and he evidently thought that he might get a permanent appointment. Waterhouse's enemies also induced the youngest of his students to sign a paper stating that his teacher was unfit. They apparently did not know that Waterhouse had corresponded with Jefferson on the subject of vaccination for almost a year while the latter was vice president. When the complaints against Waterhouse reached Jefferson's ears, he took no action, apparently believing that the doctor was competent to discharge his duties. Also, Waterhouse was supported by Benjamin Rush, Congressman and physician Samuel L. Mitchell, the governor of Massachusetts, and the secretary of the navy.[13]

Meanwhile no surgeon had been appointed for the navy yard itself. If one were selected from among Waterhouse's enemies, the man might not share his views on the need for regular medical instruction. The clinical lectures that Waterhouse had in mind for his students were similar to those in the book *Medicina Nautica* by the British naval physician Thomas Trotter. Waterhouse's choice for the position was Dr. John Randal, a middle-aged local gentleman who, he believed, had pure morals, pleasant manners, and "a peculiar turn to the therapeutic part of surgery." In addition to being a scholar, he had connections to the family of the late Samuel Adams of the Revolutionary War generation. As a "scientific surgeon," Randal would be well qualified to teach by lectures and "nice operations."[14]

At the marine hospital, Waterhouse was concerned about a dangerous surgical case that he had inherited from Dr. Eustis without any information about the patient's history. He sought the opinions of three senior medical men, Drs. James Lloyd, Samuel Danforth, and John Warren, who visited the patient and gave advice, which Waterhouse followed. The man recovered.[15]

Other matters now demanded attention. While Waterhouse praised the work of Jarvis, he felt that he did not have a system in regard to the diets and medicines of patients. In the accounts of the hospital he found a charge of $359 a quarter for spiritous liquors, apparently consumed mainly by the overseer of the liquor, who was a habitual drunkard. When it became known that Waterhouse intended to replace this man, he was confronted with a number of applicants, including one sea captain who was a member of the Boston Marine Society. Waterhouse passed over the captain and others and chose a former orderly sergeant who had served in the American Revolution. Although he was not from the class of men referred to as gentlemen, said Waterhouse, he was honest and temperate and followed directions.[16]

Next came questions in connection with the physical examination of recruits. Waterhouse found men who were prone to smallpox, and he wanted to vaccinate them. The commander of the marine detachment agreed, and Waterhouse asked Secretary Smith "if I must hereafter consider the vaccination of such subjects as a part of my duty?" If so, there would be no need to place them in the hospital, and the procedure would not delay their transfer to another station. No answer to this question has been found. The doctor apparently used his own judgment and vaccinated when he thought it was necessary.[17]

There was also the matter of the four able seamen who had been left at the hospital by the *Wasp*. These men were now well enough to be dismissed from the hospital, but the weather was inclement and the doctor thought they might be needed by a ship in the Boston area. He therefore wished to delay shipping them out and exposing them to illness.

Waterhouse used this occasion to send the secretary a copy of his earlier plans for a teaching hospital and the support he had received for the concept. As for the care of the patients, the system of dressers that he had already established could be tripled in an emergency by drawing on his students in the Boston area. He noted also that Drs. Lloyd, Danforth, and Warren had offered to help in any emergency and to be available for advice and consultation. They did this, said Waterhouse, not just out of friendship for him, but because three of four captains of the Boston Marine Society were making judgments on the qualifications of medical men. These captains were joined by "a number of young, disappointed Doctors" and had persuaded the deputy collector of the port that he had the exclusive right of nomination and appointment. Waterhouse considered the division of patients into naval and merchant seamen to be a case of "a house divided against itself." He hoped the secretary would give him as broad a basis as he could on which to build "this medical school for military physicians & surgeons." Smith was convinced, and Waterhouse was appointed physician to the marine hospital and the navy yard.[18]

Meanwhile Waterhouse had drawn up a new set of regulations for the marine hospital which became official in April 1808. He later claimed that there were no rules or orders in existence when he took over but probably meant that the earlier ones were not being enforced. His own rules showed how ideas about patient care had changed since the time of Dr. Welsh. Patients were expected to wash their face and hands and comb their hair every day. They were to be shaved every Sunday and Wednesday and given a clean shirt every Sunday, or oftener, if convenient. The overseer or steward was to visit the wards each morning to see that the men had washed themselves and to make sure that there was nothing offensive in the rooms. He was to make a similar check before bedtime to see that all the patients were in the house and that no one who did not belong there remained. Patients were to retire at 9 P.M. in the winter and 10 P.M. in the summer; lights were put out and fires allowed to burn down unless there was some special case requiring that they be maintained through the night.[19] Orders of the steward or overseer were to be obeyed, but patients had the right to appeal a grievance to the physician. Spitting on the floor or the hearth, writing on the walls or woodwork, and driving nails were forbidden. Any man who disobeyed the orders of the physician or overseer or got drunk or was guilty of theft or of committing a riot was to be dismissed from the hospital. Patients could also be dismissed for throwing away their medicine, feigning illness, or willfully impeding their cure. Card playing and gambling for money were forbidden, as were any games that were accompanied by noise that disturbed the sick. No patient was allowed to go to Boston or any distance from the hospital without permission from the physician, the overseer, or a medical student. When the physician was ready to visit patients in their wards, they were notified by the ringing of the bell.

There were also five articles that pertained to the medical staff. No seaman was to be admitted without a written certificate from the custom house certifying that he had paid hospital money into the fund. The hours of admission were 10 A.M. and 12 noon, but if a lame or weak person presented himself earlier or later, the overseer, the house-pupil or medical student, or the head nurse could receive him into the hospital and give him the low diet until the doctor could see them. But no one was to be admitted with the itch or any other infectious disorder, with the exception of venereal disease.

Nurses, who were both male and female, were to see that the patients were as neat and clean as their particular cases would permit. They were also to see that the beds, bedclothes, and wards were kept "extremely clean." In fair weather the wards were to be aired by opening the windows and doors, the length of time varying with the weather. The nurses were to see that "no nastiness of any kind" was thrown out of the windows or doors. In no circumstances were the nurses to alter the diet prescribed by the physician or allow the patients to use any diet other than that issued by the hospital. No spiritous liquors were to be brought into the wards except that prescribed by the doctor. In addition, the nurses were "to attend to the particular disgusts and cravings of the sick, and report them to the Physician." When a patient died, his effects were to be locked up and reported to the doctor, and no nurse, attendant, or other person was to take or conceal any article that belonged to a deceased patient. Cases of such theft were to be reported to the superintendent.[20]

These regulations were designed to promote order at a time when the Boston Marine Hospital was admitting an unusually large number of patients as a result of the passage of the Embargo Act, banning all foreign trade. The landlords of seamen's boardinghouses in Boston, Charlestown, and most of the other seaports in New England induced sick men to seek treatment at the marine hospital. Waterhouse reported that while he had been as circumspect as possible, he had probably been imposed upon by some of these men. To cope with the influx of patients, he instituted an outpatient service, where he gave advice and medicine to those men who could produce certificates of eligibility from the custom house. If he had not resorted to this expedient, Waterhouse believed, the hospital would have had 180–200 patients instead of 143, "yet our bill for medicine has not been higher than last quarter." As of June 29, 1808, of the 143 admitted, 3 died: 1 of consumption, 1 of "Hydro Thorax" (an effusion of water into the chest, a type of dropsy), and 1 of venereal disease. One hundred and four seamen were cured and discharged and 39 remained in the hospital.[21]

Waterhouse was happy to report that copies of his regulations had been placed in every room at the hospital and were being observed. By visiting every ward and room at least twice a week, except those occupied by patients with venereal diseases, the "directress" of the hospital was able to improve neatness, economy, and promptness. Previously items such as bedding were stolen, but under the new system only one sheet was missing. Washing and similar work in the hospital, previously done by five women, was now done by four, thus reducing expenses. A senior medical student resided in the hospital and was available to respond to the needs of patients night and day, thus gaining practical experience while being trained as a surgeon in the navy. Except for his daily ration of food, the additional service provided by this doctor was without cost.[22]

The comfort of the patients would be gradually improved, said Waterhouse, as more than 100 quick-growing trees had been planted to block the east winds and improve the appearance of the hospital grounds and cemetery. An acre of ground was devoted to a garden that Waterhouse tended for the benefit of his convalescent patients. In addition, the chapel had been cleared of lumber that had been stored there, cleaned, and opened for divine services. Each week ministers from the neighborhood conducted religious services for the patients without charge.[23]

A short time later the overseers of the local almshouse were disturbed by a notice issued by Waterhouse that the marine hospital would not admit insane seamen. The matter came to the attention of Benjamin Lincoln, the collector of customs at the port of Boston, who asked for an explanation. Waterhouse replied that in the recent past, some individuals had delivered insane people to the hospital gate in the evening and then run off, leaving him with the responsibility of trying to find the unfortunate man's late companions or delivering him elsewhere. He could not admit insane persons, he continued, because they disturbed other patients. This refusal to admit did not extend to those who were delirious or whose derangement was due to a transient cause and could be treated. He added that he did not believe that any marine hospital in the United States admitted persons who were insane. The secretary of the Treasury supported Waterhouse's decision and believed that it should be extended to incurable cases, at least until there was more money in the fund.[24]

That summer, Waterhouse applied to the collector for funds and authority to erect a new building about 25 feet square and two stories high. This would be used partly as a barn to store straw, hay, and medicinal bark, and it would also include a small room where patients with lice could be cleansed. Gallatin replied that the request could not be granted: because of the passage of the Embargo Act, customs receipts had declined, and therefore strict economy should be practiced. Later that summer, perhaps as a result of learning that unemployment at sea was increasing the patient load at the hospital, Gallatin told the collector that the building could be erected if it cost no more than $250. Apparently the building was not constructed.[25]

In the fall of 1808, James Madison was elected president of the United States, and he assumed office on March 4, 1809. Among the offices to be distributed by the new administration was that of collector of customs for the port of Boston. Henry Dearborn, who had previously served as secretary of war under Jefferson, was appointed. Waterhouse's enemies now had a new official to whom they could direct their complaints about him, and they soon seized the opportunity. Albert Gallatin was reappointed secretary of the Treasury. He advised Dearborn that no directors of the marine hospital had been appointed by the president and that therefore part of the law of July 1798 had not been put into effect. The appointment of the physician was reserved to the president, but the selection of all the other officers and servants at the marine hospital was the province of the collector, as was the making of the rules for admission. The collector determined what bills were to be paid and thus had control over possible abuses. While Gallatin felt that in practice the physician had to have enough authority to compel the obedience of his subordinates, he thought that Benjamin Lincoln, the previous collector, had "delegated more than was necessary to the attending Physician. If so, it is in your power to correct the evil whenever you please."[26]

Meanwhile new charges had been made against Waterhouse late in the previous administration which had not been resolved and which were now taken up by the new leadership. It was alleged that Waterhouse had someone on the payroll under a false name. The doctor admitted that his wife really performed the duties of the directress of the hospital, but since he was unwilling to have her paid in her married name, her maiden name was used on the payroll. Another charge was that the doctor appropriated 20 pounds of the hospital's beef for his own use. Waterhouse answered that he had lived for a year with the surgeon at the marine hospital in Rhode Island and it was the custom there for the surgeon to receive rations of bread, beef, and liquids from the hospital stores. Later on, he said it was also the practice in British hospitals. If he had considered it illegal he would hardly have risked his position and his reputation for items of such small value.

It was further alleged that the steward charged the hospital for vegetables grown in its own garden, but the investigating committee found no evidence that the doctor profited from this. It was also charged that a scavenger in the employ of the hospital agreed to receive $8 a month less than the hospital allowed; the committee found no evidence to support this. The final charge was that Waterhouse allowed wood and vegetables belonging to the hospital to be delivered to his quarters. Waterhouse responded that at Harvard he was supplied with wood by the college. He expected to receive the same from the hospital, but finding that the hospital's wood was more expensive, he again got what he needed from the college. The investigating committee found that he had not returned some barrels of wood to the hospital for which the government was charged.[27]

Before a final disposition had been made of these matters, Waterhouse's enemies continued their assaults on other fronts. In May 1809, Dr. John G. Warner wrote to Secretary of War William Eustis, formerly a practicing physician, that Waterhouse was not trained as a surgeon and had not practiced as one; neither was he well versed in anatomy. "I have seen in that hospital, persons labouring under diseases which might have been cured by a few strokes of the knife, who were wretchedly trifling with washes & salves, while their disease rapidly advanced beyond the reach of art." In the event of Waterhouse's removal, Warner wanted the appointment. He had a good practice in Boston, and the salary at the marine hospital would scarcely compensate him for the loss of his private business, but the appointment would help him to establish a medical school in Boston, for the hospital would provide opportunities for students to acquire some surgical experience. Warner promised to give a series of surgical and anatomical lectures in Boston for three or four months during the next winter and then annually which would be superior to those offered by Waterhouse. He felt sure that the patronage of Eustis would make the proposed establishment useful and the national administration popular on the local scene. Eustis's response is not known.[28]

Trouble was also brewing on the naval front. Captain Nicholson reported that when his son was stung by a wasp, he asked Waterhouse to treat him. The doctor responded that he expected to be paid for his advice and treatment of members of the captain's family. Nicholson complained to Secretary Smith that Waterhouse's predecessors, St. Medard, Jarvis, and Eustis, had treated his family free of charge. The captain wished to know whether Waterhouse's position as physician to the navy yard embraced the care of the commandant's family.

The secretary chose not to respond. Meanwhile Nicholson took his son to a private physician and later submitted his bill to the collector for payment, contending that the cost should be deducted from Waterhouse's salary. Fourteen months after his complaint, Nicholson and the navy agent received identical letters from the new secretary of the navy, Paul Hamilton, stating that complaints against Dr. Waterhouse or any other officer connected with the navy were received with "caution, and unfavorable impression[s] admitted with reluctance."[29]

Hamilton may not have been aware that Secretary Gallatin had shown the charges against Waterhouse to President Madison. The president directed that they be investigated, so Gallatin asked Dearborn to look into the matter of accounts charged to Elizabeth Oliver, Waterhouse's wife, and James Smith on charges for vegetables. At the same time, Waterhouse was served with a paper marked "Statement of facts." Before replying to this, Waterhouse apparently solicited letters from supporters. Letters from one of the justices of the court of common pleas of Middlesex County, Massachusetts, and a surgeon from Augusta, Maine, praised his work at the hospital. These were sent along with Waterhouse's explanations of the accusations against him. He also wrote to ex-President Thomas Jefferson about the charges and the fact that Dearborn apparently believed them.[30]

When President Madison saw the charges and read Waterhouse's defense, he indicated that he did not believe that the doctor could retain his position. But since he had improved the internal arrangements of the hospital, and since a removal would affect his professional character and standing at Harvard, Madison thought that he should be allowed to resign. Gallatin so informed Dearborn. Waterhouse still tried to defend his actions with Gallatin, but it was too late. The issues boiled down to his having paid his wife under her maiden name and supplied his family with provisions that had been charged to the hospital. Since Waterhouse had chosen not to resign, Dearborn was ordered to remove him. On July 25, 1809, Waterhouse was notified that he was dismissed and that he was to turn over all public property to the steward. Gallatin sent Dearborn the names of two local doctors who could replace Waterhouse. Dearborn chose the first, and David Townshend of Boston was placed in charge of the hospital temporarily. In November he received word that the president had appointed him physician of the marine hospital.[31]

Hamilton soon fell in line with the administration's position. On July 21 the secretary sent Waterhouse a one-sentence letter revoking his authority to treat seamen and marines at the navy yard. No explanation was offered. That same day, Hamilton offered the position to Dr. George Bates of Boston. For attendance on the marines and seamen at the yard who had medical or surgical needs, Bates would be paid $506 a year. Bates accepted. Hamilton may not have been aware that a candidate for the ministry named William J. Torrey had written to Waterhouse before his removal to say that a year earlier, Dr. Bates told him that he had been asked to make a statement about the situation in the marine hospital. Bates had indicated that he would send the statement requested by Washington and that it was a part of the effort to remove Waterhouse. If Torrey's information was correct, then Bates was now being rewarded. Bates was soon involved in medical duties at the yard.[32]

In 1810, while attending the men of the *Chesapeake* as well as examining recruits at the Boston rendezvous, Bates encountered cases of venereal disease. Was he entitled to a fee, as navy surgeons were, for curing such men? He raised the question with Secretary Hamilton. The answer was no. Bates also wondered if he was to charge an additional sum above and beyond his salary for attendance at the recruiting rendezvous? That query also brought a negative reply.[33]

Bates settled into his work, but a little more than a year later, he asked permission to make a voyage to Europe. In his absence, Dr. David Townsend, "a gentleman of great respectability," would discharge his duties. If the leave was not forthcoming, Bates would have to resign. Hamilton granted the request. Bates reported his return in October 1811 and continued to serve in the navy yard until he was replaced by Surgeon's Mate Charles Cotton shortly after the declaration of war in 1812. Bates considered it a disgrace that he was replaced by a junior navy doctor, and he wanted to know why. To Hamilton he wrote about his family's patriotic record in the American Revolution, adding that with the exception of himself, there was only one "Republican Physician in this place." In pointing out his allegiance to the party of Jefferson and Madison, Bates evidently did not understand that the navy wanted its own doctors, especially in a time of war.[34]

By March 1812 it was apparent to some observers that abuses had crept into the running of the Boston Marine Hospital. Adams Bailey, a steward there, wrote to Congressman Charles Turner, a war Democrat, about the conditions he observed.

> Patients that will spend from 3 to 12 months in one hospital, then go to another, and so on for years before they are discovered, and with complaints not any way bad, and with legs they often make themselves, for to get entrance into the hospitals, another class of patients who enter on board of our armed vessels for subsistence, and the same will apply to the Marine Corp, who after a few months service, they prove unfit for any, always, complaining or sick, and are sent to the hospitals (caution in engaging men ought to be strictly attended to). The Merchant sailors also impose on the institution, by sending some to the Hospital who have not been at sea for years, and others that never was [*sic*] at sea one month, and some that were taken from their poor houses, and sent to the Hospital because they formerly went to sea, there is one here now of

the last class, and has been for 10 months,—These patients that I have been describing are more than one half of foreign birth, and Captain [Henry] Caldwell of the Marine Corps of this town died this day— whether some modification of the Hospital laws prevent impositions, would not be of some consequence, is for Congress to determine, I think a saving to the funds might be made strictly observing who have a claim, to the institution and who have not.[35]

A few days later, Dearborn sent a full report on the matter to Gallatin. He reviewed the rules governing admissions and added that there were times when seamen were brought in from a foreign port in distress who were not able to give the required proof. If their story seemed credible, they were admitted. No doubt some men imposed on the officers, but not in the way that Bailey alleged. If any impositions had taken place, it was because men made errors on the side of humanity. Dearborn then gave some background on the cases noted by Bailey. In conclusion he noted that if Bailey had information on abuses, he should have made it known to the hospital authorities. So ended the complaints of an early observer of the marine hospital.[36]

There are no complete records on the total number of men treated at the navy yard or the marine hospital for the dozen years prior to the War of 1812. There is, however, a return for the hospital for a portion of this period. As of 1810, 22 patients remained in the hospital from the previous year; 150 others were admitted during 1810. Of this total of 172, 135 were discharged, 15 died, and 22 remained as carry-overs. In 1811, 205 new cases were admitted, for a total of 227, of whom 163 were discharged and 16 died, leaving 49 still in the hospital. Some of these men were from the navy and marine corps, but the exact number has not been ascertained. Such was the situation in Boston on the eve of the War of 1812.[37]

Chapter 7

Naval Health
Care in the North
and South

Elsewhere in the country the care of sick seamen left much to be desired. For both the merchant and the naval sailor, there were many ports with inadequate or improvised facilities. As was noted in the case of Boston, the passage of the Embargo Act in 1807 led to widespread unemployment in the maritime community. Unemployed men ashore needed food, clothing, and sometimes health care, but it was largely up to local and individual efforts to meet these demands. Though the repeal of the Embargo Act in March 1809 helped to improve the outlook, it was replaced by the less restrictive Non-Intercourse Act, which forbade trade with Great Britain and France. Since those countries were major markets, the new law continued to disrupt normal commercial patterns, with the result that less money was paid into the hospital fund but the demands on hospitals continued.

In the navy there was a parallel problem. The demands of the Barbary Wars had accelerated the construction of navy yards at Portsmouth, New Hampshire, Brooklyn, New York, Philadelphia, Washington, D.C., Norfolk, Virginia, and Boston. But the end of that conflict brought a return to strict economy in naval matters which slowed the completion of the yards. In both war and peace, the emphasis in the yards was on the building and repair of warships. During Jefferson's first term, the construction of large 74-gun ships was suspended, and the navy began to build small, shallow-draft gunboats that carried one or two cannon. By November 1807, 69 of these craft were completed and another 188 had been authorized by Congress. The building of the gunboats represented a change in naval strategy on the part of the Jefferson administration, and their use meant smaller

crews and a change in medical requirements. In the navy yards themselves, accommodations for the sick seem to have been considered only
after other demands had been met. As we have seen in the cases of New
Orleans and Boston, the navy tried to establish its own hospital arrangements, even if it was only a room, in order to avoid excessive reliance on
the marine hospital, whose patients were mainly from the merchant marine. With these considerations in mind, let us look at the situation in
various other ports, navy yards, and stations.

Maine was then a district of Massachusetts, and at Portland, and at
Portsmouth, New Hampshire, sick sailors were treated at the city hospital
at a fixed rate that was charged to the Marine Hospital Fund. By 1809,
Portland found it necessary to board invalids in private homes, where they
were attended by local physicians, and sometimes they were cared for by
the overseers of the poor. Prices for board and nursing were $2–$3 a week
in Portsmouth and $3 in Portland. During 1809, Portland spent $582.90 for
the care of two seamen. One was treated for a whole year and the other for
most of that time. During that same year, Portsmouth spent $171.28 on
care.

The use of private homes for boarding sick seamen was the normal thing
in Providence, Rhode Island; New London and Middletown, Connecticut;
Sag Harbor, New York; and Camden, Edenton, Washington, Newbern,
and Wilmington, North Carolina. The cost of this service ranged from
$2.00 to $3.50 a week. In Providence and New London, a physician was
under contract to provide care and medicines for $200 a year.

A resort to the local almshouse was the only option for sailors who became
sick in Newport, Rhode Island. There were separate charges for the physician, the medicines, and the hospital stores. Newport was left with the care
of one insane seaman. Alexandria, Virginia, sometimes used almshouses for
those who became ill there. Board in an almshouse cost $5 a week, whereas
in a private home it was $3.50. Medical expenses were separate.[1]

New York

In New York the sick were received at the city hospital at a fixed rate
charged to the Naval Hospital Fund. The average expense was $3.25 a
week for each seaman, and this did not include clothing, funeral charges,
or the salary of the superintendent of seamen. During 1809 there was an
average of 64 patients in the hospital, of whom 1 in 14 was a navy man,
3 "maniacs" were also cared for, 38 patients died, and a total of $10,907.61
was paid out. The nature of the diseases treated and the causes of death
are not known.[2]

One of those trying to cope with the sick of the navy in New York was Surgeon Nathaniel Weems. Assigned to duty at the naval rendezvous in 1805, he as also taking care of the crew of a ship, and of one of the midshipman at his lodgings ashore. The midshipman's illness is not mentioned, but it may have been venereal disease; Weems described his work with him as "the hardest and most disagreeable duty I have had." A surgeon assigned to shore duty received only half pay, and Weems found that his boarding expenses left him with very little money for other things. Since he was not known in the city, he could not get credit and he had few friends to whom he could turn for help. He asked Secretary Smith to authorize the navy agent to advance him $100 and allow him an additional $2 a week for extra expenses. This proved to be only a stopgap solution, and Weems resigned his commission on February 20, 1806.[3]

In the meantime the marine contingent at the New York Navy Yard required a medical officer, and Surgeon's Mate Hugh Aitken was assigned to that duty in July 1805. He started with a disadvantage since the medicine chest he had requested had not yet arrived. After six months on the job, he found himself acting as a surgeon but paid as a mate and therefore asked for a promotion. Aitken resented the fact that some physicians had been commissioned as surgeons without first serving as mates. Secretary Smith sent Surgeon Thomas Ewell to New York to be the senior medical officer in charge of the marines. Having entered the service as a surgeon, he was one of the type of doctor about whom Aitken had complained. Ewell arrived at the yard and took over the supply of medicines from Aitken. He found all of the marine guard in good health except for one man with a venereal disease, who was expected to recover soon. Aitken never got his promotion. He became ill not long after Ewell arrived, and he went on leave to Berkeley Springs, Virginia, where he died in September 1806.[4]

Maintaining the health of the marines was now the responsibility of Ewell, an ambitious man. A friend of President Thomas Jefferson, and with highly respectable family connections in Virginia and the District of Columbia, he had entered the navy with the hope of succeeding John Bullus as surgeon at the Washington Navy Yard. When the expected vacancy did not materialize, Ewell was sent to New York. Apparently Secretary Smith promised Ewell that he would have Bullus's position if the latter resigned, and Ewell reminded him of this promise a month after taking over in New York. Ewell too experienced problems living in Brooklyn on his salary. Then, six weeks into his work, he requested a leave of absence of 20–25 days and an advance of $150; his leave was authorized but not the cash advance. He then wrote to Smith that the permission to leave had arrived 20 days later than he expected and that he could not take it now. No doubt the lack of advance money was a factor. Ewell now asked Smith and the accountant of the navy if there were not some way to give surgeons on shore duty more than the customary half pay. He was told that this was not allowed.[5]

While waiting for better times, Ewell was busy translating a French book on chemistry and corresponding with Jefferson about the project. To both Jefferson and Smith he pointed out his difficult circumstances in New York and his desire to replace Bullus in Washington. Persistence paid off, and in February 1807 he was ordered to Washington to take over the duties of Bullus.[6]

Since it had long been evident that Ewell was restless in New York, Surgeon Joseph G. T. Hunt, who was on leave on Long Island, offered to take his place. Smith accepted, and Hunt took care of the marines until he was ordered to join the frigate *Chesapeake* in May 1807. Before leaving, he suggested to Smith the desirability of hiring Dr. Samuel Osborne, a former army surgeon living in the area, described as "a gentleman of very remarkable medical talents." Without waiting for the secretary to act, Lieutenant John Johnson, the commander of the marine guard, hired Osborne because he had sick men on his hands. Justifying his action to Smith, the lieutenant pointed out that whenever Ewell was absent, Osborne had acted in his stead, and, though he was considered eminent in his profession, he would work for moderate terms. Osborne wrote to Smith in his own behalf, saying he had substituted for both Ewell and Hunt in emergencies. The secretary, however, decided that he needed a regular navy doctor and ordered Surgeon Samuel R. Marshall from Philadelphia to New York. To assist him, Smith assigned Surgeon's Mate Jonathan Cowdery. Both were on duty early in August 1807.[7]

While complying with his orders, Cowdery advised Smith that he was unhappy with his situation. Describing himself as the oldest man on the list of surgeon's mates, he felt humiliated to see younger men promoted over him. He liked the navy and wanted to be of service, especially at a time when his country was having problems with Great Britain. Cowdery reminded the secretary that when he had called on him after his return from captivity at the end of the Barbary War, Smith promised him a promotion. Ten days later Cowdery again wrote to Smith, reviewing his service reminding him of his promise. The secretary promoted Cowdery to surgeon on August 24. Because this promotion was made when Congress was in recess, Smith renominated him to the president in December, and the Senate confirmed the appointment on January 16, 1808. Even better from Cowdery's point of view, the commission as surgeon was to date from

November 27, 1804. Along with his promotion and new seniority in rank, Cowdery was given sea duty. His replacement at New York was the newly commissioned Surgeon's Mate John Brown of Baltimore.[8]

Before Cowdery's problem had been resolved, the United States found itself in a situation where war seemed likely as the result of the British attack on the frigate *Chesapeake* in 1807. To prepare for the possible conflict, Commodore John Rodgers was ordered to New York to take command of the flotilla based there and place it in a state of readiness; Commodore Chauncey, in command of the yard, would be under his orders. When Rodgers began to carry out his orders, he became aware of the poor facilities for the sick. About this time, Surgeon Samuel Marshall arrived on the scene, bringing some stability and continuous professional experience to the problems at hand. Rodgers decided to establish a temporary hospital in an old mill in the yard. Marshall understood that he was in charge of the hospital, but this raised some concerns in the mind of Chauncey, who sought some clarifications from the secretary. Did Marshall's appointment mean that he managed the patients and the internal government of the hospital? Who was to approve his expenditures for medicines and hospital stores? What control did the commandant have? The secretary expressed surprise that Chauncey had any doubts about the matter. "Highly and deservedly as Docr. Marshall is respected, it is not considered expedient to make him independent of your command." The doctor was responsible for the care of the patients and the internal government of the hospital under the direction of the commanding naval officer. To make sure that all concerned understood the way things were expected to work, Commodore Chauncey was asked to mention the secretary's views to Surgeon Marshall.[9]

The temporary hospital opened on August 1, 1809. During its first four months of operation, 314 patients were treated at a cost of $301.57¼ for food. Savings were made by taking the value of the daily ration of each man (20¢) and deducting the cost for the hospital diet from this amount. This left a balance of $326.62¾ in favor of the hospital. By gradually building on this surplus, Marshall hoped that he could take care of the contingent expenses of the hospital patients. On the matter of the use of hospital stores, Marshall promised to make the necessary returns and vouchers, as the secretary might order. He also sent a table showing the number of patients and the diseases treated, but this has been lost.[10] The list provided an opportunity to call attention to the state of the building then being used as a hospital. Apparently the roof leaked, or it was not made of substantial materials, for Marshall noted that inclement weather was hard on his patients and that good accommodations were necessary for the recovery of the sick. Later he wrote a much more moving account of his time at the temporary hospital. "Frequently have I visited men infected with catarrhs, Pneumonia, Fevers and consumptions, [and] been presented with the affecting sight of beds covered with snow, or drenched in water, and at every high spring tide the river found an easy passage thro' the lower part of the house, as did the snow and rain thro' the inverted and rotten roof." For Marshall the hospital was but a way station to the grave.[11] This deplorable state of affairs was brought to the attention of both Rodgers and Chauncey. Once the administrative problems had been resolved in his favor, Chauncey brought the situation in the yard to the attention of the secretary.

> To give you some faint idea of what is called the hospital on this station, imagine to yourself an old mill situated on the margin of a mill-pond, where every high tide flows from twelve to fifteen inches upon the lower floor, and there deposits a quantity of mud and sediment, and which has no other covering to protect the sick from the inclemency of the season than a common clapboard outside, without lining or ceiling on the inside. If, sir, you can figure to yourself such a place, you will have some idea of the situation of the sick on this station.[12]

The secretary was apparently moved by this description and sent it to Representative Burwell Bassett, the chairman of the Naval Affairs Committee, which was considering a bill to establish navy hospitals. Though Congress subsequently enacted the desired law, in the short term all that could be done for the sick at New York was to authorize the rental of quarters outside the yard. Two small houses nearby were subsequently acquired and were a big improvement over the mill but still far from satisfactory.[13]

Assisting Marshall at the hospital was Surgeon's Mate William B. Hatfield. In addition to his professional responsibilities, he took on the duties of the steward and kept track of the hospital stores. In making this appointment, Marshall was under the impression that Hatfield would get additional compensation. Commodore Chauncey allowed this but the matter was referred to the secretary for a ruling. Chauncey wrote two letters urging that Hatfield receive extra pay adding that "few men in the service are more capable and deserving than Doctor Hatfield." Secretary Hamilton considered the request a reasonable one, and Hatfield was allowed $10 extra a month from the time he assumed the additional duties.[14]

By the spring of 1812, his duties at the hospital were becoming a burden to Surgeon Marshall. He did not feel well, and now, because Hatfield was on furlough, he had no one to help him. Chauncey authorized him to

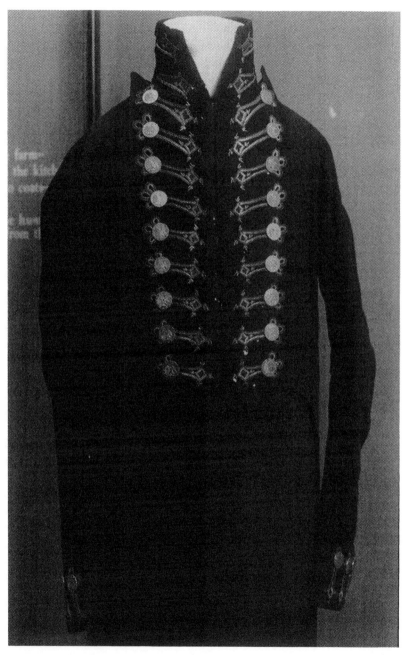

Dress Uniform Coat of Surgeon James M. Taylor, 1805–7. Collection of the Maryland Historical Society, Baltimore.

select an assistant, and Marshall chose Peter Christie, who had been a private pupil of Dr. J. W. Huyler for the previous two years and was recommended highly by him. Another endorsement came from Dr. Walter W. Buchanan of Columbia College, who noted that for several months Christie had served as the house physician and apothecary to the almshouse of New York city. His assiduity and attention to his duties had won him praise. Marshall forwarded these letters to Secretary Hamilton with his request that he commission Christie a surgeon's mate. Chauncey said that the appointment was a matter of necessity. "We have about forty patients constantly in the Hospital and nearly the same number in Vessels in Ordinary and [in the] Flotilla, and only Doctor Hunt to attend the whole as Doctor Marshall is Sick, and has been for some time past confined to his Room." Hamilton complied, and on July 8, 1812, Christie was commissioned as a surgeon's mate. By that time the nation was at war.[15]

Philadelphia

In Philadelphia the care of sick seamen was carried on in a much more organized and efficient environment. As early as 1774 the Pennsylvania Assembly passed an act to prevent the introduction of infectious diseases into the colony. Under this act a hospital was erected on Providence Island and placed under the administration of a keeper, who was to care for the sick inmates. Vessels en route to Philadelphia which had sick persons on board, carried more than 40 passengers, or had sailed from an infected port were inspected by a physician and had to have a clearance before proceeding to an anchorage in the city. The sick were kept at Providence Island until they recovered or died. During the first year of the American Revolution, Drs. Benjamin Rush and Samuel Duffield made an arrangement with the overseer of Providence Island Hospital to care for the sick and wounded of the Pennsylvania navy. He was to provide them with food and drink and wash them for the sum of 10 shillings a week each. An additional 2 shillings a week was given to him for furnishing firewood to the individual patients. Two physicians attended the sick on the island every other day. After the adoption of the Declaration of Independence in 1776, the site was renamed State Island. Less than a year later, a steward replaced the keeper as administrator of the hospital.

In 1794, Governor Thomas Mifflin recommended to the state legislature the adoption of a better system for preserving the health of the public. The result was the passage of a general health law, the establishment of a health office, and the creation of positions for 24 inspectors. By this time there was more than one hospital on the island and these were to be repaired. A health officer, a resident physician, and a consulting physician were to be permanently on duty on the island. When the outbreak of yellow fever took place in 1797, it put a strain on the ability of the board of health to deal with diseases that were or were considered to be infectious. As a result, the state legislature passed a law in 1798 that reconstructed the board and extended its jurisdiction. New buildings were to be built on State Island, and the new and old structures were to be known collectively as the Marine Hospital of the Port of Philadelphia.

Also, when yellow fever was raging, a hospital for its victims had been established at Race Street and Schuylkill Front (later twenty-second Street) which was known as the Hospital of the French Republic and later as City Hospital. Under the 1798 legislation the old board of health was abolished and a new organization known as the Managers of the Marine and City Hospitals was established. There were 12 managers, who were appointed by the mayor, aldermen, and citizens of Philadelphia, and by the justices of the peace of the districts of Southwark, Moyamensing, and Northern Liberties. The new organization had the general powers of the old board, including the right to levy a hospital tax, regulate the length of quarantine, and borrow money for public use in cases of emergency.

After a year of experience under this system, the managers decided in 1799 that new quarantine and marine hospital arrangements were needed. Accordingly they bought land on Tinicum Island in the Delaware River about 10 miles from the city. Here several buildings each measuring 60' × 22' were built to accommodate diseased and convalescent patients. There were also a house for the steward and apartments for the resident physician, quarantine officer, and other officials. Later other buildings were erected for immigrants who were not sick. The U.S. government also established an inspection station on the island for the examination and storage of goods.

The Managers of the Marine and City Hospitals were replaced by a new board of health in 1806. This consisted of five members, two of whom might be physicians. Three members were required to live in Philadelphia, one in Southwark, and one in Moyamensing. The governor appointed the quarantine master, the resident physician, and the consulting health officer. The first two had to reside on the island and the last in Philadelphia. Under this arrangement changes in the system of managing public health matters were implemented. Seamen who had come into the city with their ships or were discharged were received at the City Hospital at a fixed rate that was charged to the Marine Hospital Fund. During the year 1809 an average of 36 seamen were treated per month, and 16 died. The total expenditures for sick seamen in Philadelphia during that year was $7,592.89.[16]

Given this background and experience, it is clear that any merchant seaman or naval or marine officer or man who became ill in Philadelphia had the benefit of a well-organized and efficient system of care. Initially, as the site of the nation's capital city, Philadelphia had been much involved in the naval activities of the Quasi-War with France.

With the removal of the capital to Washington in 1800 and the signing of a treaty with France in 1801, naval activities in Philadelphia were associated with the building of a navy yard. George Gillaspy and Joseph C. Strong, who had both served as medical officers in the navy during the Quasi-War, formed a partnership to sell drugs, and they continued to practice medicine in Philadelphia. Until March 1803 they gave medical assistance and supplied medicines to the marines stationed there. After that the Navy Department relied on its own doctors to take care of the marines and sailors who became ill. These medical men were attached to the navy yard, and temporary hospital facilities were used to accommodate the sick. The indications are that only routine care was given at the yard. Serious cases went to the City Hospital or the marine hospital. Some merchant seamen and perhaps navy men as well were treated at the Pennsylvania Hospital. Various navy doctors treated sailors and marines in the Philadelphia area for short periods, two of the most notable being Surgeons Samuel R. Marshall and Edward Cutbush. The former served there in 1803 and 1805–6, and the latter in 1803–4 and 1806–13. Judging from their correspondence, both were mainly concerned about the cost of living and the support of their families on navy pay in Philadelphia and about securing a servant to help with the care of the sick at the yard.

One exception to this pattern was Cutbush's views in 1807 about the need to establish naval hospitals, including one in Philadelphia. This led Secretary Smith to write to George Harrison, the local navy agent, for his views on the subject. Harrison responded that in Philadelphia they had the best hospital in the United States, and one that was founded and supported by private and public grants. Here sick seamen and marines were received on the same terms. Poor patients were received without charge. If the secretary desired it, a brick hospital could be built which would be more comfortable for the patients.[17] Nothing came of this proposal for reasons that are discussed in chapter 8.

Though no new hospital was built, the medical scene in the navy and later at the yard changed when a member of a prominent Philadelphia family entered the service. William Paul Crillon Barton attended Princeton and graduated with distinction in 1805. He then began the study of medicine under the direction of his uncle, Dr. Benjamin Smith Barton, and received his degree in 1808 from the University of Pennsylvania.

While engaged in building a practice in Philadelphia, he became one of the surgeons attached to the Pennsylvania Hospital. In 1808 he had explored the possibility of receiving a commission as a surgeon in the navy. His application was supported by Caspar Wistar, Benjamin Rush, Benjamin S. Barton, George N. Reed, and Thomas C. Jones. He was informed that there were no vacancies at that time. The following year, Barton was informed that he could be appointed if he wished and that he would be assigned to a frigate then being equipped.[18] He accepted but asked for a delay in reporting until his contract with the managers of the Pennsylvania Hospital expired in July. He told an official of the Navy Department that he had consulted with Commodore Alexander Murray and Lieutenant William Lewis, both then in Philadelphia, about the matter, who assured him that Stephen Decatur Jr., the captain of the ship to which he was to be assigned, would be sympathetic to his circumstances. Barton received his commission as surgeon on April 10, 1809, but his rank was to take effect on June 28. He seems to have reported on board the frigate *United States,* then at Norfolk, about that time, and the first of his sick reports was dated July 7. Three days later, Decatur reported on board, and the two became friends.[19]

Barton later wrote that there was so much sickness in the *United States* that it might almost have been called a hospital ship. Fevers and fluxes caused the daily sick list to average about 40 men out of a complement of 400. He did not have enough wine, brandy, chocolate, or sugar fit to give his patients, and there were other useless or damaged articles in the medicine chest. He also lacked sheets, pillows, pillow cases, and nightcaps for the sick. Fortunately, the ship was cruising off the eastern coast of the United States and not in distant seas. Both Captain Decatur and William Henry Allen, the first lieutenant, were sympathetic to Barton's complaints. Decatur did what he could to help and Allen encouraged him to persevere. In this environment a medical reformer was born.[20]

Circumstances relating to his medical assignments created a bad image of Barton in the Navy Department. It began to form in November 1810 when Surgeon Robert B. Starke of the frigate *Essex* approached him with a request that they exchange duty assignments. Barton declined. Subsequently Captain John Smith of the *Essex* asked Barton if he would go with the ship to Europe since Surgeon Starke was 100 miles away in the country and they could not wait for his return. There was no other surgeon available at the station, Decatur gave his permission, and Barton went, seemingly without consulting the secretary of the navy. When Barton returned from Europe he was ordered to the *Essex.* He asked for permission to return to the *United States* if he had to go to sea, and, because he was now

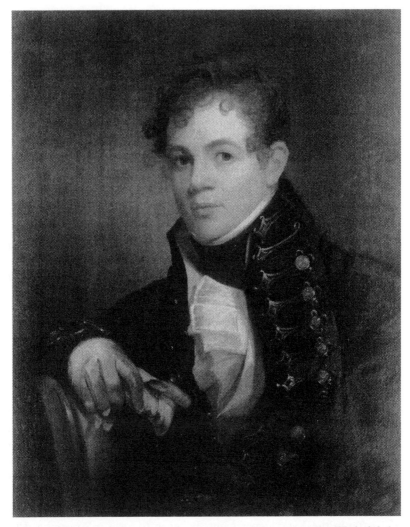

Surgeon William P. C. Barton. Portrait by Thomas Sully, Philadelphia Museum of Art: The Wilstach Collection, presented by William Barton Brewster, M.D.

ill, for a delay in joining the ship. When he had recovered sufficiently, he went to Norfolk and reported on board the *Essex.* Shortly afterward he learned that his father was at the point of death and received permission from Captain David Porter to return to Philadelphia. While there he received a letter from Porter stating that the ship would be coming north and he could rejoin it in the Delaware Bay. Barton then wrote to the secretary and requested a furlough in Philadelphia during the winter until his ship arrived. The request disturbed Secretary Hamilton.

To Hamilton it seemed as though Barton was continually coming up with excuses to avoid obeying orders. He ordered Barton to report at once to the *Essex*. In explaining his action to Dr. Benjamin Smith Barton, Hamilton said that his nephew had been indulged too much. These sentiments were communicated to Surgeon Barton and he was furious. Deeply offended by the secretary's remarks and accusations, he presented his side of the story of his various assignments and requests for postponements. On the matter of his request for a furlough, he noted that Dr. Starke had been on furlough for a year and that Drs. Harwood, New, St. Medard, Davis, and others had been on furlough for a long time. Hence he did not think he was being indulged if he asked for time to take care of some business and look after an aging and ill father. Finally he reminded the secretary that he was an educated professional man who had entered the navy voluntarily.[21]

This reply apparently mollified Hamilton. Barton rejoined the *Essex* for a winter cruise to Rhode Island. From Newport he wrote to his friend Benjamin Latrobe, the architect, and asked him to use his influence with Hamilton to get Barton a furlough for a year. He said that he was anxious to get into business to support his aged father and a large family. The surgeon also wanted to help his brother, Rhea, find some occupation. Once these matters were resolved, Barton hoped to get married and settle down. To strengthen his request, he enclosed a letter from Captain Porter approving his plans, which was to be presented to the secretary when Latrobe made his appeal. Latrobe's efforts in behalf of his friend were not successful. Barton wrote to Hamilton on his own and said that he was engaged to be married and needed a furlough to make the necessary arrangements. He also explained the financial needs of his younger brother. Meanwhile Benjamin Smith Barton had requested that his nephew be assigned to the Philadelphia Navy Yard. The job of assistant to Dr. Cutbush normally would go to a surgeon's mate, but Barton was willing to take it for the chance to remain in Philadelphia. This appeal also failed. Porter received a letter from Hamilton that amounted to a denial of Barton's request. Barton tried again in January 1812, this time asking for four or five months' leave. Receiving no reply, he wrote two more letters, which also went unanswered. In March 1812, Barton found himself ill and in sick quarters in Newport, Rhode Island. Later that month, Captain John Rodgers gave Barton a furlough of five weeks to recuperate. Then, in April 1812, he was ordered to the Philadelphia Navy Yard as an assistant to Dr. Cutbush.[22]

Meanwhile in the summer of 1811, Barton sent Hamilton a sample bottle of the lime juice then widely used in the British navy as an antiscorbutic. He suggested that the secretary let the bottle stand a day or two and then use it as he would lemonade. His friends should try it as well. Then he would appreciate receiving from Hamilton his opinion of the juice. The surgeon said that he hoped to introduce this liquid into the U.S. Navy. Hamilton's reaction to the lime juice has not been preserved. But Barton did get a favorable letter from Decatur. A bottle of juice and a copy of Barton's letter to Hamilton were then sent to Captain Rodgers with the hope that he would also send an endorsement. Rodgers obliged.[23]

In addition to his attempts to introduce an effective antiscorbutic, Barton was concerned about establishing a system of navy hospitals. At the navy yard in Philadelphia, he found 30 patients huddled in a miserable house that was scarcely large enough to accommodate 4. "So wretched was the hovel," he later wrote, "and so destitute of every necessary comfort for sick persons, . . . that every man who gathered sufficient strength, and was successful in getting an opportunity to effect his escape, absconded immediately." Barton's efforts to improve hospitals are discussed in chapter 8. Matters relating to lime juice and navy hospitals had not been fully resolved when the War of 1812 began. That conflict interrupted Barton's personal plans and gave a new dimension to his life.[24]

Baltimore

Merchant seamen and the occasional naval sailor who became sick in Baltimore were referred to a hospital under the control of the city's board of health, but the cost of their medical care was borne by the U.S. Treasury under the terms of the law for the relief of sick and disabled seamen. Later a contract was made with Dr. Tobias Watkins, who had served in the Quasi-War and was now in private practice, to provide everything except clothing and funeral expenses at a rate of 65¢ a day for each seaman from January to July 22; and at 55¢ per man from July 23 to the end of December. During 1809, Watkins treated an average of 41 seamen per month, 1 out of every 20 of whom belonged to the navy; 18 of the 41 died. Expenses averaged $4.60 a week for each seaman, and Watkins spent $588.75 that year for clothing alone for his patients. The total outlay for 1809 was $10,018.92. Unfortunately we do not know the nature of the diseases treated or the causes of death.[25]

Norfolk

For the care of seamen, Norfolk boasted a public hospital that had been purchased and supported by the federal government. In 1801 navy Surgeon George Balfour was placed in charge of the patient care at the marine hospital. A short time later he was replaced by a civilian, Dr. Philip Barraud. Attached to the hospital were a surgeon, who was paid $840 a year, and his assistant, who got $600. The steward received $8 a month, the nurses $6.50, and the matron 50¢ a day. A purveyor supplied food for the sick at a cost of 25¢ a day per seaman. The average number of sick in 1809 was 18 and the average expense was $4.47 a week for a total of $4298.07.[26]

When the navy yard was built, a two-story wooden structure was erected in the middle of the yard. Originally it was used as a storeroom for the boatswains' and gunners' supplies. Later the center portion of the second floor served as a hospital, the garret being used as a rigging loft and the lower part of the building containing the gunners' store, storekeeper's office, purser's office, and issuing room. No doubt the other activities did not make for a quiet and pleasant environment for the sick, but this hospital continued to be used for some years. Yet when one compares Norfolk to other installations, there is very little in the official correspondence on health and hospital matters.[27]

One incident is associated with Surgeon Lewis Heermann's assignment to Norfolk following his two-year furlough in Europe. During his time abroad he visited hospitals. In January 1810 he wrote to Secretary Hamilton about the need for a naval hospital at Norfolk. He complained about the mixture of merchant seamen and navy men at the marine hospital and commented on how much naval commanders objected to sending their sick there. Also, the house in the navy yard that was used as a hospital was too confined and lacked many of the comforts of a well-regulated hospital. From what he had heard from Captain John Shaw, the commander of the station, and from a former purser, there was room for improvement in the issuing of rations to the sick. If more information was desired, the surgeon was willing to come to Washington to present it. The secretary did not need an oral presentation to appreciate the situation. He was hoping to get legislation through the Congress to resolve the problems of navy hospitals. The following summer, when Captain Shaw was ordered to New Orleans, he asked Heermann to accompany him, and the surgeon sought orders from the secretary. At first Hamilton was reluctant, for it meant moving a senior surgeon already in New Orleans, but Heermann was subsequently transferred as Shaw wished.[28]

That same summer, Lieutenant Arthur Sinclair reported that the crew of the *Nautilus* had become ill from an unknown cause. The doctors thought that lead in the water taken from a cistern was the source. To test the theory, they suspended the daily ration of grog, or whiskey mixed with water, and the men got better. When the sickness reappeared two weeks later, the doctors were at a loss to determine the cause. More than half of the crew were unfit for duty, including the surgeon. Helping out during the emergency was Surgeon J. J. Schoolfield from the Norfolk Navy Yard. Since metallic poisoning had been mentioned earlier as the source of the illness, Sinclair consulted with Commodore Decatur, on whose advice he moved all the paints ashore and aired the area on the berth deck where they were stored. A gunboat was ordered from Hampton Roads to Norfolk to receive the sick men. Within three weeks all the sick who had been sent to the gunboat recovered and rejoined the *Nautilus*.[29]

Another aspect of health matters can be seen in the case of Marine Lieutenant John Gassaway of the frigate *United States,* who became ill when his ship was at Norfolk in 1810. The surgeon sent him ashore and placed him in the custody of a tavern owner until he recovered. By the time he was well, his bill at the tavern was so high that he could not pay it, and the tavern owner sued him. Gassaway's irate father wrote to Secretary Hamilton that he thought the government should pay the bill. The outcome is not known, but apparently it was unsuccessful for Lieutenant Gassaway resigned his commission in late December 1810.[30]

Personal reasons loomed large in Surgeon R. B. Stark's mind when he sought an assignment to Norfolk. In a conversation with the secretary, he was allegedly told that if Surgeon Heermann went to New Orleans, Stark would be assigned to Norfolk. August 1810 found Stark attached to the frigate *Essex* when that ship visited Norfolk. He wrote to Hamilton recalling their conversation, and receiving no reply, he wrote again. This time Hamilton responded that he could not be ordered to the Norfolk station at that time. Stark was devastated and wrote to Hamilton that he had become engaged to a young woman and hoped to marry and settle in Norfolk. The secretary relented and assigned him to the station.[31] But in November of that year, Stark asked for a furlough to transact some urgent business in the interior of the state. An an additional reason, he said, was that he had "been subject for some time past to a cough & spitting of blood—more particularly at this season of the year." He was willing to forgo pay and emoluments until called into actual service, otherwise he would have to resign. He was granted leave, but the secretary did not respond to his suggestion that he keep his commission but draw no pay. So in June 1811, Stark assumed that his offer had been rejected. He was still willing to serve in the event of war, but since this seemed unlikely at present, it would be "injudicious" for him to give up his practice in Brunswick County. Therefore Stark asked Hamilton to prepare the necessary papers so that he could adjust his accounts before resigning. This was done.[32]

Charleston and St. Mary's

Following the passage of the Embargo Act, the United States found it necessary to police the waters around the country to enforce it. The navy and the Revenue Cutter Service had this unpleasant duty. There was already a naval presence in the form of navy yards at some ports, and warships routinely cruised off the coasts. Naval units were also sent to Charleston, South Carolina, and St. Mary's, Georgia, to watch the southern border and provide security against any British interference with coastal commerce. At Charleston the marine detachment was cared for by a local practitioner, a Dr. Aitken. His bill for services was sent to Lieutenant Colonel Franklin Wharton, the commandant of the marine corps, who considered it "extravagantly high" and therefore believed that it was improper to pay it. Secretary Smith asked Nathaniel Ingraham, the navy agent at Charleston, to ascertain the usual charges for services in the area and pay the doctor on that basis. Meanwhile some new arrangements would have to be made to see that the marines were cared for by a navy doctor.[33]

As for the sailors, Lieutenant Theodore Hunt was awaiting the arrival of a surgeon's mate for the gunboat crews. Pending his arrival, Hunt was authorized to hire a civilian doctor to examine the medicines and determine which were useable. Hunt later reported that there was a considerable amount of medicine on hand. From that supply the secretary ordered that the medical chest of the brig *Hornet* be replenished. What was left over was to be delivered to the local navy agent and sold on the best terms. The money thus raised was to be used to buy other medicines and surgical instruments that were needed.[34]

The repeal of the Embargo Act and its replacement with the Non-Intercourse Act of March 1, 1809 did not mean a diminished need for a naval presence on the southern border of the United States, and hence some better arrangements had to be made for health care. Surgeon Daniel McCormick, then attached to the *Essex* in Hampton Roads, suggested to the secretary that, in view of the high cost of hospital and medical care at Charleston, the navy might consider establishing a hospital nearby on Sullivan's Island. Speaking as one who had local knowledge, McCormick was convinced that the island location would be economical and beneficial to the health of the patients. If the navy did establish a hospital there, he hoped that he would be considered for the position of surgeon in charge. Hamilton brought McCormick to Washington, where they apparently discussed the surgeon's ideas, then McCormick was ordered to St. Mary's to attend to the crews of the gunboats and marines there. To assist him, the secretary ordered the newly commissioned Surgeon's Mate Charles B. Hamilton to St. Mary's, and the two traveled together in the *Enterprise* to their assignment.[35]

After he had studied the situation, McCormick reported that a hospital on Sullivan's Island would be preferable in the summer; meanwhile he recommended renting a small house in Charleston. No instruments of any description were available, and he asked for permission to buy what was needed. As for medicines, there was an old stock of them in the custody of the navy agent, but McCormick apparently did not know their provenance. He also suggested that a surgeon's mate be attached to the gunboats stationed at St. Mary's because, despite comprehensive directions to the naval commander there, it was impossible for him "to determine with propriety, the remedies requisite in any serious care that may occur." Apparently no action was taken on this suggestion. McCormick and Hamilton were expected to take care of all medical needs at St. Mary's both on ship and on shore.[36]

As for the medical problems at Charleston, Dr. George Logan of that city was commissioned as a surgeon and assigned to take care of the seamen and marines there. By December 1810, Logan found himself operating at a disadvantage. He needed a suitable place for his clinical cases sent from the ships. When he spoke to Captain Hugh G. Campbell, the commanding naval officer, he was told that in the past patients requiring extraordinary care were sent to a private hospital. Logan then asked the secretary if he could rent an apartment near his residence where the sick could be under his immediate care. Hamilton replied that Congress was now looking at the question of building naval hospitals, and until it decided on a course of action, Logan should send his patients to a private hospital.[37]

Four months later, Logan reported that while he generally had from three to seven patients, sometimes the number was greater, and one had died. This was a marine who had been transferred from the sloop *Wasp* and expired after a lingering illness. In several instances his patients had "acute Diseases" that made them eligible for a hospital, but Logan was reluctant to move them to the only local infirmary that was available, which was run by a gentlemen of skill and respectability but, Logan believed, was primarily for Negroes and was neither as safe nor as comfortable as he desired for the seamen. With the approach of the season when fevers endemic to the region were common, he asked for authority to rent a well-ventilated apartment. Hamilton gave his permission if it could be done economically. Apparently Logan was not able to find one that met that criteria, so he decided to fix up an apartment in his own quarters. He also attended to the marines who were stationed in the city. With talk of a possible war with Great Britain in the air, he urged that a hospital be built at the navy yard. War came before anything could be done about that suggestion.[38]

Meanwhile Surgeon McCormick and Surgeon's Mate Hamilton had gone on to the St. Mary's station. In July 1811, McCormick called the secretary's attention to a sickness among the marines on Cumberland Island. "Exposure in this climate is productive of diseases, not only attended with immediate danger, but of a nature so subtle, as frequently to baffle the skill of the Physician in restoring the system to its wonted tone." The men believed that their illness was due to the drinking water, but this was excellent. Instead the sickness was due to "the putrefactive decomposition of vegetable matter suddenly exposed to the burning rays of the Sun, by the removal of sheltering trees and a large portion of under-wood." The result was the outbreak of a violent grade of "Bilious Fever" (probably malaria) characterized by intermittent attacks, some of which were of a slight nature. Two men had died, but McCormick expected to restore the rest to duty in two weeks. The sick were now kept in tents, which afforded them "miserable shelter" against inclement weather. He recommended building a small house for the reception of the sick. The only expenditure would be for timber. Also, the healthy marines were living in tents, which provided inadequate shelter, especially with the approach of the fall and the season of heavy rains. McCormick believed that it was necessary to build a barracks, but Captain John Williams, the commander of the marines, thought that it was an unnecessary expenditure. The crews of the gunboats were generally healthy, but the crowded environment made it very difficult for patients with malignant diseases. That such cases could not be transferred to a hospital ashore might prove fatal to a patient and highly dangerous to a crew.[39]

Within a month 46 marines, or a majority of the detachment, as well as both Dr. McCormick and Dr. Hamilton, were taken sick. There was no one to care for them. McCormick died on August 11, after an illness of 15 days. Captain Williams urged the secretary to send medical aid.[40] Before he heard the news of McCormick's death, the secretary had ordered Gwin Harris, the purser at St. Mary's, to consult with McCormick and Captain Williams about building a hospital on Cumberland Island. This presented Harris with a dilemma. McCormick was dead and Hamilton was too sick for duty; who could advise him about building a hospital? It happened that

Dr. Lemuel Kollock, an eminent physician of Savannah, was visiting the area, and not only did he give advice on the proposed building, but he also began attending the sick marines on a regular basis.[41]

Three weeks later, Purser Harris faced new complications. Captain Williams had received orders from the commandant of the marines to build a barracks on Cumberland Island. Harris did not deem it consistent with the wishes of the secretary to build both a barracks and a hospital and therefore deferred ordering additional timber until he heard from the secretary. This message caused the secretary pain, and he immediately informed Harris that the tents would suffice for the marines in that climate and that the priority was to build a hospital. Harris had been informed earlier that this was primarily a matter of buying the required timber, for the marines were expected to build the hospital. Harris and the marines proceeded to get a hospital built.[42]

In November 1811 a local physician, Dr. William Armstead Dandridge, a former surgeon's mate in the army, was appointed surgeon of the hospital on Cumberland Island. Meanwhile Surgeon's Mate Hamilton had recovered and asked for a transfer to less hazardous duty. His request was denied, and it was not until the spring of 1812 that he was able to get a furlough, and that only to visit his dying mother.[43]

So it was that from Maine to the Florida frontier the arrangements for the care of the sick of the navy and merchant service were for the most part makeshift and inadequate. The dislocation of commerce caused by the Embargo and Non-Intercourse acts increased unemployment among merchant seamen, caused a drop in the sums collected for the Marine Hospital Fund, and placed a strain on existing hospital arrangements. With more merchant seamen resorting to the marine hospitals for the treatment of illnesses, any dependence on those facilities became less and less desirable from the naval point of view. The lack of military discipline disturbed navy leaders because it frequently led to desertion as soon as a man was well enough to leave. Better arrangements under the control of naval and marine corps officers were needed, but to date only small and temporary hospital quarters had been established in navy yards. This was only one of the demands on the naval establishment. At the end of the Barbary Wars, resources were devoted to a gunboat building program, the completion of navy yards, and other priorities. It was only when hospital matters became urgent that efforts were made to address the problem.

Chapter 8

Washington, D.C.

During the closing months of Secretary of the Navy Benjamin Stoddert's administration, he took advantage of a loophole in the law to acquire lands for navy yards. The matter was contested by the incoming Jefferson administration, and a compromise was struck whereby the navy could keep such lands as it had but could not acquire more. In the case of Washington, D.C., the area chosen for the future navy yard had been earmarked for a marine hospital. Both Stoddert and his successor, Robert Smith, believed that the capital city should have a navy yard and that, of the lots available, those designated for the hospital were the most appropriate. So the work of preparing the yard and also of constructing a 74-gun ship was given to Captain Thomas Tingey on January 22, 1800. The act of Congress of March 3, 1801, providing for the naval peace establishment gave the navy yards the legal basis they needed. Tingey continued his work of building the base.[1]

In January 1802, Surgeon John Bullus was ordered to the Washington Navy Yard to work with Captain Tingey, the commandant of the yard, in preparing rooms for the reception of sick seamen. Bullus was ordered to acquire through requisitions on Tingey bedding and anything else he needed. The following June the secretary wrote to Bullus that he had been informed that the surgical instruments in the yard were rusty and unfit for use. Bullus was instructed to look into the matter and take whatever steps were necessary to bring the instruments to perfect condition.

Presumably this was done and Bullus was prepared when the sick began to return from the Barbary Wars. When the *Constellation* arrived from the Mediterranean, many of the crew were suffering from "Ship Fever," or typhus. The secretary ordered Tingey to see that the sick were moved from the *Constellation* and placed in the frigate *General Greene,* which had been out of active service, or "in ordinary," for some time. The *General Greene* was then to be moved out into the Potomac River at a distance from other vessels and anchored under Bullus's direction. Tingey was told that "every possible care must be taken to prevent a communication between the different ships, until the sick were restored." The captain was also to furnish Bullus with whatever attendants, bedding, or other necessities for the *General Greene.*[2] So it was that the *Greene* became a temporary hospital ship.

When navy ships went out of active service and were placed in ordinary at the yard, it was the custom to assign the care and maintenance of each ship to a small number of warrant and petty officers, seamen, and marines. While the goal was preservation, the activities of these groups was not without danger. For example, fires were maintained in each ship for warmth and cooking, and they posed a danger to every other ship in the yard. Much time was spent in cleaning up the dirt in these vessels. In addition, it was hard to assemble all the men from all the ships at a central point in the yard when they were needed. Existing arrangements allowed an excess of idleness, which led to drunkenness and fighting. In January 1804, Lieutenant John Cassin, who was then in charge of the yard, recommended changes to the secretary which were incorporated into an amendment to the Peace Establishment Act passed by Congress on March 27, 1804.

Under this act officers and men would be attached to the yard for general service and assigned as necessary. The master of the yard would assign men to visit the ships in ordinary once a day to inspect them and to keep them clean, as well as to report any problems. The men did their cooking and slept in the ship in ordinary to which they were assigned or in a house built for the purpose. It was believed that this arrangement alone would bring about a great saving in fuel and diminish the danger of fire. Savings would also result from eliminating the need for 9 sailing masters, 28 petty officers, 30 seamen, and 8 guards of marines. Among those retained were 1 surgeon and 1 surgeon's mate, who were to receive the same pay, rations, and emoluments as army medical officers of the same ranks.[3]

The reduction in the work force proved to be temporary, for by the end of 1804, cutbacks in the number of ships on active duty resulted in an increase of those in ordinary from seven to nine. The care of these vessels and other responsibilities necessitated the addition of 108 men to the yard force in 1805. New rules governing the administration of the yard were drawn up by Captain Tingey, who was again the commandant, and approved by the secretary of the navy. These rules were applied to all navy yards. For medical men and most other people with specialized skills, the chain of command was short: from the secretary through the commandant, then through the clerk of the yard, who dealt directly with the surgeon. Grievances, suggestions, and appeals of decisions followed the reverse order.

Along with the growth of the work force came an increase in the number of marines, who were needed to guard the materials being assembled to construct ships and erect buildings. Tingey recommended that a company of marines be assigned to this duty. A site for the marine barracks was chosen in 1801 by Lieutenant Colonel William W. Burrows in consultation with President Jefferson and Secretary Smith. As commandant of the marines, Burrows was given $20,000 to start the construction of a new barracks. But the economic constraints imposed in 1802 limited the marine guard to 1 sergeant, 1 corporal and 15 privates. The lack of funds in 1802 and 1803 meant that all work on docks, wharves, and buildings was suspended. Things began to change in 1803 when Jefferson designated Washington, D.C., as the home port of the navy and the place for all vessels in ordinary. The Barbary Wars also brought an increase in activity in the yard. In 1803 the marine force grew to 13 officers, 26 noncommissioned officers, 16 musicians, and 146 privates. By 1804 occupancy of the barracks could begin. Those still waiting to move in lived in rented quarters nearby and helped with the construction work. The increase in the number of marines meant that there were guards for the ships and the yard as well as music for ceremonial occasions.

Both the commandant of the yard and the commandant of the marines had their own views of their prerogatives. The marine insisted on maintaining control over his men, which meant that the duties of marines at the yard had to be worked out in a cooperative atmosphere and often with the direct involvement of the secretary of the navy. Because of this touchy situation, there were two separate hospital arrangements at this and every other navy yard, as we have already seen in the cases of Boston, New York, Philadelphia, and Norfolk. One hospital was for the navy officers and men attached to the yard; the other was for the marines. Hence the surgeon and his mate had to divide their time between the two. They also had to be available to any workman who was injured or taken sick in the yard, and in 1805 the civilian work force was increased by 105 men.

Because Washington was the place where ships going out of active service were maintained until needed again, Surgeon Bullus had to be concerned about the medical supplies of the whole navy, including those ships involved in the war with the Barbary pirates. Faced with the problem of furnishing medical chests to ships at irregular intervals, and based in a city that was still being built, Surgeon Bullus had made his own arrangements to get what he needed. He had established a small apothecary shop at the corner of Pennsylvania Avenue and Ninth Street for the convenience of the public and hired James S. Stevenson to run it for him. Bullus acquired medicines and instruments and kept them at the store, thus having a convenient source of supply when the navy needed medicines.

Later, Bullus urged the secretary to establish a system of furnishing medical supplies modeled after those then in use in Europe. Such a system was headed by an appointed medical purveyor. When supplies were purchased, the purveyor would inspect them to assure that first-quality goods were being sold at fair prices. Thus the doctors could not blame the medicines for their own lack of success with some patients. It would be the duty of the purveyor to maintain stores of medicines and instruments and make regular reports to the Navy Department on what had been received and issued. When a ship was placed in ordinary or dismantled, its surgeon would give the purveyor a report on what had been received and used and what remained. The purveyor would acquire instruments from sources abroad or in the United States. Bullus's suggestions had merit, but nothing was done about them. Bullus believed that until such a system was in place, his apothecary shop was necessary to supply the navy and the public with good medicines on short notice. So, when he left for New York, he sold his apothecary store to Stevenson and urged the Navy Department to continue to buy its medical supplies there, for quality items could be had at reasonable prices. Stevenson also asked the secretary to continue to purchase its medical supplies from him, and for a time this arrangement seems to have continued.

In June 1807, Bullus went to the Mediterranean to inspect the supply situation. It had been expected that he would become the navy agent for the squadron, but the end of the war with Tripoli meant that there was no need for one, and he returned home in December 1807. While Bullus was gone, it looked as though he would have to be replaced as surgeon at the Washington Navy Yard, and Secretary Smith told Surgeon Thomas Ewell at New York that if Bullus resigned, Ewell would get the appointment. So Ewell was brought to Washington in the summer of 1807. When Bullus returned in December, it was clear that new arrangements would have to be made. Thus on February 8, 1808, Bullus was appointed as the navy agent at New York, effectively ending his career as a medical officer. Ewell remained in Washington.

Ewell began to familiarize himself with his new surroundings and looked into the practice of procuring medicines. He was to receive by inventory a list of the government's medicines and instruments in the custody of Bullus. For his services in taking charge of them and issuing them to warships, Ewell was allowed an additional $400 a year. Investigating the supplies of medicines at the yard, he found them all in a heap and spent some time sorting, arranging, and placing them in proper containers. Many had been stored in white glass bottles that were easily broken. Ewell recommended that in the future they be ordered in black glass bottles, which he described as "ten times as durable and three times as cheap." Those that were damaged or contaminated by contact with poisons were thrown out.[4] Also in a deplorable state were the medical instruments. There were parts missing from many of those that were in cases; others were separated into different parts; still others were in a store in the navy yard; and some were mixed with trash in a stairwell. Ewell brought them all together and tried to assemble sets so that they could be examined by a cutler. Shortly afterward, Ewell learned that the keeper of public stores at the navy yard had on hand a considerable quantity of hospital stores. In view of this, it seemed prudent to use what was on hand before purchasing anything new.

With necessary supplies in hand, Ewell devoted his attention to the hospital. He described it to the secretary as "wretched" and strove to improve it. The immediate needs were for new mattresses and four dozen plain cotton sheets. Old mattresses had new covers sewn on them and surgical instruments were repaired. The secretary said that it was his desire "to erect a national hospital as will afford the sick and disabled seamen and marines all essential comforts."[5] Ewell was asked to send a report of his professional observations and opinions on the defects in the present hospital establishment and the advantages of creating a new one. Within two months, Ewell was able to report that there were not sufficient restraints in place to prevent the grossest abuse of every article in the hospital. A properly regulated hospital, he continued, would be more comfortable for the sick and would cost half as much as the present system.

The secretary had other things on his mind when he received this recommendation, but Ewell was impatient for change. Within a month he found a house in a healthy location near the yard which had a reasonable rent. At that time the navy was renting a house in an unhealthy location for use as a seamen's hospital. The marines kept their sick at a hospital in the barracks, which was crowded and presented a problem even for healthy men. With a new house, the two hospitals could be combined to provide better care and save on rent. Ewell consulted with Colonel Wharton of the marines and Captain Tingey of the navy. To the secretary he pointed out that the marines and the navy bought their hospital supplies separately and that in many instances, those used by the marines were of an inferior quality. He asked permission to buy from anyone who could furnish quality items on the cheapest terms. He estimated that he could save the navy $500 a year if his patient load did not increase.

While the matter of a more competitive arrangement for purchasing drugs was being considered, Ewell drew up a copy of regulations for the new hospital and sent them to the secretary. He informed Smith that Captain Tingey, Colonel Wharton, and his own surgeon's mate, John Harrison, had approved them. Dated November 1, 1807, the regulations gave the surgeon authority over his patients until they recovered. While they were in the hospital, the surgeon could make such arrangements among them as he considered expedient, as long as they were not unlawful. It was the duty of the surgeon to superintend the hospital, prevent or correct all abuses, provide written orders for the patients whenever necessary, visit the hospital twice daily or more frequently if necessary, keep accurate accounts of all transactions, medical practice, and the expenses, and from time to time report to the commanding officers of the navy and marines on the men under his care. In addition, the surgeon's mate was to attend at the hospital whenever required to do so by the surgeon, visit the sick men at the barracks and navy yard, and report on those who needed to be transferred to the hospital. The hospital appeared to be off to a good start, and relations with Great Britain at that time suggested that it might soon be heavily used.

Four months later, Ewell asked the secretary for permission to appoint a steward for the hospital. He explained that in the earlier hospital for seamen, a female nurse had been employed at a wage of $15 a month. Later Tingey replaced her with a seaman from one of the ships in ordinary at the yard who was allowed to draw an extra ration for this service, thus costing the government $24 a month. Now that the marine corps and naval hospitals were combined, there was a greater demand on the chief nurse and hence a person of better character was required. For $25 or $30 a month, Ewell said, he could hire a young man to perform all the duties of the nurse and help with the preparation of the medicines. Since this would be a convenience, Ewell asked for permission to hire a male nurse instead of using a sailor. Smith agreed that a nurse was indispensable, and he authorized hiring one at $25 a month if a suitable person could not be found at a lower wage.

It is not known whether this was done, but prior to receiving the secretary's reply, Ewell again wrote that with the approach of "a sickly season" and the number of men stationed at different places in the yard, he needed another surgeon's mate to help him. He asked for Robert French, who had received his commission two months earlier. If this assignment was made, it was of little help to Ewell, for French resigned in April 1809. Another matter of concern to Ewell was his allowance for house rent. Pointing out that his suggestions about the hospital had saved the navy money, he reminded the secretary that he himself was paid less than the mechanics who worked in the yard. He needed to have his income increased "because it is customary for regular physicians to live in the best of circumstances, and because the chances of successful investigations will be increased by an increase of comfortable provision."[6] There was little that the secretary could do to help him. The surgeon's need for money forced him to seek additional funds through other means—with unfortunate results, as we shall see. Meanwhile developments in Anglo-American relations had brought a new sense of urgency to the problems with hospitals and to medical care in general.

War clouds had gathered as a result of an attack on the U.S. frigate *Chesapeake* by the British warship *Leopard* in U.S. waters on June 22, 1807. Prior to sailing, the *Chesapeake* had enlisted four deserters from the British service, and the *Leopard* followed the U.S. ship after it left Hampton Roads. About 10 miles off the coast, the British commander insisted on searching the U.S. frigate for deserters. When this demand was refused, he opened fire, killing three men and wounding six men and two officers in the *Chesapeake*. Totally unprepared to fight, the *Chesapeake* fired one gun for the honor of the flag before capitulating. Four members of the crew, who had formerly been in the British navy, were removed. Surgeon Joseph G. T. Hunt and his mate cared for the wounded.

The *Chesapeake* returned to Hampton Roads, where news of the attack created a sensation. For a number of years, British warships had stopped U.S. merchant ships on the high seas and impressed members of crews into its naval service, but this was the first time a public vessel had been forced to give up men. The American public was outraged, and the State Department demanded an apology and reparations. On July 2, President Jefferson issued a proclamation that closed U.S. ports to all armed British ships.

Worried that the *Chesapeake* crisis might lead to war, and conscious of the shortage of experienced medical personnel and hospital facilities, Surgeon Cutbush did what he could to share his knowledge and insights. In 1808 he published a small book entitled *Observations on the Means of Preserving the Health of Soldiers and Sailors*. In this, the first book published by a U.S. Navy medical officer, Cutbush discussed methods of preventing as well as treating sickness. His rules of prevention were: (1) keep the sick dry and properly ventilated; (2) keep the bodies and clothing of the crew clean; (3) avoid cold, fatigue, and intoxication; (4) in winter keep the crew warm by means of fires; (5) preserve an exact and regular discipline; and (6) furnish the crew with wholesome provisions and water. When a contagious disease appeared in the ship, Cutbush recommended six actions: (1) separate the sick from the well and prevent unnecessary communication between the two; (2) keep the ship clean, dry, and properly ventilated; (3) avoid exposing the men to cold, fatigue, and intoxication; (4) dispel moisture between decks by fires in the stoves; (5) avoid depressing the spirits of the men by unnecessary severity in discipline; and (6) frequently whitewash the berth deck with lime.

On the matter of washing decks, especially those where the men slept, Cutbush quoted with approval the words of the British naval surgeon Thomas Trotter against "too frequent and indiscreet drenching of decks," particularly in a cold climate. Trotter claimed that such practices had killed thousands in the British navy.[7] Related to his concern about keeping living spaces dry and warm, Cutbush recommended that Americans place their kitchens and ovens between decks, as the Dutch and the French did, instead of in the forecastle, thus rendering the area between decks more salubrious and comfortable. Another useful practice would be to have the sides of the beams of the berth deck whitewashed and slaked with lime once a month.

In an attempt to give medical men who were new to the navy a sense of proper procedure, Cutbush described a sick call on a ship and offered advice on the duties of the naval surgeon.

> He should have a small dressing box containing all his common dressings, which should be carried to the gun-deck, when he prescribes, at a regular hour every morning; for example, after the gun deck has been cleaned, which in all regulated ships is finished by eight o'clock. He should send the loblolly boy fore and aft [on] the gun and berth decks with a small bell, to give notice to those who are slightly indisposed, to venereal patients and those with ulcers to attend him at the mainmast, where he should have his table and prescription book.[8]

When it came to hospitals, Cutbush focused particular attention on discipline and the authority of the hospital surgeon.

> In order to preserve peace in the hospital, his command over the men should be absolute, as though they were under their respective officers. To quell riotous behaviour, some severity is at times absolutely necessary, however repugnant it may be to the feelings of the surgeon. Punishment in a solitary cell, or by fixing a clog to the leg, will in most cases answer the purpose, except the offender be destitute of every feeling,

which a soldier or sailor ought to possess. To avoid improper conduct, convalescents should not be detained longer in hospitals than is absolutely necessary.[9]

Cutbush's effort appears to have been well received in the Navy Department, but by the time it was published, the threat of war over the *Chesapeake* incident had abated and diplomatic means were now being employed to resolve the issue. In the navy a sense of hostility and a desire for revenge burned strong but there was little anyone could do.

Meanwhile concern about a possible war induced Congress to pass a law in January 1809 authorizing an increased naval force. The president was given the authority to put into active service as many of the ships as he thought necessary. To man these, he was authorized to add up to 300 midshipmen and to enlist up to 3,600 seamen and boys for two years. Authority was also given to increase the number of marines by 1 major, 2 captains, 2 first lieutenants, 185 corporals, and 594 privates. The men were to be enlisted for five years.[10]

While these preparations were prudent, in neither law was there any provision for increasing the number of medical men. Secretary Hamilton went ahead and did so, but then the navy found itself with some doctors on its rolls to whom no duty could be assigned until the president put more ships into active service. No one knew how long this might be. Hamilton wanted to be ready for emergencies, but by leaving newly commissioned officers in an inactive status, he created problems for his successors. On the other hand, the removal of the immediate danger of war gave the secretary additional time to investigate what could be done about hospitals.

In February 1810, Secretary Hamilton wrote to Burwell Bassett, the chairman of the naval committee of the House of Representatives, and discussed the need for naval hospitals within a larger framework. He began by pointing out that there were basic inequities in the pensions of marines and sailors in comparison to those of men in the army. As for hospitals, to date the men of the navy had paid into the Marine Hospital Fund the sum of $55,649.29, but few had received any benefits. Great inconvenience and embarrassment resulted when seamen and marines were placed in marine hospitals because there was little in the way of discipline, with the result that three out of every five convalescents deserted. Hamilton urged the establishment of hospitals exclusively for the men of the navy.

To pay for these hospitals and increase the funds currently available, Hamilton proposed that the balances of money due to deserters be paid into the fund, as well the money owed to men who died without heirs. The cost of grog forfeited by men for minor infractions of discipline and all

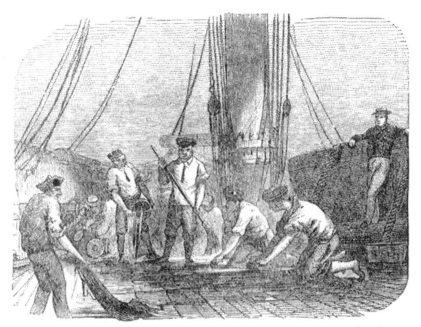

Sailors Scrubbing a Deck, circa 1840. Smithsonian Institution, Washington, D.C.

losses of pay as the result of courts-martials could also be transferred. Additional money could be raised by deducting 20¢ a month from the pay of officers. He also believed that the monthly deduction from the pay of officers, seamen, and marines could be raised to 50¢. Still other sums might be realized by raising the cost of the slop clothing sold to the men. The value of the rations normally drawn by the men would be applied to the fund when they were in the hospital. Also, individuals who were disabled would be asked to choose between receiving a pension and going into a naval hospital for life.

When it came to staffing hospitals, the secretary also had low-cost solutions. Disabled officers could be used as the governors; widows of seamen killed on active duty could be employed as nurses; the children of deceased seamen would be taught reading, writing, and arithmetic; and midshipmen could be taught navigation there.

Congressman Bassett introduced the requested legislation, and when Cutbush read about this in the Philadelphia newspapers, he immediately wrote to the secretary. Cutbush pointed out that he had served 12 years in the navy and had been in charge of the naval hospital in the Mediterranean. Hence he thought himself qualified to be placed in charge of one of the new hospitals. Hamilton replied that if the pending bill passed, Cutbush would be considered.

While the bill was in committee, Hamilton and Thomas Turner, the navy accountant, responded to requests for information. After Hamilton had forwarded information on navy hospitals, he received a letter from Captain Isaac Chauncey in New York noting that the sick at that station had to be sent to private homes. Hamilton sent an abstract of the letter to the committee. The secretary of the Treasury estimated that the sum available for transfer from the Marine Hospital Fund to the navy was approximately $75,000 but that $20,000 of this had been pledged to Charleston whenever a marine hospital was built there.

Democratic congressman John W. Eppes of Virginia looked at the estimates for the navy for 1810 and 1811. He wanted to know why they were higher in the latter year. Hamilton replied that with the decision to employ the brig *Oneida,* and with a greater number of gunboats, an additional 241 men were placed on the rolls. Also, the cost of a barrel of flour had increased by $4, and the estimates for medicines for 1810 had proved too low and an additional $12,000 had to be transferred because of unexpected costs in New Orleans.

The House of Representatives passed the naval hospital bill in February 1811 and sent it to the Senate. Hamilton was called upon to supply information to that body on the amount of hospital money received and spent on the navy. While the Senate was deliberating, Chaplain Andrew Hunter wrote to the secretary requesting that the duties of navy chaplains be extended to include visiting the sick at stated times. Hamilton's response is not known, but the question of the chaplain's role in regard to hospital patients would emerge again in subsequent years.

The act establishing navy hospitals became law on February 26, 1811. It named as commissioners of navy hospitals the secretaries of the Treasury, War, and Navy departments, and $50,000, the unexpended balance in the Marine Hospital Fund was placed at their disposal. All fines imposed on navy officers, seamen, and marines were to be paid into the Naval Hospital Fund. The commissioners were to select suitable sites for hospitals, erect the buildings at the least cost and according to a design that allowed for future additions if needed. At one of these hospitals the commissioners were "to provide a permanent asylum for disabled and decrepit navy officers, seamen and marines." The secretary of the navy was to prepare the regulations for the government of the hospitals and send them to Congress at the next session. Finally, the law provided that whenever a naval officer, seaman, or marine was admitted to a navy hospital, he was to be allowed one ration per day while there, the cost to be deducted from

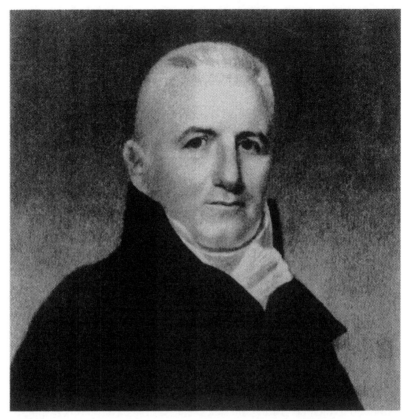

Surgeon Edward Cutbush. Naval Historical Center, Washington, D.C.

the account of each man. If the patient was a pensioner, then the cost of the ration was deducted from his pension. So it was that some of Hamilton's ideas were incorporated into the final law.[11]

The secretary took advantage of this legislation to accelerate improvements in health care. Since the situation of the sick at the navy yard in New York had earlier been brought to the attention of the secretary and the Congress, Hamilton wrote to Surgeon Marshall on March 7, 1811, and ordered him to meet with Captain Chauncey and John Bullus, the navy agent, and choose a site for a new navy hospital. Then Bullus was to designate some neutral and unofficial person in whom he had confidence to go to the owner of the property and inquire about the cost of buying 6–10 acres of land. This information was to be sent to the secretary. Once the site of the new hospital had been chosen, Marshall was to consider himself its surgeon and prepare a system of internal regulations. The secretary also requested suggestions on how the new navy hospitals should be organized and administered from Surgeon George Davis, who responded promptly with a lengthy report. It was apparent that Davis had some very clear ideas about what should be done. He was not alone in his views.

Once the news of the Senate's passage of the naval hospital act reached Philadelphia, Cutbush wrote to Charles Goldsborough, the chief clerk of the Navy Department, and asked for details. He expressed the hope that his service and experience would be considered when it came to establishing the hospitals. A day later he wrote to Hamilton, reviewed the highlights of his career, and asked to be considered for duty in a new hospital. Hamilton responded by asking Cutbush to prepare a system of regulations for the hospitals during the coming summer and advising him that he and surgeons Marshall and Davis would be ordered to Washington during the coming summer to consult together and formulate a system of rules. Cutbush replied that he would be happy to draw up the regulations requested. As for the design and arrangements of the hospitals, he suggested that the secretary consult a French work by Jacques René Tenon, *Mémoires sur les Hôpitaux de Paris,* published in Paris in 1788, which contained plans of both large and small hospitals as well as information on the internal arrangements.

For reasons that are not clear, Cutbush, Davis, and Marshall were not called to Washington that summer. Most likely it was because not all the suggestions for regulations had been received. It was not until late in October that Surgeon William P. C. Barton sent in his suggestions, which, he said were based on observations of English marine hospitals that he considered to be "perfect institutions of their kind."[12]

Hamilton also asked George Bates, who had worked in the Boston Marine Hospital before taking leave to study medical practices in Europe, to send his observations on the management of British and Portuguese hospitals. Bates did so and promised to send the secretary any additional information he might wish.

When the various ideas and suggestions were in hand, Hamilton needed medical men on whom he could rely to sift through them and draw up the most practical regulations for navy hospitals. For this task he brought Surgeons Davis, Cutbush, and Marshall to Washington, where they met with Ewell. Hamilton submitted their report to Congress, as required. A copy was sent to Surgeon Barton, who expressed his approval. Before much progress could be made in implementing the suggestions, however, the nation was at war.

Chapter 9

The War of 1812 at Sea

On June 4, 1812, the House of Representatives declared war on Great Britain by a vote of 79 to 49. The Senate passed the declaration of war on June 17 by a vote of 19 to 13, and the following day President Madison approved it. The declaration was the result of years of frustration over the failure to resolve outstanding issues. Involved in a long war with Emperor Napoleon I of France, the British sought to subdue him through economic pressure, and U.S. commerce was a victim of the British blockade as well as of Napoleon's efforts to retaliate with his own economic measures. But the blockade was not the only source of problems with Great Britain. Americans were outraged by the practice of impressment, or the taking of sailors from merchant ships to man the Royal Navy. When this practice was applied to the frigate *Chesapeake,* a warship, the resulting furor had nearly led to war. Diplomats did not settle the *Chesapeake* affair until 1812. In the meantime the navy experienced the sensation of settling an old score when Commodore John Rodgers in the frigate *President* exchanged cannon shots with the British corvette *Little Belt* in the darkness off the U.S. coast on May 16, 1811. Thirteen of the British crew were killed and 19 wounded in the exchange. In the *President* the only casualty was a wounded boy. The defeat and humiliation were a source of pleasure to many Americans, especially to those in the middle and southern states.

While violations of neutral rights were a major cause of U.S. discontent, reports of British activities among the Indians were also a concern to settlers in the West. Some expansionist-minded individuals may also have seen a war with Britain as an opportunity to move against Canada or

Spanish-held Florida. British troops were then involved in efforts to liberate Spain from French rule.

As for the question of neutral rights, Congress and the president tried to use the Embargo and Non-Intercourse acts to force Britain to amend its policies. When these failed, Congress passed Macon's Bill no. 10, which prohibited all British and French armed vessels, except official packet ships, from entering U.S. ports. Gradually members of Congress came to see that the choices open to the nation were war or economic ruin; in the circumstances war seemed to be the lesser evil. It seemed highly probable that U.S. forces could seize a portion of Canada and use it to force the British into serious negotiations to resolve the outstanding issues. The irony was that war was declared just as Britain repealed its oppressive Orders in Council, which had done so much to damage U.S. commerce and the sense of national pride.

The delay between the vote of the House and that of the Senate gave navy officers a little time to make preparations. An hour after the receipt of the declaration of war and his orders, Commodore John Rodgers sailed from New York in the *President*, accompanied by the frigates *United States* and *Congress* and the sloops of war *Hornet* and *Argus*.[1]

At 6:00 A.M. on June 23, a vessel was seen to the northeast and Rodgers's squadron began a pursuit. The *President*, 44 guns, opened the encounter with its chase guns, and the first shot was reportedly fired by Rodgers himself. It struck the rudder of HMS *Belvidera*, 36 guns, and lodged in the wardroom. Several effective shots followed, but at the fourth discharge the gun burst, killing 1 midshipman and wounding 14 men, including Rodgers. The explosion threw the commodore into the air, and when he fell, he broke his leg. The accident delayed other firing and allowed the *Belvidera* to open a counterattack with its stern guns. One British shot killed a midshipman and 2 men in the *President*. Then, by lightening the ship, the *Belvidera* was able to escape to Halifax, Nova Scotia. The exchange cost the *Belvidera* 2 killed and 22 wounded. Total casualties in the *President* were 3 killed and 19 wounded. The *President* was the only ship in the squadron that took part in the action, and its surgeon and mates cared for the wounded.

Rogers's squadron continued to cruise until within a day's sail of the mouth of the English Channel, when they stood to the south, passed Madiera, and reached Boston on August 31. Rodgers wrote to the secretary that he had returned home quickly because scurvy, "that wretched disease," had appeared among the crews of the squadron to an alarming degree.[2] Rogers also had 80–100 prisoners who had been taken from British merchant ships captured in the course of the cruise and who were sent to Commodore Bainbridge at the navy yard. Those prisoners requiring medical treatment were sent to the marine hospital. The sick of the navy were treated at the navy hospital in the yard.

When Rodgers arrived in Boston, he heard the news of the victory of the *Constitution*, 44 guns, under Captain Isaac Hull over HMS *Guerriere*, 38 guns, on August 19, during which the latter lost 15 killed and 62 wounded, plus two dozen who were missing, presumably carried overboard when the masts were shot away. Casualties in the *Constitution* were 7 killed and 7 wounded, who were treated by Surgeon Amos A. Evans and Surgeon's Mate John D. Armstrong. Once the fight was over, Armstrong went on board the British ship to help Surgeon Irvine with his wounded. An effort was made to tow the *Guerriere* to port, but with five feet of water in the hold and heavy seas, this became impossible. Also, the British crew got into the ship's liquor supply and, emboldened by the alcohol, refused to man the pumps. Hull had no choice but to destroy the ship, but before this could be done, the men and their possessions had to be transferred. One of those assigned to this task was Midshipman Henry Gilliam. Contemplating the deck of the *Guerriere*, he saw "pieces of skulls, brains, legs and blood in every direction and the groans of the wounded were enough to almost make me curse the war." But remembering that he was serving a republic that was fighting for its liberty against the subjects of a king, he concluded that the losses were the decrees of fate and his mind was put to rest.[3]

During the transfer of prisoners and their possessions, Captain Hull moved among his crew. He saw Surgeon Evans of the *Constitution* and Surgeon Irvine place a young seaman named Richard Dunn in a position to have his leg amputated at the knee. Dunn did not cry out but muttered to the surgeons: "You are a hard set of butchers." Hull tried to console the boy by promising that he would look after him. Two days after the operation, Dunn complained of a stinging pain in the stump and some spasms in the abdomen. To relieve the pain in the stump, Evans wetted it with laudanum and gave the patient laudanum mixed with wine. The abdominal cramps were sometimes accompanied by an inability to urinate. The surgeon applied warm fomentations to the abdomen and gave Dunn a dose of laudanum, after which he was able to pass urine. On August 24, Evans removed the dressings from the stump and examined it. It appeared to be healthy, but there was a considerable discharge from it. Dunn suffered pain every time the wound was dressed. While having a bad dream the following night, Dunn somersaulted from his cot and landed on the deck. Some adhesions were opened but he sustained no other injuries. He continued to be treated for pain in the stump and a lack of sleep.[4]

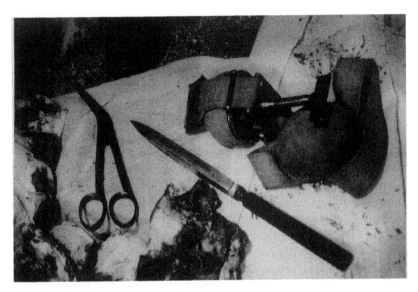

Surgeon's Instruments from the USS *Constitution*. **USS** *Constitution* **Museum, Boston.**

Another of Evans's serious cases was Lieutenant Charles Morris. He received a musket ball in the abdomen about an inch above the umbilicus which came out of the ileum. Poultices were applied to the wound, and the patient was bled and given sulfate. His bowels were cleared by an enema, and he was given cool and diluted drinks. Morris was in pain and his abdomen was swollen, but he was able to retain food. In succeeding days he had a little fever and some appetite. The application of poultices was continued. Five days after he was wounded, he had little fever or pain. The wound discharged a little pus. Morris's bowels were kept open by enemas. His appetite was good, and he was given arrowroot, chicken broth, and a light diet. For two days after this, he was costive and was given a small amount of "oil of racine" (Ricini, or castor oil), which produced a copious discharge. The operation of this medicine was checked and his stomach settled by giving him laudanum and oil of mentholatum mint. On August 27 his wound began to discharge small particles of cloth from the previous dressings. By this time he was considered well and on the way to recovery.[5]

Seaman Daniel Lewis had been dangerously wounded by a blow to the cranium which produced concussion. In addition, he had been struck in the arm by a musket ball. The scalp wound appeared to be small and there was no indication of any external depression or fracture. Lewis was bleeding from one ear. Surgeon Evans bled him and gave him an ounce of

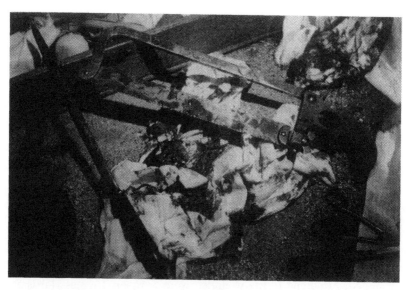

Detail of Surgeon's Instruments from the USS *Constitution*. USS *Constitution* Museum, Boston.

sulfate magnesium. Lewis complained of great pain in the head and nausea. His arm wound was treated with a simple cerate and poultice. For the next two days, Lewis appeared much better and the poultices were continued. On August 23 he still had pain in his head and sickness in his stomach, but his stomach did not reject food. The scalp wound had healed, and the arm wound was better and had no discharge.[6]

Surgeon Evans's other cases were less serious and the healing process was continuing. On August 30 the *Constitution* reached Boston and the wounded were transferred to hospitals ashore. The British were sent to the marine hospital and the men of the *Constitution* to the hospital in the navy yard.[7]

The news of the *Constitution*'s victory prompted a great outburst of celebration in Boston and elsewhere in the nation. Hull's triumph helped to offset the bad news of the surrender of the army garrison at Detroit and the unhinging of the defense of the western borders. But within two weeks of Hull's arrival came the reminder of another defeat at sea. In July 1812, the *Nautilus,* 14 guns, under Lieutenant William M. Crane, was overtaken by a British squadron and taken to Halifax. The *Nautilus* was the first regular naval vessel of war to be taken by either side in the war. During the chase that preceded capture, Crane hurt his leg by accident. He received no treatment for it while he was a captive.

He and his men, along with some other captured American sailors, were returned in a cartel ship that reached Boston on September 11. On the return trip the cartel ship was to carry the men of the *Guerriere* to Halifax. But Crane told Commodore Rodgers that six men of the *Nautilus* had been detained at Halifax on the grounds that they were British subjects, and Vice Admiral Herbert Sawyer, the commander there, had sent them to England for trial. When Rodgers heard this, he stopped the cartel ship and removed 12 of the *Guerriere's* crew. He sent word to Halifax that he would treat them as justly as were the 6 removed from the *Nautilus*. [8] Fortunately, this unhappy note in regard to prisoners did not continue for the rest of the war.

While en route to a rendezvous with the *Constitution,* the *Wasp,* 18 guns, under Master Commandant Jacob Jones, overtook a convoy under the protection of HMS *Frolic,* 18 guns, and after a spirited encounter on October 17, the *Frolic* surrendered. Fewer than 20 of the crew of 110 in the British ship escaped unharmed; in the *Wasp* 5 men were killed and 5 wounded. Attending to the wounded were Surgeon Thomas Harris and Surgeon's Mate Walter N. New. Before the battle, Lieutenant Alexander Claxton had been confined to bed by illness, but in anticipation of the action, he came on deck. Although too weak to be with his division, he nevertheless served a purpose, as his calm bearing during the fight apparently inspired all hands. While the Americans were repairing their battle damage, HMS *Poictiers,* 74 guns, arrived on the scene and the *Wasp* was forced to surrender. About a month later, Jones and his men were paroled and made their way to New York. How the wounded were treated during the interval between capture and parole is unknown. As in the case of most of the actions at sea during the war, few details survive about the individual casualties of battles.[9]

New laurels were being won at sea by Captain Stephen Decatur in the frigate *United States,* 44 guns. After a brief action on October 25 west of the Canary Islands, HMS *Macedonian,* 49 guns, was forced to surrender. Out of a crew of 300, it lost 36 killed and 68 wounded; 3 of the dead were men who died of their wounds. Captain John S. Carden of the *Macedonian* estimated that of the remaining wounded, 32 had slight wounds and would probably recover; another 36 had severe wounds from which the captain believed they could not recover. In the *United States* 7 were killed or died of wounds, including 1 officer; and 5 were wounded. Surgeon Samuel Trevett Jr. and his mate, Samuel Vernon, of the *United States* and their British colleagues treated the wounded. Decatur put a prize crew on the *Macedonian* and sent it to New England. When it reached Newport, Rhode Island, the wounded put a strain on facilities. Lieutenant Oliver

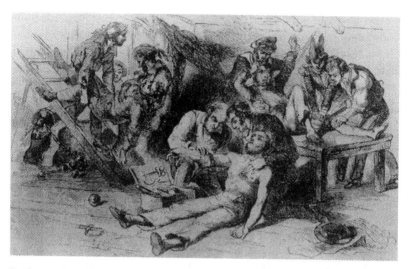

Cockpit of the British Frigate *Macedonian*. Library of Congress, Washington, D.C.

Hazard Perry had rented a few rooms for use as a temporary hospital, but this was not enough, and the overflow had to be sent to the gunboats. All the sick and wounded were under the care of Dr. Edward T. Waring of Newport.[10]

Victory and glory such as Decatur's were not the lot of Lieutenant George Washington Reed of the brig *Vixen*, 12 guns. While cruising in the West Indies, the *Vixen* was chased by HMS *Southampton*, 32 guns, and captured on November 22, 1812. Both vessels were subsequently wrecked in the Bahamas, but the officers and crews survived. The Americans were taken to Jamaica, and here Reed died of a fever, presumably yellow fever. The rest of the officers and crew survived and were later exchanged.[11]

New victories at sea raised the spirits of many of the people on the home front. While off the coast of South America, near Bahia, the *Constitution*, now commanded by Captain William Bainbridge, overtook HMS *Java*, 38 guns, on December 29, 1812. The *Constitution* dismasted its opponent and left it unmanageable. In the British ship 57 were killed and 83 wounded including Captain Henry Lambert. By comparison, the Americans suffered 9 killed and 26 wounded. One of those hurt was Bainbridge, who had been struck in the thigh by a musket ball and suffered several contusions from wooden splinters. The medical staff in the *Constitution* consisted of Surgeon Amos A. Evans and his two mates, John D. Armstrong and Donaldson Yeates.

The *Java* was too badly damaged to take into port, so it was set on fire and blown up. But the destruction meant that accommodations in the *Constitution* were severely strained because in addition to its crew, the *Java* was carrying nearly 100 supernumeraries, military and naval officers who were en route to India. A few days later, Bainbridge unloaded his prisoners at San Salvador. In his official report on the loss of the *Java*, Lieutenant W. H. D. Chads praised the treatment they had received at the hands of Captain Bainbridge. Later, Surgeon T. C. Jones of the *Java* complained that the British wounded were treated with callous indifference and that he was unable to attend to them while in the *Constitution*. These charges were not known to Surgeon Evans until sometime later, and he published a rebuttal in a Washington, D.C., newspaper in March 1814.[12]

As for the treatment of the U.S. wounded, Surgeon Evan's prescription book provides some details. Bainbridge's splinter wounds responded quickly to applications of soft dressings, but the injury from the musket ball presented some problems. At first it looked like a splinter wound. The ball had entered the quadriceps muscle a few inches above the knee. Evans was unsure of the direction it had then taken but presumed that it went downward. In succeeding days the wound continued to drain. On January 8 the doctor decided to enlarge the wound and in doing so found a piece of copper with irregular edges from the ship's railing which had been imbedded in the flesh. Once this was removed and the edges of the wound brought together, Bainbridge quickly recovered.

Others were not so fortunate. Lieutenant John C. Aylwin had been struck in the shoulder by grapeshot, which injured the clavicle and scapula bones. His breast and back were discolored by internal bleeding that had been absorbed. The wound was treated with warm poultices. It ceased bleeding on January 29 but then again began to bleed freely. Aylwin developed a fever and died that day.

Seaman Peter Furanse's case was also difficult. He had been severely injured by a piece of grapeshot that struck him below the middle of the leg and lodged in the Achilles tendon. The ball was removed, the leg splinted, and warm poultices applied to the wound. Furanse was purged and placed on an "antiflogistic regimen." Nevertheless he became an extremely complicated postoperative case for Evans. On January 30, Furanse discharged a large amount of pus from his wound, and eight days later he died.

Another fatality was that of Seaman Joseph P. Chevers, whose arm was amputated. His condition steadily deteriorated and he died on January 27.

Some of the more successful cases involved amputation of the arm or leg. One of the more worrisome was that of Seaman John Clements, whose leg was shot off above the ankle. The leg was badly lacerated, and Evans took it off below the knee. For days after the operation, Clements complained of considerable pain. He had a little fever and was treated with a cathartic and given an anodine. On the fourth day he had a secondary hemorrhage and lost a great deal of blood before it was discovered. Evans removed the dressings and bathed the stump but could not find the source of the bleeding. He again dressed the wound, and he checked it twice in succeeding days and found no further signs of bleeding. The discharge from the stump was rather irritating. Clements was still in pain and his pulse was "quick, jerking and irregular." He was given opiates and occasionally treated with wine and a nourishing diet. Throughout his treatment of Clements, the surgeon complained of a lack of warm water in the ship. When the *Constitution* reached Boston on February 17, 1813, the wounded were transferred to the hospital in the navy yard.[13]

The year 1813 saw more encounters at sea. In February the *Hornet,* 18 guns, and HMS *Peacock,* 18 guns, clashed for 15 minutes off British Guiana before the British ship yielded to superior force. The British lost 4 killed and 29 wounded, 3 of whom subsequently died. The *Hornet's* loss was 1 killed and 2 wounded. Also, 3 of the *Hornet's* crew and 9 of the *Peacock's* drowned when the latter ship sank after the battle. Medical help for the wounded was provided by Surgeon's Mate Samuel M. Kissam and his British counterpart. The *Hornet's* commander, Captain James Lawrence, now found himself with a total of 275 men in a ship with only 134 gallons of water. Provisions were also running low. There was no friendly port nearby where the captives could be released, so Lawrence headed for the United States. He reached Holmes Hole, on Martha's Vineyard, Massachusetts, on March 19. The wounded were transferred to the hospital at Boston.[14]

By the spring of 1813, the British had gradually imposed a blockade of U.S. ports, but it had not been extended to New England. Nevertheless, activity in and out of the port of Boston was being closely watched by HMS *Shannon,* 38 guns, and HMS *Tenedos.* Captain Philip Broke of the *Shannon* was waiting for the frigate *Chesapeake,* 38 guns, to emerge. He sent Lawrence a challenge to fight ship to ship in a fair contest and sent the *Tenedos* away. Lawrence never received the Englishman's challenge, for Bainbridge sent it to Washington as an item of interest. The *Chesapeake's* captain was also eager to fight despite the inexperience of his crew. So, on June 1, the *Chesapeake* sailed and headed for the British ship. The *Shannon* opened fire when its adversary was 50 yards away, and within a few moments Lawrence was wounded and his sailing master killed. When it became clear that the ship could not maneuver properly and that there was no evidence of organized resistance, the British boarded the *Chesapeake*

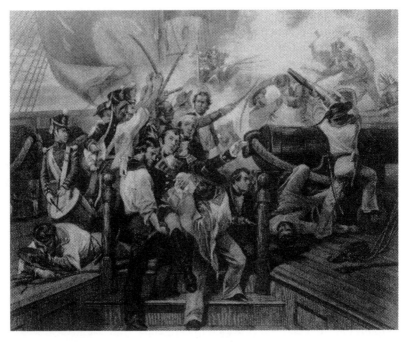

Death of Captain Lawrence in the *Chesapeake*. Library of Congress, Washington, D.C.

and hauled down its flag. Within the space of 15 minutes, the British lost 24 killed and 58 wounded. The *Chesapeake*'s losses were 61 killed and 85 wounded. The captured ship and its men were taken to Halifax.

En route to that port the surgeons of both ships worked to treat the wounded. Lawrence died before the ship reached port, and 12 other Americans also died of their wounds. At Halifax the wounded were transferred to hospitals ashore and the healthy went to a prison camp. Although the loss of the *Chesapeake* was a disaster, Lawrence's words to his men as he was carried below became a source of inspiration in the navy: "Don't give up the ship. Fight her till she sinks."[15]

One of those who was not inspired by the *Chesapeake*'s fight was Commodore William Bainbridge at the Boston Navy Yard, who apparently gave vent to his feelings when he encountered a veteran of the controversial battle. Henry Hyde was wounded in the fight, captured, and taken to Halifax with the other prisoners. Later exchanged as a prisoner, he arrived in Boston and was hospitalized at the navy yard for about three weeks. He then went to see Bainbridge about a pension and pointed out that his wounds had deprived him of the use of his legs. According to Hyde, Bainbridge responded that the men of the *Chesapeake* were a damned set of cowards and kicked him out of his office. Afterward, Hyde was attached to the flotilla based at the yard, but he maintained that he was unfit for any service. Appealing to the secretary, he asked for his discharge and a pension of $6 a month, or half of his pay. He does not appear to have been successful, for his name has not been found in the pension files.[16]

Another fight against unequal opponents took place in British waters and involved the brig *Argus,* 18 guns. The command of this ship had been given to Lieutenant William Henry Allen, one of those who had shared in Decatur's triumph over the *Macedonian.* As the *Argus* was made ready for sea in New York, various officers reported on board, among them Surgeon James Inderwick, who began keeping a record of his cases in the ship starting in May 1813. He had received an A.B. degree from Columbia College in 1808 and was a student in that institution's medical school during 1808–9, taking courses in anatomy and chemistry. Apparently he received a master's degree somewhere else and then pursued additional medical studies, perhaps in association with a physician. He was the house surgeon at the New York Hospital for a year beginning in February 1812. On June 18 the *Argus* sailed. Although he joined it in May 1813, Inderwick was not commissioned as a surgeon until July 24, 1813, when the ship was at sea.[17]

Allen's orders embraced two objects: the first was to carry William H. Crawford, the newly appointed minister plenipotentiary to France, and his entourage to that country. This was accomplished at the port of L'Orient between July 12 and July 20. The second mission was to attack enemy commerce in the English Channel. This Allen proceeded to do. Between July 24 and August 14, 19 prizes were taken. On the latter date the brig HMS *Pelican,* 18 guns, caught up with the *Argus* off the coast of Wales, and an intense fight followed.

Four minutes after the battle began, Allen was struck in the knee by a cannon shot. He tried to continue to give firing orders for a few minutes, but he was soon exhausted by a loss of blood. He was carried below and placed in the care of Surgeon Inderwick. Within a few minutes the second in command, Lieutenant William H. Watson was carried below after being struck in the head by grapeshot. After 45 minutes of exchanging shots, the *Argus* was helpless and the British were preparing to board it. With his head bandaged, Lieutenant Watson returned to the deck and surrendered the ship. The victory cost the British 2 killed and 5 wounded. U.S. losses were 6 killed and 12 wounded, of whom 5 later died. One of the dead was Allen. Surgeon Inderwick amputated his leg at the thigh about two hours after the battle, but the patient's condition did not improve, and four days after the battle, Allen died in the hospital at Mill Prison, near Plymouth, England. Other members of the crew were in the same prison, including Surgeon Inderwick. On August 16, he noted in his journal: "Our wounded are in a distressed condition. The riotous behaviour of the captors is such that they have no rest whatever and are frequently trodden upon and bruised by them." It was not a very happy way to begin a period of captivity. Inderwick and most of his shipmates remained prisoners until 1814.[18]

Accounts of captures and defeats at the hands of the British made for discouraging reading, but good news came in early September. The *Enterprise,* 14 guns, engaged HMS *Boxer,* 12 guns, off Portland and captured it after a short fight. The commanding officers of both ships were killed. British losses were put at 21 wounded and 20–25 killed, the exact number unknown because some of the dead were thrown overboard. American casualties were 1 killed and 13 wounded, 3 of whom subsequently died. In the *Enterprise,* the only medical man in attendance was Surgeon Bailey Washington. The wounded were taken to Portland, in the Maine district, where they came under the care of Surgeon Samuel Ayer. News of the victory helped to restore the confidence of the Americans, which had been shaken since the loss of the *Chesapeake.*[19]

Meanwhile in October 1812, a squadron under Commodore William Bainbridge had sailed from the United States. It consisted of the frigate *Constitution* and the sloop of war *Hornet,* 18 guns, which were to rendezvous with the frigate *Essex,* 32 guns, sometime after it left Delaware Bay. Captain David Porter in the *Essex* failed to overtake the other ships, so he decided to cruise on his own, hence the *Essex* became the first U.S. warship to round the Cape of Good Hope and sail into the Pacific Ocean. After taking on supplies at Valpariso, Chile, Porter headed for the Galapagos Islands, a favorite rendezvous for British whalers. Here he captured 12 of them. One was converted into a warship mounting 20 light guns and was named *Essex Junior.* In October 1813 the two warships and the three prizes went to the island of Nukahiva in the Marquesas group, where the crew overhauled, refitted and reprovisioned them.[20]

Porter had now been at sea for over a year, and the majority of his crew remained healthy. When the *Essex* put to sea there were 22 men on the sick list, 7 of whom had venereal diseases; 5 others were suffering or recovering from debility; 2 were convalescing from influenza. The sick list also contained single cases of such ailments as contusion of the elbow, sore ankles, swelling of the knee, an ulcerated leg, and "Saint Anthony's fire." The last term usually referred to a gangrenous form of ergotism, a disease contracted by eating the ergot fungus on rye or other cereal grains. The "fire" referred to painful skin infections, gangrene, and neurological distur-bances. A month later, when the ship reached Port Praya in the Cape Verde Islands, only 3 men were reported sick. Of these, 2 were regarded as incapable of duty, 1 because of a liver disease and the other because of paralysis on one side accompanied by an inability to speak or to help himself. Shortly after the ship left Port Praya, the latter died.[21]

For most the time at sea, Porter's crew enjoyed good health. Much of this good record has been attributed to his concern about cleanliness. Lime and sand were used at regular intervals to clean the decks without water. Each day the ship was freshened below decks by using a wind sail to divert fresh air down the hatchway and by sprinkling the area with vinegar. Every morning all parts of the ship were fumigated by pouring vinegar on red-hot shot. The surgeon, Robert Miller, objected to the use of vinegar on the grounds that it was corrosive. Porter refused to discontinue using it until had proof of its harmful effects. It at least changed the smell of things for awhile. But in late January or early February 1813, Porter discontinued fumigating with vinegar and began issuing it as a part of the ration in the hope of warding off scurvy. Otherwise his cleanliness rituals were carried out in his own ship and those captured from the British.

During the day the sick were brought up to the gun deck, where their messmates slung their hammocks in a place that was cool and out of the way. At sundown they were moved below deck again. Healthy men were allowed to sleep on the gun deck in good weather instead of in the dark and confined area of the berth deck.

Porter's men were issued a half-gallon of water a day for drinking and washing and were told to bathe daily while in Port Praya. Presumably this was what a later generation would call a sponge bath. Later, while in the Pacific, Porter had to cut the water ration to two quarts per day, and this restriction in hot weather was a hardship. Yet there were only two men on the sick list, one with chronic debility and the other with painful neck muscles, and both could report to their stations if needed.[22]

From his journal it is apparent that Porter understood the value of limes and oranges for the health of his crew, and he called the prickly pear "a sovereign antiscorbutic." He tried to limit the amount of salted provisions the men had to eat, acquiring, wherever possible, pigs, chickens, and other live animals for fresh meat. In the Galapagos Islands he stored many live turtles in the hold for later consumption. His attention to such matters no doubt contributed to the fact that he had only one case of scurvy in his crew, and that emerged after his men had been living on an island for weeks. After pondering why a seaman of about 40 years of age and a slender build would come down with this disease amid an abundance of vegetables and fruit, Porter could only conclude that it was because of "a lethargic [and] melancholy disposition," which prevented him from taking part in the amusements of the crew. Believing that the man could not recover, Porter left him on the island of Nukahiva. Porter could also note with pride the health record of his prisoners. He eventually had 333 on his hands, and when many of them came into his custody, they were suffering from scurvy. But when he left the Marquesas, only a few still had slight cases of that disease.[23]

In the course of its cruise, the *Essex* had 10 deaths that were not related to combat, including those of two officers. One was a lieutenant who died in a duel; the other was the surgeon, Robert Miller, who suffered from consumption. Six were seamen or petty officers, and two were marines. One of the marines died as a result of "excessive fatigue" and the other from a "pulmonary complaint." Of the six seamen or petty officers, the death of one who was partly paralyzed has already been noted. Two others died as the result of falls from aloft, and the fourth, a gunner's mate, died from an accidental gunshot wound. There was one seaman for whom no cause of death was listed by Porter, and the sixth was a quarter gunner who died of violent convulsions and while foaming at the mouth. After the death of Dr. Miller, the medical duties in the ship were performed by acting Surgeon Richard Hoffman and acting Surgeon's Mate Alexander Montgomery.[24]

A new and exciting adventure for both the officers and men began when the ships anchored off Nukahiva. The interval proved to be an unforgettable experience. When they arrived on October 25, 1813, they found a lush island with white, sandy beaches, handsome, well-formed natives, and attractive and friendly women and girls. They also found a U.S. naval officer, a sailor, and an English beachcomber. On his own authority, Porter annexed Nukahiva Island to the United States and became involved in intertribal wars. One American received a spear wound in the neck during an attack on a village during which five natives were killed. But for the most part the rest and recreation were appreciated by all the Americans, especially the sailors. When Porter left the island, he said that he had no sick in his ship.[25]

Believing that he had done as much damage as possible to British commerce in the Pacific, Porter intended to leave the area, but he had hopes of further enhancing his record by defeating a British warship. Upon learning that a British squadron under Commodore James Hillyer, RN, was seeking him, Porter sailed for Valpariso, where he was sure the British would visit. He was correct. On the morning of February 8, 1814,

HMS *Phoebe*, 36 guns, and HMS *Cherub*, 18 guns, came in and anchored. After refitting, the British ships cruised off the coast while waiting for Porter to emerge from a neutral port. Porter hoped he would be able to fight the *Phoebe* alone, but Hillyer would not oblige him. Having no desire to fight in an unequal contest, Porter tried to escape. A heavy squall tore off his main-topmast and drowned four or five sailors. He then anchored in what he alleged were technically neutral waters, but the British attacked him there on March 28, 1814.

With the *Cherub* off her bow and the *Phoebe* off her stern, the *Essex* took terrible punishment. Porter wrote later about the state of his ship after two hours of fighting, "I was informed that the cockpit, the steerage, the wardroom and the berth deck could contain no more wounded; that the wounded were killed while the surgeons were dressing them, and that unless something was speedily done to prevent it, the ship would soon sink from the number of shot holes in her bottom." All the carpenter's crew had been killed or wounded and only that warrant officer remained. Flames could be seen coming from each hatchway. Faced with a hopeless situation, Porter hauled down his flag in surrender. Out of a crew of 255, the Americans lost 58 killed or dead from wounds and 66 wounded. Another 31 were reported missing and presumably drowned when they tried to swim ashore. Porter praised his medical officers, as well as his chaplain, David P. Adams. Their attention and indefatigable efforts saved many of the wounded. British losses were 5 killed and 10 wounded. Most of the damage had been done to the *Phoebe*.

The survivors of the *Essex* who were not injured spent the early days of their captivity caring for the wounded, assisted by the women of Valparaiso through the cooperation of Captain Hillyer. A short time after the loss of the *Essex*, the *Andrew Hammond*, one of the prizes that Porter had taken, converted to a cruiser, and placed under the command of Marine Lieutenant John Gamble, was captured by the *Cherub*. The *Essex Junior* was disarmed, neutralized, and used to carry the surviving Americans to the United States as prisoners of war. Two of the men from the *Essex* had wounds that were not healed enough for them to travel, so they were left behind. The rest reached New York on July 5, 1814.[26]

Meanwhile the United States had suffered other losses. The *Constellation* was blockaded near Norfolk by a British force, and several attempts were made to send boats of armed men in to capture or destroy it. These were repulsed, but in one of the actions in February 1813, Captain John Southcomb was wounded in five places and captured along with two of his wounded men. The friends of the captain were concerned about him and received permission to send a cartel ship to the British commander to request his return. The mission was entrusted to Surgeon's Mate Hyde Ray. When he reached the British squadron he learned that Southcomb had died of wounds the previous evening. The British released the two other wounded men, and they were sent back to Norfolk in the cartel ship. Ray waited until the British built a coffin for Southcomb and returned to his command with the body.[27]

On June 1, 1813, the Norfolk flotilla under Commander Joseph Tarbell chased two British barges back to their ships in Hampton Roads. Fifteen boats in two divisions attacked HMS *Junon*, 38 guns, which responded with a few guns. But HMS *Barrosa*, 18 guns, was nearby and attacked the U.S. boats with effective fire and inflicted damage. One American was killed and two wounded before the contest was broken off.[28] Later in that same month, the British planned to attack Craney Island at the entrance to the Elizabeth River. With the island and its 700 defenders and a battery in their hands, the British were within easy reach of the *Constellation* anchored in the river. But the entrance to it was also protected by a line of gunboats. The British attack on Craney Island on June 22, 1813, was beaten off by the force of army, militia, sailors, and marines. British losses were 40 killed, wounded, and missing.[29] There was another action in the Norfolk area in July 1813 where Midshipman James Sigourney was killed and 10 others killed or wounded while defending the tender *Asp*, one of the many small vessels that were armed and fitted out to defend various bays, inlets, and rivers. The British boarding party in boats lost 4 killed and 7 wounded. The *Asp* was captured and set afire but later saved.[30]

In the North, July 1813 brought the news that gunboat no. 121, operating as a part of the Delaware flotilla, was captured by eight armed boats from the British frigate *Junon*, 38 guns, and the sloop *Martin*, 18 guns. Before being overwhelmed, the Americans killed 7 and wounded 12 while suffering 7 wounded themselves.[31] The British blockade kept a squadron under Captain Stephen Decatur from getting to sea. The frigates *United States* and *Macedonian* and the sloop of war *Hornet* first tried to get out by way of Sandy Hook, New Jersey, and failed. Decatur planned to make his next attempt by way of Long Island Sound. If he got to sea, he anticipated that his ships would have to operate far from home for some time, and with this in mind, he decided to take two female nurses with him in the *United States*. The women were the wives of two of his seamen, and they were carried on the books as supernumeraries beginning May 10, 1813. Decatur's immediate need for nurses may have been in connection with a group of British prisoners whom the *United States* was taking to New London.

One would assume that the surgeon was consulted about this arrange-

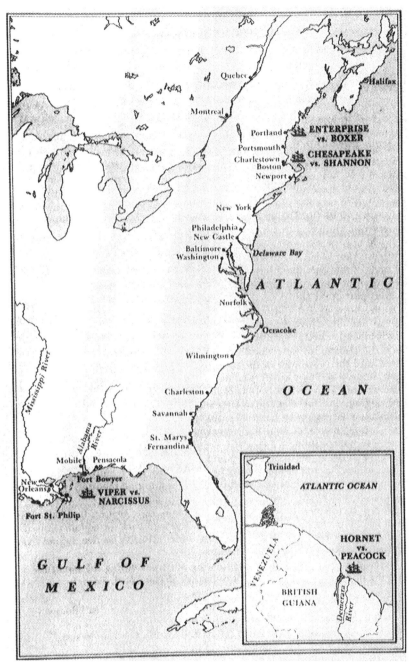

Map of the Atlantic and Gulf Theaters during the War of 1812, by
William Clipson. In William S. Dudley et al., eds., *The Naval War of
1812: A Documentary History*, 2:6.

ment, for Decatur had good relations with his medical officers, but there is no mention of the surgeon's views. In any case, the women were in Decatur's ship when his squadron sailed from New York on May 24, 1813. The squadron passed through Hell Gate, and during the next five days, Decatur learned all he could about the disposition of the blockading squadron. When he discovered that there were two British ships southwest of Montauk Point, on Long Island, he decided to put to sea while an escape route was open. When the British ships saw Decatur's squadron off Block Island, they tried to cut off any escape route to Connecticut, but the Americans managed to elude their pursuers and reached Fisher's Island, off New London, on May 26. A close blockade of that port was now imposed. While waiting for a chance to slip through, Decatur kept his ships in a state of readiness. It was while the *United States* was in New London that John Allen, the husband of one of the nurses, fell overboard and drowned on October 28, 1813. The widow, Mary Allen, asked for and received Decatur's permission to return to New York. It is not known what happened to the second nurse, Mary Marshall. She may have left the ship when Mary Allen did, or she may have stayed on board until her husband was transferred to the *President* in May 1814. Though Decatur's experiment in taking female nurses to sea with him ended after only a brief period, the innovation stands as a useful reminder of his thinking. The experiment was apparently carried out without the knowledge of the secretary of the navy.

On November 14, 1814, one of U.S. ships, the *Hornet*, 18 guns, slipped through the blockade, captured a merchant ship en route to New York, and then operated successfully in the South Atlantic. Its last victory took place three months after the war officially ended. For the rest of Decatur's squadron, however, all hopes for a breakout from New London ended in the spring of 1814. Decatur was transferred to the frigate *President* at New York, and most of his men went with him. The men of the *Macedonian* were transferred to the *Great Lakes*.[32]

In the South, 1814 began with an attack on a U.S. ship. The *Alligator* (formerly gunboat no. 166) was fired upon on by six enemy boats while at anchor at Cole's Island, south of Charleston, on January 29, 1814. The commander cut his cables, escaped, and inflicted damage on the enemy. U.S. casualties were two killed and two wounded. Subsequently, while in Port Royal Sound in July of that year, the ship capsized in a squall and 23 men were drowned; 12 others were rescued. Weather was a major cause of losses on the St. Mary's station. In the course of the war five other gunboats were lost in storms. By comparison, the New Orleans flotilla lost the support ship *Etna* in a storm in 1814, and 30 men were drowned.[33]

As the year progressed, there were more reverses at sea. On June 22, 1814, the brig *Rattlesnake,* 16 guns, was captured by the more powerful HMS *Leander,* 50 guns. July brought news that the brig *Syren,* 14 guns, had been seized by HMS *Medway,* 74 guns, after a long chase off the west coast of South Africa.[34]

Meanwhile the government had decided to build sloops of war to cope with the smaller ships of the British. These were put into service as soon as they were ready. One was the *Peacock,* which under Captain Lewis Warrington was making a reputation at sea. Off Cape Canaveral, Florida, on April 29, 1814, Warrington found a three-ship convoy under the protection of HMS *Epervier,* 18 guns. He attacked, and after a 45 minute battle, the British ship surrendered, its casualties 8 killed and 15 wounded. In the *Peacock* there were no deaths and only 2 wounded. Caring for the wounded was the responsibility of Surgeon William A. Clarke and his mate, John Cadle, assisted by their British colleagues. Warrington and his prize sailed for Savannah and reached that port on May 2. Here his wounded were transferred to accommodations ashore and his prisoners were taken into custody.[35]

The sister ship of the *Peacock* was the *Wasp,* 22 guns, under Captain Johnston Blakeley, who captured the sloop of war HMS *Reindeer,* 18 guns, after a fight of nearly half an hour in June 1814. The *Wasp* had 5 killed and 21 wounded, 6 of whom subsequently died. In the British ship the loss was 23 killed and 42 wounded. The *Reindeer* was destroyed the next day. Burdened by his prisoners and the wounded, Blakely headed for the nearest friendly port. At L'Orient, France, he was welcomed, his ship repaired, and his captives and casualties transferred ashore. Refitting the ship took seven weeks, and it is possible that in that interval some of his wounded recovered and rejoined the ship. On August 27, Blakeley set sail again in search of new prizes. Within three days he had taken and destroyed three merchant ships. In September the *Wasp* fought and sank HMS *Avon,* 18 guns, which suffered 33 killed and 34 wounded out of a total of 118 men. The *Wasp* lost 5 killed and 21 wounded. A short while later, Blakeley captured the *Atalanta* and sent it to Savannah with a prize crew. Sometime early in 1815 the *Wasp* was lost; supposedly it foundered in a gale.[36]

On the European front the forces allied against Napoleon had made significant gains in the war. The French suffered huge losses in the unsuccessful effort to subdue Russia, and in 1813, British forces liberated Spain. As a result of these gains, Britain now had troops and ships that could be released for service against the United States. In 1814 there was a series of attacks on points on the U.S. coast, two of the most serious of which were directed at Washington, D.C., and Baltimore.

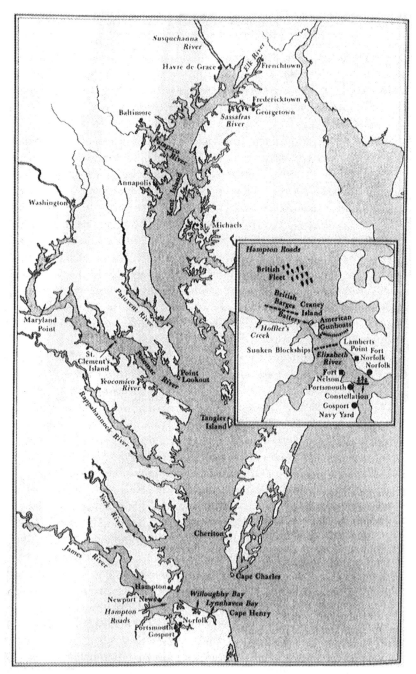

Map of the Chesapeake Bay Theater during the War of 1812, by William Clipson. In William S. Dudley, et al., eds., *The Naval War of 1812: A Documentary History*, 2:312.

A flotilla of gunboats under Commodore Joshua Barney, based at the mouth of the Patuxent River, 60 miles below Baltimore, was to guard the Chesapeake Bay and the approaches to these cities. An attack by British barges on June 8 was driven off by Barney's men. Reinforced by 30 men from the *Guerriere,* Barney's flotilla attacked another enemy force at the mouth of St. Leonard's Creek on June 26 and forced it to withdraw. The Americans lost an acting midshipman and 3 men; another 7 were wounded. Barney then left the mouth of St. Leonard's Creek and took his flotilla up the Patuxent.[37]

One of those serving on a barge with Barney's flotilla who was injured and disabled in some unknown fashion about this time was a seaman named David Townsend. There being no medical help in the flotilla, he was sent home to his brother in Baltimore. He arrived there early in July and died a few days later on July 10. Dr. L. B. Martin, a civilian physician who attended Townsend, said that his death was doubtless due to a lack of early medical and surgical care.[38] The nature of gunboat duty while away from a port was such that it was usually difficult to supply direct medical assistance.

In August 1814, when the British landed troops at Benedick, Maryland, and marched toward Upper Marlboro and an accompanying naval forces moved up the Patuxent, Barney was trapped. He left a few men behind to blow up the boats when the British approached and with the rest headed for Washington. They subsequently gave a good account of themselves in the Battle of Bladensburg on August 24. Barney was wounded and captured, and two of his officers were also wounded and two were killed. Barney and the other wounded were treated by British army surgeons and later by those of both the army and the navy of their own country. After the defeat of the U.S. forces at Bladensburg, the British captured Washington and burned a few public buildings before returning to their ships. The British squadron then ascended the Potomac River and captured Alexandria before returning to Chesapeake Bay.

Next on the agenda was Baltimore, but the attempt failed as a result of a clash between British troops and the Maryland militia at North Point and the subsequent unwillingness of the British commander to attack Americans in entrenchments. A naval effort to reduce Ft. McHenry on the Patapsco River also failed. The British withdrew and moved down the coast in search of other targets. Naval officers serving ashore participated in the defense of Baltimore but apparently did not sustain any casualties.[39]

It was at New Orleans late in 1814 that the next major British attack took place. Contesting their approach to the city were five U.S. gunboats on Lake Borgne under the command of Lieutenant Thomas Ap. Catesby Jones.

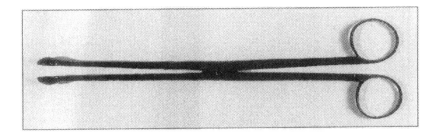

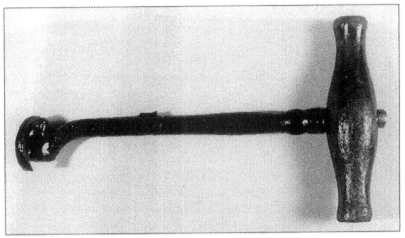

Medical Instruments from Commodore Barney's Gunboats: *top*, Cross-Legged Forceps (8-in. length); *bottom*, Dental Tooth Key (6-in. length). Calvert Marine Museum, Solomons, Md.

They met in battle on December 14, 1814, and the Americans were overwhelmed by superior force. Jones and the British commander were severely wounded. The British lost 17 killed and 77 wounded, among them their commander, Captain Nicholas Lockyer. U.S. losses were 6 dead, 35 wounded, including Jones, and 86 captured. The U.S. wounded were treated by their captors. Continuing their advance, the British reached Villere's plantation on the Mississippi eight miles below New Orleans.

Here they camped on the night of December 23. That evening the schooner *Carolina*, 14 guns, under Lieutenant J. D. Henley anchored out of musket range and fired on the camp. The British suffered heavy losses and took shelter behind a levee. After about half an hour, the British heard new fire from an inland direction above them. It came from troops under General Andrew Jackson, the commander of the defense of New Orleans.

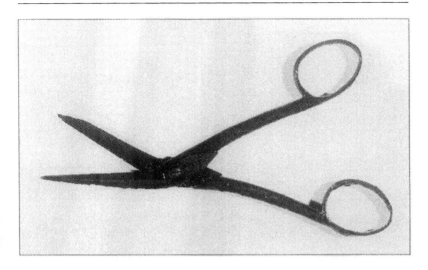

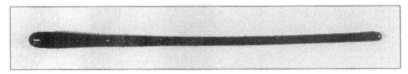

Medical Instruments from Commodore Barney's Gunboats: *top*, Surgical Scissors (5½-in. length); *bottom*, Director and Scoop (5⅜-in. length). Calvert Marine Museum, Solomons, Md.

The *Carolina* ceased firing so as not to hit Jackson's men. After a night battle lasting about an hour the Americans withdrew, taking 66 prisoners with them. U.S. and British losses were 213 and 228, respectively, killed, wounded, and captured. None of the U.S. casualties was from the ship. The *Carolina* continued to fire into the British camp during the night, as did Major Thomas Beale's New Orleans Sharpshooters. Finding that the *Carolina* was unable to move upstream because of adverse winds, on December 27, the British set the ship afire with hot shot. Seven men were killed or wounded in the ship.

The remainder of the crew escaped to the U.S. lines, where they served with Jackson's men in the subsequent battle. Captain Daniel T. Patterson, the naval commander at New Orleans, placed Lieutenant Henley in charge of a battery that he placed on the west side of the river. The only naval vessel left was the *Louisiana*, 16 guns, which was positioned to protect Jackson's flank and harass the enemy troops with its guns. The navy thus contributed to Jackson's victory over the British on January 8, 1815. New

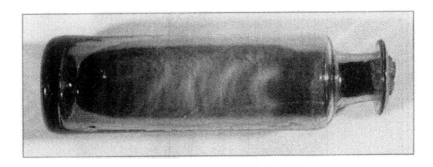

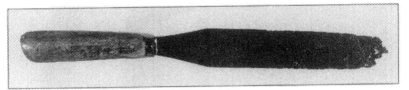

Medical Instruments from Commodore Barney's Gunboats: *top,* Pharmaceutical Bottle (5¾-in. length, 1⅛-in. diameter); *bottom,* Apothecary Mixing Spatula (10-in. length). Calvert Marine Museum, Solomons, Md.

Orleans was saved. Naval men also harassed the retreating British and took some prisoners. One of those who received a special acknowledgment from Jackson was Surgeon Lewis Heermann for the "very able manner" in which he superintended the general hospital while the regular director, Hospital Surgeon David Kerr, was on duty at Jackson's camp. With the approval of Commodore Patterson, Heermann was one of three medical volunteers with the army.[40]

Meanwhile back in New York, the *President,* 44 guns, under Captain Stephen Decatur, was still waiting for an opportunity to get to sea. It got its chance on the night of January 14, 1815, during a heavy storm, and it sailed. The commander of the British blockading ships anticipated this move and the probable course that the Americans would take. Accordingly, HMS *Endymion,* 50 guns, attacked the *President.* After two and one-half hours of battle, the *Endymion* was deprived of its sails and could not move. It had 11 killed and 14 wounded. The casualties in the *President* were 24 killed and 55 wounded. Two other British warships now overtook Decatur and he surrendered. He and his men were taken to Bermuda, where the wounded received additional care. The Americans were later paroled.[41]

Near the end of December, the *Constitution* was able to sail from

Boston and escape through the blockade. When it was about 200 miles off the coast of Madeira, it encountered two British ships, the frigate *Cyane*, 34 guns, and the sloop of war *Levant*, 20 guns. In the battle that followed, Captain Charles Stewart of the *Constitution* captured both ships. British losses were 12 killed and 26 wounded in the *Cyane* and 23 killed and 16 wounded in the *Levant*. The Americans lost 3 killed and 12 wounded. Their care was entrusted to Surgeon John A. Kearney, assisted by his mates, Benjamin Austin and Artemas Johnston, as well as by the medical men of the British ships. Stewart sailed to Port Praya, where he tried to land his prisoners, but the arrival of a strong British force led him to put to sea again. The British ships chased the *Levant* back into the harbor, where it was forced to surrender. Stewart succeeded in getting the *Constitution* to Maranhão, Brazil, where he landed his prisoners. Later, while in Puerto Rico, he heard that the war was over and sailed for New York, arriving there in mid-May.[42]

Meanwhile on March 23, 1815, the *Hornet*, 18 guns, fought a battle with HMS *Penguin*, 18 guns, off Tristan da Cunha. Twenty-eight minutes later the *Penguin* was captured. The British lost 14 killed, including the ship's captain, and 28 wounded; the Americans lost 1 killed and 10 wounded including the captain and the first lieutenant. Subsequently the *Penguin* was scuttled. The *Hornet's* surgeon, Samuel M. Kissam, was charged with the care of the wounded and was assisted by the captured medical men of the *Penguin*. The *Hornet* was chased by HMS *Cornwallis*, 74 guns, but escaped. When the *Hornet* reached San Salvador, its captain learned that the war was over, and he too sailed for New York.[43]

On June 30, 1815, the *Peacock*, under Captain Lewis Warrington, captured the *Nautilus*, 14 guns, a schooner of the East India Company. A few days later, learning that peace had been declared, Warrington gave up his prize.[44]

The various actions at sea, in bays and harbors, and on shore in which navy men participated resulted in casualties of at least 227 dead and 381 wounded, plus a minimum of 355 drowned. U.S. surgeons and mates cooperated with their British opposite numbers in the care of the wounded after the battles. Most of the wounded who survived a battle were transferred to hospital facilities ashore usually within a few days. Here we lose track of them, and it is not possible at this late date to determine how many ultimately recuperated. It is believed that a fair number did recover, but many of these were eligible for pensions and were thus lost to the navy. Yet there were undoubtedly others who deserved pensions but for one reason or another did not get them or got them many years after the injury.

One example is Seaman John Wentworth of the *Constitution*. On August 10, 1812, he was injured when a gun carriage ran over his foot. One of his toes was "sloughy & gangerous," and he was placed on the sick list until the fight with the *Guerriere* on August 19. Wentworth did his duty at his prescribed station during the battle and did not report himself as sick or injured after it. What effect this injury had on his subsequent health and performance is not known. Thirty-four years after the incident, he applied for a disability pension. At that late date it was difficult to determine what amount of disability, if any, was due to his injury.[45]

Also lost to the navy and to their loved ones was an unknown number of men who died as the result of accidents. The most dramatic of these were the loss of the frigate *Epervier,* the sloop *Wasp* and the schooner *Alligator,* with a total death toll of 285. Also, on almost any voyage in war or peace, some men fell to their death from aloft or overboard. Where logbook or medical records survive, these accidents can be dated and recorded, as has been noted in earlier chapters. But one must leap from the known to the speculative in trying to determine the statistics of deaths due to injuries at sea in the War of 1812. My estimate is that they probably totaled about 50.

Chapter 10

The War of 1812
Ashore

The war placed fresh demands on naval hospitals, many of which were barely adequate for peacetime requirements. Also, few surgeons or surgeon's mates on active duty had any kind of wartime experience. Among those who had experience during peacetime were some who desired to leave the navy. One was Surgeon's Mate Samuel Gilliland of the *Constitution*. Poor health made him request and receive a three-week leave of absence, during which he called upon Secretary Hamilton to ask if he could resign, citing as reasons his health and the desire of his parents that he leave the service. Hamilton asked for a written request, which was sent. The doctor also indicated that he had found professional opportunities that were appealing in Gettysburg. Hamilton accepted Gilliland's resignation and wished him prosperity in his private business.[1] To replace doctors like Gilliland, Hamilton had to seek new and usually younger medical men.

Among those ready to take advantage of any opportunities was Samuel Whittelsey of Watertown, New York. He wrote to Gideon Granger of Connecticut, who had been Jefferson's postmaster general, asking that his son William be given an appointment as a surgeon's mate in the navy. The former cabinet member was informed that the young man had been "pursuing a regular course of study in Physic and Surgery for several years." Now that his education had been completed, he sought an appointment in the navy. Granger forwarded the letter to the secretary of the navy with an endorsement that the father was one of the country's "respectable citizens." On July 10, 1812, Whittelsey was appointed a surgeon's mate.[2]

The war made it necessary to put the gunboats at the various ports in a state of readiness, and they needed medical men to care for the crews. For the gunboats stationed at Portland, in the Maine district, Commodore Bainbridge at Boston appointed Dr. John Merrill, a local man, as surgeon. When he inspected the gunboats, he found that there were no surgical instruments or medicines among the government's supplies. Fortunately he had his own instruments, and he bought the medicines he needed from the local apothecary. Bainbridge's prompt action met the immediate needs of Portland, and the secretary appointed Dr. Herman W. Clarke of Dover, New Hampshire, as a surgeon's mate to assist Merrill. But the secretary had other ideas about the senior position: he appointed Dr. Samuel Ayer as surgeon and ordered him to Portland. Merrill was informed that his appointment had not been confirmed by the Senate and that his duties would end when Ayer arrived. So after nearly 10 months on the job, Merrill was replaced. The nature of his medical activities during that time are not known.[3]

Medical men were also assigned to the navy yard at Portsmouth, New Hampshire. One of these was an experienced practitioner, Surgeon Robert L. Thorn, who had been in the navy since 1806. It is not known how extensive his duties were, but for most of the civilian population, Portsmouth was a healthy town. Except for shipbuilding at the navy yard, the war appears to have had little impact on the community.[4]

Another New England community that experienced the war largely from the sidelines was that at the navy yard at Boston. The victories of the *Constitution* early in the war were occasions for celebration by both the naval and civilian citizenry, but the British blockade of the New England coast and the growth of opposition to the war in Massachusetts greatly restricted naval activity in the area. Therefore the marine and naval hospitals were largely concerned with routine health cases and the examination and care of prisoners of war, who were carried in cartel ships to and from Halifax, Nova Scotia. For Americans returning home, Boston was the logical place to carry out exchanges in the northeast. The hospital at the Boston Navy Yard was the place where surgeons could examine those injured in battle and determine what constituted a just claim for a pension. They could also decide which men were suitable for service in other areas once they had recovered from their time in captivity. Finding men willing to serve in the war could be difficult in New England. From surviving correspondence it appears that many navy medical men were bored by routine duties and wanted transfers to a more active and challenging environment. From the point of view of the secretary, he had to defend far more coastline than his resources permitted, and he could never be sure that an area that was quiet at one point in the war would remain so throughout the conflict.

Political, diplomatic, and financial aspects of the war all played a role in determing how the secretary of the navy was able to respond to the demands of the war and the needs of the service. An offer from the czar of Russia late in 1812 to mediate between the United States and Great Britain led to the appointment of Albert Gallatin, the secretary of the Treasury, as one of the negotiators sent to Europe. In his absence, Secretary of the Navy Jones was asked to manage the Treasury as well as his own department. Jones accepted the challenge and early in 1813 sent to the House of Representatives a report on the nation's finances. With it he included a list of nine direct and indirect taxes that Gallatin believed were necessary to balance the budget and maintain the credit of the country in 1814. Debates in Congress ensued over what was to be taxed and how the burden was to be distributed over various sections of the nation. These arguments not only divided Federalists and Republicans but also pitted Republicans against one another. In the end, about three-quarters of the Republicans in both houses voted for the taxes they could support and abstained from those they could not.

In his capacity as acting secretary of the Treasury, Jones drew up a budget for the army and navy that required maximum economy and efficiency from March through December 1813. The taxes voted by Congress were beginning to be collected by the end of the year, but Jones estimated that they would raise only about two-thirds of the money required. The remainder of the funds needed would have to come from a loan. Jones estimated that $29,350 would be needed. After nearly three weeks of debate, the House authorized a loan of $25 million.

As a result of these factors, economy in government spending was the watchword for most of the year. The demands of two cabinet posts prevented Jones from introducing reforms in the navy. Discouraged and suffering from personal financial losses, he wanted to resign from the administration in December 1813 but was induced by Madison to stay for another year. The lack of adequate funds for the war and the distractions of the secretary of the navy had an impact on health care, and we must now examine the way installations on shore were affected.

New York City was a case in point. If the British should decide to move against that city, much would depend on the frigates supplemented by the gunboat flotilla. But even without a specific British threat, there were concerns about the health and readiness of the naval units at New York. Because of his own illness, Surgeon Samuel Marshall appointed Dr. Peter Christie as his assistant. He wrote to the secretary and expressed the hope that Christie would commissioned as a surgeon's mate. Endorsing this sentiment was Dr. Giles Smith, who wrote of Christie's services in the New

York City almshouse; Richard Simmons also wrote a letter of recommendation. Christie was commissioned as a surgeon's mate on July 8, 1812.[5]

Another young man who wanted to join was Andrew B. Cook, who asked Surgeon Samuel R. Marshall to examine him on the various branches of medical science. Marshall found him fully qualified and wrote to Hamilton asking that he be appointed a surgeon's mate. Supporting letters came also from Dr. McNeven of New York and former Congressman Gurdon S. Mumford of that state. Cook was appointed as a surgeon's mate on December 21, 1812. This is the only known case of a candidate requesting an examination before that procedure became the norm in 1824.[6]

Meanwhile the requirements of several naval stations were being brought to the attention of the secretary. Commander Jacob M. Lewis had been appointed by Captain Isaac Hull to the command of a flotilla of gunboats which was to protect New York City. But both the sick and the prisoners being held at the New York Navy Yard were being transferred to the gunboats, which were becoming a combination of prison ship and hospital. The number of patients and prisoners soon became so great that there was not enough room, and many of the sick died for want of proper medical attention. Lewis appealed to both Commander Charles Ludlow, the commandant of the navy yard, and Dr. Marshall, the surgeon of the base, for assistance. Neither responded. When later asked about this by the secretary, Marshall replied that he already had too many patients. "The bunks are so close as to be nearly in contact, 13 of these men are affected with the prevailing epidemic which has proved to be so very marked on board the John Adams. The two small houses are now occupied by the sick and are (although the best that could be obtained) too contracted and in other essential respects unsuitable for the purposes to which they were applied."[7]

So, with no additional help forthcoming from his medical staff and with 70 sick men on his hands, Lewis turned to the New York City physician Dr. Joshua Parsons. Earlier Parsons had served with Lewis and had been captured and taken to Halifax. He had only recently been exchanged when Lewis appealed to him for help. The doctor accepted and went to live on a gunboat. According to Lewis, the doctor performed the work of three surgeons in ministering to the sick in the gunboats. Subsequently Surgeon's Mates C. B. Hamilton and Hermon M. Clarke were assigned to the flotilla. Lewis asked that Parsons be assigned to the New York station. The commander admitted that he had already placed Parsons' name on the ship's books because it was the only way he could be paid. Dr. Robert C. P. Barton took charge of the hospital at Spermacati Cove at Sandy Hook. Commander Lewis's action in making an unauthorized appointment did not come to the attention of the secretary until some months later. When he found out, Jones was outraged. He asked the commander by what authority had he assumed the prerogatives of the Senate and terminated Parsons' appointment. Later the secretary made the New York flotilla subordinate to Commodore Decatur in New York.[8]

What effect, if any, did these problems have on the health situation in the navy on the New York station? The historical record provides no clear answers. Surviving statistics from the fall of 1813 to June 1815 show that for the 30 gunboats employed for most of that period, the complement of officers and men ranged from 24 to 43 each. Out of that number there were only 14 deaths. Two of these were the result of drowning and one man was killed in action. No cause of death is recorded for the others, although some presumably died in the temporary hospital at Spermacati Cove. In addition, there were deaths among the 697 men attached to the flotilla but not assigned to any particular ship. Between October 1813 and June 3, 1815, this group sustained 14 deaths, of which 3 were drownings. For the remaining 11, no cause of death is recorded, but 9 are listed as dying at Sandy Hook and only 1 of these is noted as being at the hospital there. There are also 584 entries on the muster rolls of those who were attached to vessels in ordinary at the New York Navy Yard or to the yard itself, and 13 deaths are recorded. One of these was that of Surgeon David Hatfield, who died on May 13, 1815, or shortly after the end of the war. No cause is given for his death or for the others, except for two drownings. Of the 13 deaths, 6 are listed as having taken place in a hospital. This same muster list shows that another 12 men deserted while they were in the hospital.[9]

The continuing demand for medical supplies underscored recurring problems in getting them promptly. Early in the war, Surgeon Samuel Marshall called on Secretary Hamilton with some thoughts on how the situation might be improved. Marshall suggested that he be appointed the purveyor of medical supplies at New York. He was probably familiar with the operations of the War Department's purveyor of public supplies in Philadelphia and wanted to adapt the idea to the needs of the medical department. Apparently Hamilton indicated that he would look into the matter; encouraged, Marshall looked forward to receiving the secretary's thoughts. When nothing was forthcoming, Marshall concluded that matters associated with the war had distracted the secretary and prevented him from responding, and he therefore felt it was appropriate to send the secretary additional information on how the proposed office would work.

Under this system the purveyor would see that the government got what it wanted at a fair price. He would keep abreast of price fluctuations in drugs, determine what quantities would be needed for at least a year, and contract for the necessary supplies. As Marshall visualized it, the purveyor would examine and approve all bills presented for drugs, surgical instruments, and medical stores. Presumably these bills would then be forwarded to the Navy Department and from there to the Treasury for payment. When ships returned from a voyage and were laid up in a navy yard, the purveyor would receive all the medicines and surgical instruments and determine what should be preserved for future use. He would report his findings to the secretary and dispose of any unwanted items in a way to prevent loss of public money. If these measures were followed, said Marshall, ships could be put into commission and supplied with medicines at a much lower cost than was now the case.

This time Marshall's suggestions got the secretary's full attention, probably as a result of the developing problems with Surgeon Ewell at the Washington Navy Yard (see chap. 8). Hamilton thought Marshall's ideas had merit and gave him the responsibilities he sought, but in a limited area. Marshall was authorized to take charge of all medicines and surgical instruments belonging to the navy at New York and any that might be sent there from other places for public use, as well as those from ships laid up in ordinary. Medicines to be preserved were to be turned over to the local navy agent. All perishable drugs and those liable to damage were to be sold. Regular records were to be kept of all medicines received and used, and an accounting must be made to the accountant of the navy. For this work Marshall was to receive $500 a year. So it was that an experiment in the better control of medicines was launched in New York.[10]

Philadelphia and New Castle

At the Philadelphia Navy Yard, Commodore Alexander Murray discussed with Surgeon Cutbush the medical arrangements for the gunboats that would operate in Delaware Bay. It was anticipated that there would be 20 gunboats and 400 men, exclusive of officers. The gunboats would probably be divided into two divisions, either each having a surgeon's mate or possibly together sharing one surgeon and one mate. A small medical chest had been ordered for the use of each division, but there was a shortage of some articles, such as tourniquets. Since the gunboats did not have accommodations for the sick, and since operations could not be performed in them, Cutbush naturally wondered what would be done with the sick and wounded. If they were sent to the navy yard at Philadelphia, several days would pass before an operation could be performed. Or would they be landed at some convenient spot on Delaware Bay? The secretary had to decide and issue the necessary orders.[11] Hamilton replied promptly that

Cutbush was the best judge of what should be done in regard to supplies and accommodations for the sick. He was to exercise "due economy," but he should consult with Commodore Murray about his needs and then take steps to procure what was necessary. On this basis, Murray and Cutbush organized things as best they could.[12]

Cutbush immediately set out for New Castle, Delaware, to establish a temporary hospital for the sick of the gunboat force stationed there. He found that the owners of vacant houses were reluctant to rent them for that purpose. Eventually a small house was obtained which could accommodate only 15 men, and the doctor now set about preparing it to receive patients. Cutbush was obliged to make a round trip from Philadelphia to New Castle that took 48 hours—time away from his patients. He urged the secretary to send him two assistants, one to remain in Philadelphia and the other to serve at New Castle. As things now stood, Dr. Barton's was no help to him, for his time was wholly taken up with the examination of men in Philadelphia who were to serve in the *Constellation*. Cutbush urged that the seamen enlisted for such service be shipped to Washington rather than be crowded together on a gunboat awaiting orders. Eventually crowding would impair their health.

Describing his own caseload, Cutbush said he had a number of men sick with what the seamen called "Ladies Fever," or what later generations would call a venereal disease. Since this disease was not related to their duties, Cutbush thought that the men ought to pay something to the hospital fund for the treatment they received. Apparently his suggestion was not acted upon. The surgeon further said that he still had one man from the *Wasp* under his care, and he was called upon to examine men who enlisted in the marines.[13]

Hamilton assigned Surgeon William P. C. Barton to assist Cutbush in Philadelphia, and he promised that a surgeon's mate would soon be sent for service at the temporary hospital. In the meantime, to care for the sick at New Castle, Hamilton suggested that Cutbush approach a local civilian practitioner, Dr. Allan McLane, who was highly recommended, and offer him the position of surgeon's mate. Cutbush did so and reported that the doctor would be willing to do the duty but not to join the navy. Hamilton therefore authorized paying him the wages of a surgeon's mate.[14]

The medical help promised by the secretary turned out to be Surgeon's Mate William L. Whittelsey, who arrived in New Castle on November 12, 1812. Cutbush was extremely disappointed in what he saw and complained to the secretary. Whittelsey was "a youth of about 18 years of age. What his acquirements are I know not, but conceive from his age that he is not capable of acting in any situation alone." Cutbush sent him to Philadelphia until he knew the wishes of the secretary. Commodore Murray thought that the services of Dr. McLane might be dispensed with, the sick at New Castle could be transferred to Philadelphia, and Whittelsey might be useful in helping to care for them. He would act under Cutbush's orders and would acquire "professional information" in the process. This was done, but the following July, Whittelsey was transferred to the cartel ship *Perseverance*.[15]

Things did not work out as planned with Surgeon Barton either. He resisted serving under Cutbush at New Castle, and the latter complained to the secretary. Hamilton replied: "Dr. Barton must act as your mate, he is subject to your order!" But the reality was that Cutbush, the senior man, had to supervise the affairs at New Castle while Barton remained in Philadelphia. Apparently Barton used political influence to stay where he was.[16]

With the coming of winter, the gunboats were laid up, and Cutbush anticipated closing the New Castle hospital until spring. But in November, Captain David Porter of the *Essex* dropped off nine invalids at the hospital. In a letter to Cutbush he said that none of the men would ever be of any use to the service and that if time and circumstances had permitted it, he would have discharged them himself. The arrival of these men posed problems for Cutbush. They needed clothing, and he was not authorized to issue any. From the purser of the *Essex* he had requested a copy of the men's accounts but had not yet received it when the ship sailed. Should the hospital at New Castle be kept open for them? Commodore Murray thought that if they were not going to be discharged, it would be better to send them to the navy yard at Philadelphia. The secretary agreed.[17] Cutbush also forwarded to the secretary the names and illnesses of the men from the *Essex*, along with his comments on their cases. Of the nine, two were old cases of syphilis, a third man suffered from a diseased testicle, and a fourth had a "Stricture in the Urethra." Two were found to have scrofula, and another was diagnosed as having a "Scrophulous Abscess." The ninth man had a rupture, which he said was the result of an injury in the line of duty, and he was therefore entitled to a pension.[18]

The men were transferred to Philadelphia, and it soon became apparent that not all their problems were medical. Cutbush complained to Hamilton that two of the sailors from the *Essex* were "the most hardened villains" he had ever seen in the service. They were in the habit of leaving their sick quarters at night and climbing the fence to go in search of alcohol. When they returned in an intoxicated state, they resisted the guards on duty. Cutbush was fearful that one of these encounters might result in bloodshed. Attempts to punish these men by chaining them and confining them in "the black hole" in the yard had not brought about any change in attitude. Therefore Cutbush asked for the authority to discharge any men who violated the rules of the hospital and the base. Hamilton did not want to discharge them until he had their records from the *Essex,* and these were not forthcoming. He therefore authorized Cutbush to use his own judgment in discharging men for the good of the service. In such cases the balances due to the men could be ascertained.[19]

Meanwhile Surgeon Barton continued to examine recruits and work on his book on naval hospitals. Then, in February 1813, Secretary William Jones told him that Commodore Decatur had requested his services and he should report to that officer in New York. Barton at once wrote to Decatur expressing his unwillingness to go to sea and his determination to avoid such service. Decatur forwarded this letter to the secretary and apparently expressed sympathy for Barton's position. Jones told Decatur that while he was inclined to be sympathetic in matters involving the reasonable convenience of officers, he could not yield to the "claims and pretensions" of Dr. Barton. "If young gentlemen in his situation were suffered to decline active service, at such a crisis as this in order to enjoy a sinecure on shore, the good of the service would be rendered subservient to personal interest & indulgence." Jones therefore asked Decatur to forward a letter to Barton, which said that Barton's reasons for declining sea service were not sufficient and that he was to reply whether he would report to Decatur or resign. Barton went to New York as ordered, but he did not acquiesce. Jones was forced to yield, apparently as the result of political pressure, and with great reluctance on March 16, 1813, he ordered Barton back to Philadelphia.[20]

Later in that year, when Cutbush was transferred to Washington, there was speculation about who would succeed him at Philadelphia. One who was eager for the position was Dr. Barton, and he enlisted the aid of his uncle, Dr. Benjamin F. Barton, who wrote to Attorney General Richard Rush, a fellow Pennsylvanian, about the matter. But Barton had antagonized Jones, and the secretary had no disposition to appoint him. A more worthy candidate was Surgeon Samuel D. Heap. First appointed in 1804 as a surgeon's mate, he was promoted to surgeon in slightly less than eight months. He had served in the Mediterranean, at New Orleans, and at Boston. Hearing that Cutbush had been transferred to Washington, Heap applied for the position in Philadelphia. Jones gave him the job, and Heap took up his new duties on July 11, 1813.[21] For the remainder of the war the medical staff in Philadelphia had only to concern itself with the routine care of the men in the area. The war was felt more in other locales.

As for Barton, the brief interval between the departure of Cutbush and the arrival of Heap left him temporarily in charge of the patients. An increase in the number of sick made it necessary to rent a house adjacent to the yard and procure additional supplies. This was done on the authorization of Commodore Murray, the commandant of the yard, but without the knowledge of Secretary Jones, who reacted with displeasure to what he saw as a presumption of authority. Barton was able to explain his actions, but when Heap arrived, the secretary told him that Barton was no longer attached to the navy yard. Jones said that it was improper for a surgeon to be employed to do the work of a mate. Barton was placed on half pay awaiting orders for another assignment and remained in that status for the rest of the war.[22] Later, in the spring of 1814, when Heap asked for and received leave to go to New Orleans, he recommended that his assistant act in his stead. This was acting surgeon's mate C. M. Reese, who had been helping out since the departure of Surgeon's Mate Whittelsey. Heap noted that Reese had recently graduated from the University of Pennsylvania with great credit, and he was qualified for the required duties. The secretary chose not to act on this suggestion and ordered another officer to Philadelphia.[23]

Washington, D.C.

In Washington there was concern about hospitals and the care of the sick in the area. Benjamin H. Latrobe had intended to develop plans for the proposed navy hospital, but he found himself distracted by other obligations. Surgeon Ewell was insistent that Latrobe help him develop his own plans for improved facilities. Latrobe also had to appear twice as a witness in court proceedings, and he advised committees of the House and Senate on the proposed alterations to the halls of Congress. He had also promised the trustees of Lexington University that he would design a building for them. As a result of these distractions, the plans for the naval hospital did not reach Secretary Hamilton until late June 1812.[24]

When William Jones took over as secretary of the navy in 1813, he asked for a copy of the plans, and Latrobe obliged. When it later developed that there was no money for the proposed hospital, the matter dragged on. In 1814, Surgeon William P. C. Barton published a *Treatise on Marine Hospitals,* which presented the results of his own research and thinking on the subject. Latrobe continued to work on his own ideas, and in January 1815 he sent a new set of drawings to the secretary and apparently met with him and the secretary of the Treasury, Alexander Dallas, to go over the material.[25]

While the design of the hospital was slowly taking shape, the day-to-day needs of the sick at the Washington Navy Yard were the concern of Surgeon Thomas Ewell, a who had been a fixture there since 1807. Ewell's chronic need for money for personal needs caused him to become involved in an ill-conceived project to manufacture gunpowder. The powder he delivered proved unsatisfactory: among other things, it ignited too slowly. Problems related to a powder contract led to a controversy with the chief clerk of the Navy Department, Charles Goldsborough, as well as with the secretary, and it led to Ewell's forced resignation as surgeon on May 5, 1813.[26]

When the news of Ewell's impending departure became known, several people applied for the post. One was Surgeon's Mate John Harrison, who also heard a rumor that the position was to be given to his colleague, Surgeon's Mate Henry Huntt. Harrison had been at the yard for nearly nine years, in contrast to Huntt's year and a half. Deeply disturbed by the rumor, and without making an effort to determine its validity, Harrison complained to the secretary of the navy. Naval officers and others, he wrote, could testify that he had been a slave to the duties of his situation. "I have been at my Post upon all occasions ready & willing at all times and at all hours to render any assistance or services that were required." He then noted that he continued to see men younger than himself promoted. It turned out that neither Harrison nor Huntt got the job because an officer with a better claim to the position than either of them exerted influence in high places.[27]

That applicant was Surgeon Edward Cutbush, who pointed out to President Madison that he had been in the navy since 1799 and that various secretaries had promised him the post at the Washington Navy Yard but a combination of circumstances had previously prevented his appointment. He believed that the position should now be given to him. This time he was successful. On the very day that Ewell resigned, the secretary wrote to Cutbush telling him to come to Washington as soon as convenient and assume charge of the hospital establishment in the city.[28]

When Cutbush took over his new duties, his medical colleagues were busy coping with the health problems of men who had formerly been attached to the frigate *Adams,* which was a part of the Potomac flotilla that guarded the river approach to Washington. The men were now living in the old frigate *New York* at the yard, which was in a filthy state. They began to suffer from colds accompanied by sore throat, redness of the eyes, and a pain in the right nipple. Within 48 hours they had a fever, an increased pain in the breast, and frequently delirium. Several days later the pains in the breast had increased so much that the patients were in a constant state of agony. As treatment, Surgeon's Mate Henry Huntt first gave doses of calomel and tartic emetic, applied a large blister to the breast, and then immersed the patient in a warm bath. About the third day he would begin his treatment with calomel and opium and alternate with wine, bark, and Virginia snakeroot. Snakeroot was frequently used with Peruvian bark in treating intermittent fevers or the later stages of fevers. At night the patients were given a painkilling drug. Huntt found that if the patient survived for six or seven days, he recovered. In two cases, however, the patients complained about great pain in the right nipple accompanied by a cough and difficult respiration. Huntt thought they had pleurisy and he bled them. Afterward the patients experienced cold in their extremities, a faltering pulse, and violent delirium. Within a few hours both were dead.

By mid-June, Huntt had 140 cases of what he considered to be pneumonia. Patients started out with symptoms of typhus, which changed quickly into typhoid. His pattern of treatment now was to give an emetic first, which had a good effect, and follow this with nitrous ether and laudanum, given every two hours, and a blister applied to the chest. A day or two later the bark, snakeroot, and wine were freely administered until the patient recovered. When he had time to do so, Huntt gave pills of calomel and opium and found them to be very successful.

In those instances when the onslaught of the disease was sudden, accompanied by difficulty in breathing, cold skin, a feeble pulse, and a loss of energy, Huntt was afraid to use any evacuant but resorted to stimulants. Wine, brandy, and aromatics were freely given, then a hot blister was applied to the chest, and hot applications to the extremities. It was Huntt's view that few patients could stand the normal purgatives. When they complained of pain or uneasiness in the bowels, he gave a gentle purge. By following this method of treatment, he had the satisfaction of seeing 134 of his 140 patients recover.

About mid-May 1813, while Huntt was still treating sailors from the *Adams*, the same type of illness struck the men of the *Viper*, at the yard. These men had been given the privilege of leaving the navy yard and had got drunk. When sickness struck them it was frequently accompanied by persistent vomiting and diarrhoea, as well as a cold and clammy sweat. Huntt was convinced that the disease was contagious. Twenty-two men were stricken and seven died. Autopsies were performed on four. Huntt found that except in one man, the thoracic and abdominal viscera showed no appearance of the disease. In one case the left lung was greatly diseased. But Commodore Tingey later informed Huntt that this man had suffered from a pulmonary infection for some time.[29]

For much of the war the medical problems at the Washington hospital were fairly routine respiratory and digestive disorders. But in 1814 the British began a series of raids on the U.S. coast. In August they defeated a

U.S. force at Bladensburg, Maryland, and marched into Washington, where they burned the Capitol, the White House, and other buildings before returning to their ships. Marines and men from Commodore Barney's flotilla participated in the Battle at Bladensburg, and some were wounded. When the secretary heard about them, he ordered Cutbush to send Surgeon's Mate Harrison to the battlefield to examine and report on the wounded. The secretary understood that Barney's men were in bad shape. One of them had had his leg amputated. Jones believed that if possible the men should be moved to Washington. If they could not, they should be attended and comfortably provided for until they could travel. Cutbush did as ordered and informed the secretary that Harrison had returned to the yard with five of the wounded. The rest could not be moved without endangering their lives and were under the care of Surgeon's Mate John O'Connor of the army. If the secretary thought Harrison should be in attendance there he should issue an order to that effect. Cutbush used the occasion to report to the secretary the situation at the naval hospital. He now had 37 patients including officers, and 24 of these had wounds. He dressed the wounds of each man twice a day and attended to the sick. These duties were becoming almost impossible for him to perform alone, and he desperately needed an assistant. He had been on duty at the hospital for ten days without rest. A surgeon needed time to reflect on the condition of his patients under his care, he said. The secretary, sympathetic to Cutbush's plight, replied that Surgeon John A. Brereton was in the vicinity and would join Cutbush the next day. A surgeon's mate would also be ordered to assist him.

The need for help became more acute when Cutbush received word from an army surgeon that the hospital at Bladensburg was to be dismantled and the patients and doctors moved elsewhere. Hence the four patients from the marines and Barney's flotilla who remained would have no medical men to attend them. Cutbush said that he had no authority to provide quarters or medical attendance for these men. The secretary promptly gave him this authority. Not only were the wounded at Bladensburg to be made comfortable and provided for, but Cutbush was to consider his orders as embracing all cases in the vicinity of Washington. Those persons with serious wounds who could not be moved to the city were to be placed in convenient accommodations and given necessary comfort and medical care. Meanwhile the secretary had received a letter from a civilian practitioner, Dr. U. Wedderburn of Alexandria, who was also taking care of some of the wounded. Cutbush was to write to inform him what he should do in regard to such cases and certify his charges for medical assistance and supplies at a rate he considered to be just.

Acting on these orders, Cutbush sent Surgeon's Mate R. C. Randolph to Bladensburg to take charge of the two men who were too badly wounded to be moved. He also sent Harrison to the Montgomery County Courthouse to attend two patients housed there, one who had had his leg amputated and the other suffering from a fever. The surgeon himself was still treating 37 patients in the naval hospital, the marine barracks, and in their quarters, but some relief was in sight. Barney's men would be ready to leave the hospital within a week, and Cutbush asked the secretary for guidance on what to do with them. Jones replied that they should be sent to Baltimore under the supervision of their own officers, who were now at the hospital. If the officers were not able to travel, then Commodore Tingey was to appoint an officer to accompany them.[30]

With the passage of time the wounded recovered, Cutbush's caseload dropped, and the focal point of the war moved to New Orleans. By that time, Cutbush and his superiors were again involved in paperwork relating to pensions and other claims for compensation. According to the records of the Washington naval hospital, there were 121 admissions in 1813, of which 15 died. In 1814 there were 90 admissions and 10 deaths. In addition, the doctors attached to the navy yard attended to the needs of 18–20 families of persons attached to the yard.[31]

Norfolk, the Carolinas, and Georgia

Treating routine illnesses and doing what they could for the distressed was the lot of most of the navy medical men at Norfolk during most of the war. Battles near the city in 1813 resulted in a small number of casualties. These men and the regular sick were cared for in the makeshift hospital on the second floor of a frame structure in the navy yard. At the beginning of the war, Captain John Cassin had his office on the ground floor of this building, and he regularly had problems: every time Surgeon Joseph J. Schoolfield washed the floor of the hospital, the water would drip through the ceiling and wet Cassin's books and papers. Clearly both the hospital and the captain needed better arrangements, but it was easier to find another office for Cassin than a hospital for Schoolfield.[32]

In the Carolinas and Georgia, the makeshift arrangements of the prewar period were continued, with some changes. The declaration of war made it necessary to try to do something about the medical situation there. Friends had recommended Dr. E. D. Morrison of Newburn, North Carolina, for a position. He came to Washington, where, in the absence of the secretary, he talked to Charles Goldsborough, the chief clerk, who appointed him as a surgeon's mate and allegedly told him that when the secretary returned, a surgeon's commission would be sent to him. When Morrison arrived at Newburn, the local navy commander ordered him to attend to men in the gunboats at Ocracoke Inlet, where he found himself doing the duties of both a surgeon and a mate. In addition, Master Commandant Thomas N. Gautier, the naval officer in command at Wilmington, North Carolina, asked Morrison to look after the gunboat men at Beaufort, where there was no surgeon. Because of the distances involved, Morrison had to rent a horse and spend time on the road.

During the winter, while Morrison was in Ocracoke, the men in gunboat no. 147 at Beaufort became ill. Several had dysentery and others were suffering from pleurisy. When one man died of pleurisy, the gunboat commander hired a local civilian physician, Dr. James Manney, to care for the sick and supply medicines at a cost of $30 a month. This news was not well received at the Navy Department. Probably the same was true of the news that Morrison was using his servant to do the duties of surgeon's mate and his requests for expense money and a promotion. When asked for an explanation Morrison pointed out that he was covering two stations that were nearly 100 miles apart. As he saw it, he was doing the work of two surgeons and was paid as a mate. In addition to his medical duties, he had had to travel to South Carolina to get Sailing Master George Evans out of jail, where he had been confined for his involvement in a duel. Jones wanted to dismiss Morrison but received favorable reports about his work, and so his solution was to station him at Wilmington and authorize the navy commander to hire an acting surgeon's mate for Ocracoke. In June 1813, Jones ordered that there be three gunboats at Wilmington, one at Beaufort, and two at Ocracoke. Master Commandant Gautier was told by Jones that he was to exercise the utmost vigilance in guarding against abuses and regulating expenditures. As a result the situation there was stable for the remainder of the war.[33]

At Charleston, South Carolina, the summer of 1812 brought the annual outbreak of fever. It killed several prominent persons but was less severe than in previous years. At the marine barracks in Hampstead, near Charleston, Surgeon George Logan's patient load varied from 7 to 13 over a two-month period. Only 1 marine died, and that was from "a pulmonary Disorder" and not fever. Among the seamen there were 4 or 5 cases each on the guard vessel and in the sick quarters ashore, but only a few at the navy yard. No deaths occurred, but a purser who was extremely ill was moved to quarters on Sullivan's Island, where his condition gradually improved.[34] One unusual case involved a seaman named Robert Allison, who was diagnosed as having scurvy and was transferred from the brig *Argus* to the hospital at Charleston. There he was cured of scurvy but developed dropsy. He was tapped and about eight quarts of water were reportedly removed from his legs before he died in October 1812.[35]

In November, Logan and his family nearly lost their lives when a house adjoining theirs caught fire at night and flames prevented their escaping by a stairway. Their cries for help eventually brought aid, and they were rescued by ladder from a balcony. Logan reported to the secretary that he had lost his instruments, commission, medical diploma, and virtually all that he owned. Only a set of trepanning instruments, which were at another location, were saved.[36] While Logan was trying to replace his losses, medical help arrived in the persons of surgeon's mates Horatio S. Waring and Oliver Le Chevalier. Logan expressed to the secretary his great satisfaction with both. Waring was assigned to Logan, and Captain John H. Dent, the local navy commander, sent Le Chevalier to a guard vessel near Sullivan's Island. Le Chevalier regularly consulted with Logan about difficult cases.[37]

During the previous 18 months, it had been the custom for Logan to take under his immediate care all of the clinically sick and those who needed to be moved to sick quarters. This was an inconvenience, and the need for a hospital was sorely felt. Reports on these cases were regularly sent to Captain Dent. When Jones became secretary in 1813, he approved the arrangements so long as they gave relief to the sick at the least possible cost to the government. But later in 1813, as an economy move, the marines were transferred to quarters in the navy yard and their barracks at Hampstead were used for the sick of the navy.[38]

At the end of 1814, new arrangements became necessary when the barracks were transferred to the army. The corporation of Charleston agreed to make two large rooms in the city hospital available for the sick of the navy; the steward of the hospital would keep order among the patients and direct a nurse and a cook on matters relating to their health care. In lieu of rent, the Navy Department agreed to pay a moderate sum each quarter to the steward. Logan rejoiced that these arrangements would give more comfort and safety to the invalids, and it was also more economical. The surgeon moved nine of his clinically sick patients into the hospital at the end of December, expecting the number to increase in the winter months. Sick seamen were also cared for on gunboat no. 9. Originally built at Charleston for use in the Tripolitan War, it had been modified by building a roof over the deck to create, in effect, a berth deck. Here the seamen had the benefits of fresh air but were protected from rain and sunlight.[39]

Farther south, on the St. Mary's station in Georgia, things became difficult after Surgeon William Dandridge died in July 1812. At that time,

Surgeon's Mate William Baldwin had over 20 sick men to care for, and he could not do justice to all. When he got through that crisis and was promoted, he asked for the services of a mate. Since February 1813 a local physician, Dr. Seaborn Jones Saffold, had been acting as his mate, and he should get the appointment. In addition to being qualified, Dr. Saffold was a native of the area. The secretary did not adopt this suggestion and instead sent Surgeon's Mate Hyde Ray to St. Mary's. This arrangement did not work out, and in August 1814 Safford received a commission as a surgeon's mate.[40]

Baldwin also suggested to Jones that gunboat no. 3 be modified to accommodate the sick, so that they might be cared for less expensively than on shore. Before this suggestion could be evaluated, the secretary's attention was directed to the amount of money that had been spent by Master Charles F. Grandison in outfitting the sloop *Troup* at Savannah. Investigations by Captain Hugh Campbell showed that the ship was unfit to be a cruising vessel, and Grandison was dismissed from the service. The *Troup* was stripped, and the secretary's suggestion that it be used as a hospital ship was adopted. In mid-October 1813, Captain Campbell reported that during the previous three months there had never been fewer than 30 patients in the ship, but now the number had risen to 45. He did not state the nature of the illnesses. But he did note that between sickness, desertions, and the discharge of men whose enlistments had expired, there were too few able-bodied men on the station to navigate a schooner that the secretary had ordered to Wilmington, North Carolina.[41]

Meanwhile the secretary had received a complaint about the denial of health care. Lieutenant Alexander Sevier of the marines asked Baldwin for medical help for his men at Point Petre, Georgia. Baldwin refused on the grounds that he had never received any orders in regard to the marines on that station. Sevier asked the secretary for advice on how he should proceed. It became the practice of Jones not to respond to such letters but to refer them to the writer's commanding officer, for he believed they should be dealt with on the local level.[42]

Help was also needed at Sunbury, Georgia, where six armed barges were on guard. Secretary Hamilton offered the post to Dr. Joseph M. Troup of Darien, Georgia, giving him the option of a temporary appointment while the navy was deployed off Sunbury or a permanent commission as a surgeon. Troup decided to do neither but to continue to act as a civilian. By the end of December 1812, the cost of the hospital establishment at Sunbury had become so high that the sick were sent to Savannah. There all the officers except one were very ill, including Master Charles Grandison, the local navy commander. Therefore Grandison appointed John Posey an acting surgeon's mate, but the appointment was revoked by the secretary. Instead Surgeon's Mate Joseph W. New, a veteran of the Tripolitan War, was given the assignment. The situation in Sunbury became so expensive that Grandison transferred all the sick to Charleston, thus reducing expenses from $200 to $6 a month.[43]

So it was that each of the naval installations had its own arrangements for dealing with health care, and for many of them the war brought at least one period that strained the existing facilities. In the early months of 1813, the financial situation of the U.S. government became so strained that it was necessary to curtail operations in various places. But in 1814, British activities along the coast led to efforts to strengthen positions that seemed to be threatened. Fragmentary records tell little of the nature of the illnesses treated at the various naval installations and about the number of deaths. But the information that does survive suggests that many surgeons and their assistants had enough to keep them busy even if combat wounds were not among their problems.

Chapter 11

The War of 1812
on the Lakes

The outbreak of the war caused a concern about the border defenses on Lake Erie and Lake Ontario. Control of these waters became even more important after Detroit fell to the British in the first weeks of the war. Commodore Isaac Chauncey, who was given the task of building ships to defend both lakes, turned over his command of the New York Navy Yard to Captain Samuel Evans and proceeded to Sacket's Harbor on Lake Ontario to take on his new responsibilities. Men had already been sent ahead to begin transforming the location into an important base.[1]

To assist him on the medical front, Chauncey turned to Dr. Walter W. Buchanan of Columbia College, who had served in the navy during the Quasi-War with France. In the intervening years he had held a professorship at Columbia and had a contract with the Corporation of New York to attend at the almshouse. With the United States again at war, Buchanan indicated a willingness to serve in a medical capacity. Chauncey was quick to take him up on his offer and, acting on the authority given to him by the secretary of the navy, appointed Buchanan a surgeon on September 21, 1812. Buchanan settled his affairs and made his way to Sacket's Harbor, where he was soon joined by other medical men.[2] In addition to its naval activity, Sacket's Harbor was a place where army units were assembling in anticipation of a campaign against the British forces in Canada. Buchanan was placed on an equal footing with the hospital surgeons of the army. A hospital was established ashore and Buchanan attended the navy sick there as well as in the ships. Generally the sick were treated on shipboard, and the more serious cases were sent to the hospital.

On November 10, 1812, the squadron under Chauncey's command at-

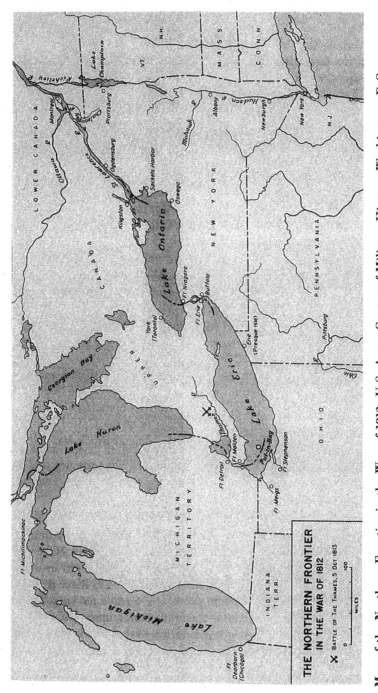

THE NORTHERN FRONTIER
IN THE WAR OF 1812

X BATTLE OF THE THAMES, 5 OCT 1813

0   100
MILES

Map of the Northern Frontier in the War of 1812. U.S. Army Center of Military History, Washington, D.C.

tacked the British ship *Royal George* and the batteries at Kingston. During this action the guns of some of Chauncey's ships were dismounted and shots were fired through the sails. Two received damage to their hulls. One man was killed and eight others were slightly wounded and treated on their individual ships.[3] In this action as well as other operations by Chauncey's squadron, Surgeon Buchanan was afloat. In anticipation that the British would retaliate and attack Sacket's Harbor, Chauncey issued a general order on December 4, 1812, forbidding any officer or man from sleeping out of his ship without a recommendation from the doctor and written permission from himself. Subsequently orders were issued that in the event of an attack, all fires, including those in the hospital, were to be extinguished.[4] Months passed, however, and the expected attack did not come.

During the winter months the ice on the lake prevented any naval activity, and to all intents and purposes, the war was in abeyance. But cold weather brought discomfort and sickness. In the case of officers, Chauncey usually granted them leave to recuperate among their friends or family. For the enlisted men winter meant an increase in the number on the sick report. The care of the sick seamen and marines was made more difficult when Buchanan's two assistants, Surgeon William Caton and Surgeon's Mate Andrew B. Cook, became ill themselves. As a result, Buchanan attended to the hospital and the squadron without assistance for much of the time. Also, a new medicine chest was needed, and Chauncey sent Buchanan to Albany to get one; payment was to be made by the navy agent.[5]

By late January 1813, the number of sick marines had increased to such an extent that Chauncey was obliged to ask Brigadier General Richard Dodge of the New York State militia, who was then in command of the military force, for a sergeant, a corporal and 15 privates to act as sentinels for the squadron. Sickness continued to take its toll of the marines. By early March death and sickness had so reduced them that Chauncey had only 39 who were fit for duty. He said that the vessels on both Lake Erie and Lake Ontario required 300 marines in addition to those used as guards, and he asked the secretary to send him 200 more by spring.[6]

By March 12 the military forces had been increased by the arrival of troops under General Zebulon Pike. These and other troops under General Henry Dearborn were embarked on Chauncey's ships and transported to York (later Toronto), the capital of Upper Canada, where they landed on April 27. The Americans attacked and captured the town with the loss of 40 killed, including Pike, and over 200 wounded. The victors burned the the Parliament building, the residence of the lieutenant governor, and part of a barracks. The government printing presses were destroyed and some £2,000 taken from the public treasury. There was also some destruction of the property of individuals. After this the U.S. troops were taken to the Niagara River, where they were expected to move against the British forts in that area. Chauncey then brought his ships back to Sacket's Harbor. The treatment of the wounded during the operations against York caused Surgeon Buchanan a great deal of strain and fatigue, with the result that he was confined to bed for just over four weeks.[7]

Buchanan had scarcely recovered when he and his two assistants, Caton and Cook, had new demands made on their professional skills. Early in the morning of May 29, 1813, British troops under Sir George Prevost landed at Sacket's Harbor. They were met by U.S. regular army troops and militia, who, after the initial engagement, fell back to blockhouses and a fort, from which they disputed further British advances. While the British were coping with a blockhouse flanked by a log barracks and some fallen timber, there was confusion in the shipyard behind this defensive position. There a navy lieutenant, on being told that the battle was lost, set fire to the ships, naval barracks, and storehouses. The army commander was appalled to find a fire raging at his rear, but his troops held fast. Sir George Prevost decided against incurring further losses by continuing his attack, so he reembarked his forces. The U.S. troops offered no challenge to the departing British. Prevost's losses for the day were 48 killed, 195 wounded, and 15 missing. The Americans suffered about 100 casualties. But Sacket's Harbor, as well as the U.S. squadron, had been saved.[8]

Chauncey's squadron was absent bombarding British positions on the Niagara River prior to an army attack that captured Ft. George. A fresh attempt to invade Canada ended with the U.S. defeat at Stoney Creek. Meanwhile Chauncey learned of the attack on Sacket's Harbor and went in pursuit of the British squadrons, but it eluded him. The arrival of the British squadron with reinforcements after the defeat at Stoney Creek demoralized Dearborn's troops, and they retreated to Ft. George. Chauncey returned to Sacket's Harbor and to the work of rebuilding the base.[9]

Illness continued to weaken Chauncey's forces. In July 1813 he reported that the number of sick in his command varied from 10 to 20 percent and was frequently at the higher figure. At the time of this writing, his flagship, the *General Pike*, had more than 25 percent of its crew on the sick list. The following month Chauncey reported that more than 80 of the crew of the *Madison* were sick.[10]

It was anticipated that sooner or later the rival squadrons under Chauncey and Captain Sir James Lucas Yeo would meet in combat to determine which side would have supremacy on the lake. On August 7, 1813, Yeo's force moved up on the slightly superior U.S. squadron that was anchored off Ft. Niagara. Maneuvers and countermaneuvers followed. Chauncey's squadron was largely made up of schooners that were difficult to sail. That evening two of the U.S. schooners were struck by a squall and sank with an estimated loss of 53 lives. Two others were captured.[11] For two days the rival commanders watched each other's forces, but neither wished to risk battle. In the months that followed, each commander voiced a desire to meet in combat, but it was not to be. The lack of a decisive battle for the control of Lake Ontario worked in favor the British attempts to protect Canada from invasion. But the continued existence of a U.S. squadron also acted as a deterrent to British plans to carry the war to U.S. soil. Nevertheless, the lack of any significant naval activity tended to undermine the morale of ambitious officers and made them request assignments elsewhere.

In the meantime, Chauncey had pushed preparations on Lake Erie. He visited the navy base at Black Rock, near Buffalo, in December 1812, and the following month he transferred it to Presque Isle, which was located on a small bay across from the town that was subsequently known as Erie, Pennsylvania. Logistic considerations were the motivation for this change. It was easier to ship guns and supplies by road and water from Pittsburgh or Philadelphia to Presque Isle than to to carry them from New York to Black Rock or Sacket's Harbor. Master Commandant Oliver Hazard Perry was placed in charge at Presque Isle with instructions to supervise the completion of efforts to build a squadron in order to challenge British control Lake Erie. By the time Perry arrived near the end of March 1813, two brig corvettes, a clipper schooner, and three gunboats were already under construction. In addition to rushing ship carpenters to the area, the Navy Department was also busy assembling officers and men for Perry's squadron. Among the medical officers was Surgeon's Mate Usher Parsons, and the medical story of events at Presque Isle and on Lake Erie can best be seen through his letters and journal from those years.[12]

After studying medicine in Boston under Dr. John Warren, in February 1812 Parsons obtained a license from the Massachusetts Medical Society and began to explore opportunities for starting a practice. Discouragement over the small number of desirable openings available, as well as the outbreak of war, made Parsons consider a commission in the army. His application to the War Department was not accepted because, Parsons believed, he did not have enough friends to support it. He then learned that there might be opportunities in the navy. Accordingly, he wrote to his Congressman, Josiah Bartlett, and asked him to take his application to the Navy Department. Bartlett was happy to oblige. At first the secretary was inclined to return it on the grounds that there were no vacancies, but as he read the letters of recommendation, he was impressed. The secretary then ordered that Parsons be placed on a waiting list, and he told Bartlett that it was probable that his constituent would be called into service.[13]

Hearing that the frigate *John Adams*, then at Boston, was without a surgeon's mate, Parsons made a hasty trip to that city. When he arrived, the ship had already sailed, and he returned discouraged to Dover, New Hampshire. A few days later he received a letter from the secretary advising him that he had been appointed a surgeon's mate. Instructions were sent to Parsons about signing and returning his oath and about having a uniform made in anticipation of an active assignment. August brought him orders to report to the *John Adams* at New York. Parsons set out by stagecoach, reached New York about September 1, and joined the ship a few days later. Captain Isaac Chauncey visited the *John Adams* on September 20 to call for volunteers for a special assignment. Parsons promptly volunteered, and he soon found himself with a contingent of officers and sailors headed for Lake Erie. They began their journey with a trip up the Hudson River to Albany. The group had not traveled very far before the medical talents of Parsons were in demand. By the time they reached Albany, he had three men on the sick list for unspecified ailments. At Albany they followed the Mohawk River west. Midshipman Samuel Swartwout became ill and was left in the care of the Dutch settlers in Amsterdam.

When the naval contingent was near Utica, there was a great deal of disruption both in and around the column. The sailors had made enemies of farmers and townspeople by stealing from them. Also, the wagons carrying the men's possessions were uncovered, exposing them to damage from the weather and dust as well as to theft. This state of affairs made for discontent among the officers, sailors, and the wagoneers. The antics of the sailors were also putting a strain on discipline. Amid all of this, Parsons lost the keys to his medical chest and narrowly avoided a challenge to a duel by a midshipman over some perceived offense. Beyond Utica things improved. The wagoneers were paid off and new ones hired. Here also the road divided: one road led to Lake Ontario and on to Sacket's Harbor; the other, the one that Parsons and his group took, led to Buffalo and Lake Erie. On October 16, they reached the naval station at Black Rock, where they became part of the command under Lieutenant Samuel Angus.

Parsons had scarcely settled into his new environment when he was obliged to deal with various health complaints of sailors, most of them apparently due to fevers, which he treated with a solution of nitric acid and water. Other men suffered from dysentery, and he gave them large doses of calomel. Apparently all the sailors eventually recovered.

While some of these men were still convalescing, there were wounded soldiers to care for from the Battle of Queenstown Heights. This battle was the result of General Stephen Van Rensselaer's plan of a double attack. While one body of men was to cross the Niagara River and capture the village of Queenstown, another group of regular army men was to be taken by boat to Lake Erie and landed in the rear of Ft. George. If Ft. George and Queenstown were captured, it was believed, the British line of communication would be cut and their shipping driven from the mouth of the Niagara River. The Americans would have a foothold in Canada from which other attacks could be launched. In preparation for the double attack, regular army troops and the New York militia were assembled at Lewiston, across the river from Queenstown Heights. Additional regulars and militia were in Buffalo, as well as 250 sailors and 400 Indians.

However only the attack on Queenstown took place on October 13. Only a part of the force got across the river, captured the heights, and beat off two British counterattacks. The New York militia was supposed to reinforce them, but the men refused to cross the river. In the end the Americans on the heights were overwhelmed by superior British forces. Ninety Americans were killed, 900 surrendered, and an undetermined number were wounded. The wounded made it back across the river, where they were treated in both army and navy hospitals.[14]

The large number of patients meant that navy medical men at Black Rock had to divide their time between their camp and a lower and upper hospital. On one day, Parsons treated 49 patients. He found that the care of the sick was taking all of his time. As their condition improved, the wounded were moved from the navy camp to a naval hospital, and then to an upper hospital, where they came under the care of the army. When a patient died, Parsons usually conducted what we would consider a limited autopsy to examine the wound or source of infection and the surrounding tissues, thereby enlarging his knowledge of the effects of disease and wounds.[15]

By this time, Brigadier General Alexander Smyth, the army commander at Buffalo, had decided that the forts and redoubts on the Canadian side of the lake should be destroyed before the main body of the army could attempt a crossing, and a group of volunteer soldiers and sailors was assembled. The attack took place on November 28, 1812, and the men making it immediately came under heavy fire. Within a few minutes the positions were carried. Guns were spiked and barracks were burned. Lieutenant Samuel Angus led 27 navy men in the attack, accompanied by a volunteer aide to General Smyth and navy Surgeon's Mate Joseph Roberts, who took a prisoner. When Angus found that most of his men were killed or wounded and that the anticipated reinforcements did not arrive, he gathered together the remnants of his force, including the wounded and some prisoners, and retreated across the lake. The affair cost the navy 4 killed, 12 wounded, and 1 captured. Angus sustained injuries to the head, which aggravated earlier damage suffered during the Quasi-War. Chauncey learned of the action when he arrived at Black Rock for an inspection on December 21. He was full of praise for Angus and his officers and men but thought that the dead had been sacrificed to little purpose. One immediate result was that Chauncey was left short of officers, and he made two of his midshipmen acting lieutenants.[16]

No sooner did the medical men have the wounded under control than they were confronted with an alarming outbreak of pleurisy. In the experience of Parsons, the only remedy for the disease was repeated bleeding, and amid his duties he found time to write a letter to the *Buffalo Gazette* setting forth his views on the treatment. A few weeks later he was gratified to receive a letter from a physician in Danville, Pennsylvania, complimenting him on his newspaper piece. The pleurisy cases began to decline by January 18. But the incidence of other ailments increased. In late December there were three cases of pneumonia. These showed improvement after a few days, but there was a fresh outbreak on January 9. There were also a few cases where the symptoms resembled typhoid fever. In late February, Parsons noted in his diary that while the number of men on the sick list was about 25, there were not 2 with ailments to which the same treatment could be applied.[17]

At noon on St. Patrick's Day, the British began firing cannon into the U.S. camp killing one man and wounding two or three. One of the wounded had to have his arm amputated, and Parsons did the job. The recovering man was then added to his patient load.[18]

During one month, Parsons saw the number of sick for whom he was responsible rise from 33 on March 25 to 51 on April 4, then decline to 33 by April 15 and to about 25 by mid-April. Parsons was too busy to record either what their complaints were or his methods of treatment. Many cases seem to have been related to dysentery. It was during this same period that one man died of suppurated lungs, and one from cholera morbus. Another, who had been ordered to Presque Isle, died en route. The cause of his death is not noted. Still another died of diarrhea.[19]

Summer brought new problems. The men were very unhealthy, but the nature of the illnesses is not known. Probably there were more cases of diarrhea, dysentery, and fevers. The number of sick men reached 70 on July 6. Perry himself became afflicted with "lake fever," but he continued to force himself to do his duties in getting his ships built. To care for the sick, a new hospital was opened in the county courthouse in Presque Isle.

This was a plain, two-story brick building with a cupola which was located in what is now the West Park section of Erie. Sails were stored in the upper rooms of the building and the downstairs space served as the hospital.

Later the number of men on the sick list made it necessary to establish two additional hospitals, one at the point of Misrey Bay and the other near Garrison Hill. These were probably tent hospitals or simple wooden structures designed to provide some shelter from the elements.[20] Meanwhile Perry had made great progress in building his squadron. When his ships were completed, he faced the problem of how to get them over the sand bar and into the lake. After all ballast had been removed, floats, or camels, were placed on each side of the ship and filled with water; when the water was pumped out, the vessel was lifted over the sand bar. By this means, Perry got the brigs *Lawrence* and *Niagara* into Lake Erie while the British squadron was away briefly in early August. The long-awaited manpower for his squadron arrived from Sacket's Harbor on August 10. With them came Commander Jesse D. Elliott, who became Perry's second in command, and who was placed in charge of the *Niagara*.[21]

Since June, Surgeon's Mate Parsons had been visiting and treating the sick men attached to the squadron, and once the *Lawrence* was in the lake, he was assigned to it. When the squadron made a practice cruise to the west end of the lake, Parsons became very ill but nevertheless had to care for a number of sick crewmen. Most of these men were inexperienced. General William Henry Harrison sent 30 or 40 army volunteers to help fill out the crews. Perry later claimed that his squadron had less than 100 first-class seamen and only 40 of these knew anything about guns. Among those who did were some veterans of the *Constitution*. But regardless of whether they had been to sea, all had to adjust to a new environment on the lakes. Meanwhile, one soldier who was acting as a marine died. For a brief period, Perry himself was sick with what was described as "bilious remittent fever." Many of the men had the same ailment.

In spite of these handicaps, the month of training proved to be most important for the history of the war on Lake Erie. Acting on General Harrison's suggestion, Perry now made Put-in-Bay, near present day Port Clinton, Ohio, his base. This enabled him to maintain close contact with Harrison's army and watch for the British squadron under Captain Robert H. Barclay. Proximity to the army also enabled Perry to replace the men who were sick. It has been estimated that ultimately Harrison supplied about 40 percent of the sailors and marines of Perry's squadron. Included in this figure were several officers and one doctor, W. T. Taliaferro.[22]

While Perry was preparing for battle, Parsons had to cope with growing numbers of sick men. Between September 2 and 5, his patient load rose from 26 to 57. Four days later he had the sole responsibility for the care of 87 men because the other medical men attached to the squadron were absent or ill. On the day that Parsons noted his enlarged patient load in his diary, Perry called his line officers together for a conference in which he explained the role that each ship would play in the coming battle for the control of Lake Erie.[23] More problems lay ahead for Parsons.

Just before dawn on September 10, the *Lawrence*, 20 guns, hoisted a signal that the enemy squadron had been sighted five or six miles away. Perry had already decided that his ship would engage Barclay's flagship, the *Detroit*, 19 guns. Other U.S. ships were assigned specific British ships to attack. As the squadrons moved toward each other, Perry saw that the *Detroit* was in the lead, and he ordered the *Niagara*, 20 guns, to shift its position in the line so that the two flagships could engage each other. It was Perry's strategy to bring all the short-range guns in his squadron to bear on the enemy and deny them the advantage of their long-range cannon. As the battle developed, most of the ships of the British squadron disregarded the other U.S. ships and concentrated their fire on the *Lawrence*.

The first shot from the *Detroit* fell short, but the second killed an American. Perry's first broadside fell short. For nearly two hours the *Detroit* and the *Queen Charlotte*, 17 guns, engaged the *Lawrence*. Perry's flagship took a terrific pounding: its rigging was shot away, its spars were splintered, its sails were reduced to tatters, and many guns were torn from their mountings. All of Perry's line officers were killed or wounded, as were about 80 percent of the crew. When the *Lawrence*'s guns became silent, the *Niagara* moved toward the front of the line, and a boat came from the *Lawrence* bearing Perry and four of his men. Perry transferred his flag to the *Niagara* and resumed the fight, and other U.S. ships became involved. About 2:40 P.M. the *Detroit* surrendered. The other British ships followed suit or were captured while trying to escape. Perry then returned to the *Lawrence* to accept the surrender of his foes. He stepped onto a deck that was slippery with blood and was met in silence at the gangway by a few who could walk and could be spared from other duties. On the deck were the bodies of 20 officers and men. Everywhere in the ship the groans of the wounded were heard.

Throughout the battle, Parsons had been valiantly tending the wounded of the *Lawrence*. Out of a crew of 150 men, 31 were sick before the battle. During the battle 7 were killed and 63 wounded. Working steadily, Parsons was able to put tourniquets on the wounds that were bleeding most freely and dressed about one-third of the wounded while the battle was in progress. He amputated six legs, and afterward these men were laid out on the berth deck. Here four of them died from cannon balls coming through the hull or from their wounds. Cannon balls also passed through the cockpit while Parsons was operating and came close to killing him and his patients. In general, he did what was immediately necessary to save a life. He gave his charges cordials, or alcoholic liquors, and anodynes, which contained opiates, and thus killed their pain and allowed them to sleep. In later years he realized that by delaying the operations until the patient's system had recovered from the shock of the injury, he had saved many lives.

Although the battle ended on the afternoon of September 10, there was no slackening of the demands on Parsons and little time to sleep. He was the only navy medical man on duty in the U.S. squadron. The next morning he resumed his work. Before breakfast he dressed the amputated leg of one of the men who had survived the previous day's operation and battle. He found that the adhesive plaster he had used on the stump was bad and he had to put in two sutures. After breakfast he amputated another leg. In this case, as in the one of the previous day, Parsons found that he had not applied the tourniquet tightly enough before he made his incisions. He made the necessary adjustments and continued. His next case involved the amputation of an arm. The patient had suffered a compound fracture of the humerus and the loss of some of the integuments. The doctor could not apply a tourniquet and had to resort to compression on the first rib to stem the flow of blood. After the bone was cut, he found that the artery had retracted so much that it took him 15 minutes to locate and secure it. The wound was then covered.

By Sunday, September 12, Parsons had finished dressing all the wounded in the *Lawrence,* and he turned his attention to the 23 who were hurt in the *Niagara.* The surgeon of the ship, Robert Barton, was still sick with fever and had not been able to attend to the men. To Parsons the most interesting case here was a quartermaster who had been wounded in the head. He removed several pieces of bone and a piece of leather (from the man's hat) from the cerebellum. While the patient was undergoing a trepanning operation, he began to sink. Parsons completed his work and dressed the wound as promptly as he could. Five days later the man died.

On Monday, September 13, the effects of his intensive labors caught up with him and he became ill. He called in the two British surgeons from the captured ships and conferred with them. They helped out with the U.S. wounded as well as their own. Parsons was highly pleased with them, as well as with the news that his amputation patients were doing well. The casualties of the battle for the Americans were 27 killed and 96 wounded; 22 of the dead and 61 of the wounded were in the *Lawrence.* According to Commander Barclay, the British losses were 41 killed and 94 wounded.

The next day officers from General Harrison's army came on board the

Lawrence, and an army surgeon helped Parsons with his patients. On Wednesday another army doctor, probably a militia officer, named Tull, made the rounds and conferred with Parsons about the treatment of the wounded, and Parsons felt well enough to prepare an official report on the wounded. News of the health of the men in the other ships in the squadron came from acting Surgeon Samuel Horsley, who was in low spirits, for while he was in the *Lawrence,* his illness had meant his missing a great battle. Parsons himself was not well and was unable to attend to all of his duties until 10 days after the battle. The army continued to lend a hand. On September 21, General Harrison came on board the *Lawrence,* bringing with him Hospital Surgeon John R. Martin, who consulted with Parsons about his most serious cases. The wounded of all the squadron were assembled on the *Lawrence,* which was used to transport them to Presque Isle. According to a later report, one of the patients died en route. We do know that 14 days after the battle, the wounded of the squadron were taken ashore at Presque Isle and placed in a large but unfinished courthouse. Here they remained until they recovered. Parsons continued to treat them until the end of the year, assisted by Dr. John C. Wallace, the first practicing physician of the city. Wallace had served as a medical officer in the army under Generals Anthony Wayne and James Wilkinson in the campaign against the Indians in 1794 and later in Kentucky. Early in the War of 1812, he commanded the local militia regiment. As a medical man with the longest experience in the area, he undoubtedly brought much expertise to his patients. Of the 96 wounded under the care of the two doctors, only 3 died.

In later years, Parsons offered this analysis of why so many of the wounded survived: "The recovery of so great a proportion of the wounded may in a great measure be attributed to the following causes: *First* to the purity of the air. The patients were ranged along the upper deck, with no other shelter from the weather than a high awning to shade them. They continued in this situation for a fortnight, and when taken on shore, were placed in very spacious apartments, well ventilated. *Secondly,* to the supply of food best adapted to their cases, as fowls, fresh meat, milk, eggs, and vegetables in abundance. The second day after the action, the farmers on the Ohio shore brought alongside every article of the above description that could be desired. *Thirdly,* to the happy state of mind which victory occasioned. The observations, which I have been able to make on the wounded of three engagements, have convinced me that this state of mind has greater effect than has generally been supposed; and that the surgeon on the conquering side will, *caeteris paribus,* always be more successful than the one who has charge of the vanquished crew. *Lastly,* to the assistance rendered me by Commodore Perry and Mr. Davidson. The latter gentleman was a volunteer soldier among the Kentucky troops, and engaged to serve on board the fleet during the action. After the action he rendered the wounded every aid in his power, continuing with them three months. And the Commodore seemed quite as solicitous for their welfare as he could possibly have felt for the success of the battle."[24] These reasons, as well as the aforementioned delay in operating on cases, resulted in a mortality rate of a little more than 3 percent.

After the battle, Perry shifted his flag to the *Ariel* and the captured British vessels *Queen Charlotte* and *Detroit* became hospital ships along with the *Lawrence*. The wounded were transported to Presque Isle. Parsons went ashore to treat the men transferred to the hospital in the courthouse. He was assisted by Dr. John C. Wallace, and they worked together at the courthouse hospital from November 1813 to January 1814.

In his reports on the battle of Lake Erie, Perry was full of praise for Parsons, and this was in large measure responsible for the doctor's promotion to surgeon in April 1814. Months before the promotion was officially confirmed, he was again ordered to the *Lawrence*. Leaving his quarters at the hospital at Presque Isle on January 19, he reported to his ship. Yet he still continued to care for some cases ashore, including a few civilians.[25]

Insights into the practice of medicine at Presque Isle after the Battle of Lake Erie can be found in the trial of Surgeon J. G. Roberts in December 1814, who was charged with neglect of duty, neglect of his patients, the want of proper respect and decorum to the commanding officer of the station, and unofficerlike conduct toward a midshipman. On the first charge, it was stated that Roberts was sent to Pittsburgh to get an assortment of medicines for the hospital. Instead he let the apothecaries give him several hundred dollars' worth of medicines that were useless or unsuitable for a naval hospital, as well as items that were damaged or unfit for use. Usher Parsons testified that among the items procured were two boxes of damaged chocolate and four female catheters. Under questioning, Parsons said that if they had to move any women or children, the female catheters might be useful. Dr. John C. Wallace, who was in charge of the naval hospital at Presque Isle, testified that in addition, Roberts had acquired worm medicine and $500 or $600 worth of damaged or useless medicines.

The second charge, that of neglect of his patients, brought out the information that the captured British vessels *Queen Charlotte* and *Detroit* had been converted to hospital ships. Surgeon's Mate John C. Richardson lived on board the ships with the patients and knew what was necessary for their comfort and recuperation. He reported to Roberts that some of the men needed bedding and clothing, but these items were not furnished. In his testimony for the defense, Lieutenant Edmund P. Kennedy said that some articles of clothing were not on hand when first requested and that the delivery of bedding might have been delayed by rain. Richardson said that instead of visiting his patients every day, Roberts frequently let two or three days go by, and so he, Richardson, rather than the surgeon, had to prescribe for the patients. Additional damming testimony came from Lieutenant Thomas Holdup Stevens, the commander of the *Lady Prevost*. He said that during the winter and spring of 1814, when Roberts was acting surgeon, he had so neglected the sick that in two instances Stevens was obliged to send patients ashore to prevent their suffering. The court also heard testimony that on one occasion Roberts told a patient that his life was not worth saving. In addition, Roberts was charged with threatening Surgeon's Mate Richardson and Surgeon Robert R. Barton if they reported his neglect of duty.

The third charge of unofficer like conduct had to do with Roberts allowing a midshipman to kick him without resisting. Since the midshipman died before the trial began, the court did not pursue the charge. Except for having two officers testify in his behalf, Roberts did little to defend himself. The court found him guilty of the first and second charges and sentenced him to a six-month suspension and the forfeiture of pay. By the time the verdict was rendered, the war was over. Roberts resigned from the navy on May 30, 1815.[26]

A discussion of Roberts's case has taken us beyond the war, and we must now return to the strategic situation on the Niagara front. Perry's victory gave the Americans the control of Lake Erie and focused attention on the quest for the control of Lake Ontario and the war on the Niagara frontier. In the spring of 1814, the British squadron blockaded Oswego and Sacket's Harbor. When Chauncey tried to shift guns and other supplies from Oswego to Sacket's Harbor by boats moving along the shoreline which were protected by riflemen and friendly Indians, they were attacked by 200 seamen and marines from the blockading force. Although surprised, the Americans rallied, killed 18 and wounded 50 of the enemy, and forced the surrender of the remainder. This loss of men weakened the British and they ended their blockade. During the summer of 1814 the U.S. army captured Ft. Erie and won a foothold in Canada. But without the control of Lake Ontario, they could not move against Ft. George. In the end, sickness among the American troops forced the withdrawal from Ft. Erie and the Canadian side of the Niagara River.[27]

Although the naval battle for the control of the Lake Ontario never took place as Chauncey and others expected, the medical staff had to care for a number of sick men. Surgeon Buchanan asked for and received extra compensation for his services. In late November 1813 it occurred to him that he had never received a confirmation of his appointment from the secretary of the navy. He brought the matter to Chauncey's attention, who, in turn, took it up with Washington. In fact, the Senate had confirmed Buchanan on December 21, 1812, and the secretary had notified him the following February, but the letter was lost. This was reassuring news to Buchanan, as were the efforts of the secretary to see that Chauncey had enough medical help.[28]

Perhaps it was the experience of not having formal notice of his commission that made Buchanan feel insecure. He complained to Chauncey in December 1813 that falsehoods were circulating in the area that were detrimental to his reputation. Chauncey expressed surprise that there was anybody in the squadron who would do such a thing and assured Buchanan that his professional talents were so high as to need no encomium from the commodore. Nevertheless, Chauncey said that he was "much flattered" by having the doctor serve with him. Presumably Buchanan's feelings were soothed by this statement of support.[29]

A more serious threat to Buchanan appeared at Sacket's Harbor on June 1, 1814, in the person of Surgeon George Davis. Appointed in 1799, Davis was one of the senior surgeons in the navy. It will be recalled that he accepted an appointment as the U.S. charge d'affaires at Tunis in 1803 and that he subsequently served as the U.S. consul at Tripoli. Apparently he did not resign his navy commission when he became an officer of the State Department and no official insisted that he do so. After his diplomatic service, he was on leave for a time, but the wartime demand for surgeons brought him back into active service, and he was sent to help Chauncey.

When he arrived at Sacket's Harbor, he was under the impression that he would succeed Buchanan as hospital surgeon, although his orders did not state that. Chauncey wrote to the secretary that while Davis had the earlier commission, he had not served as a doctor for the past 12 years. Buchanan, on the other hand, had served as a surgeon in 1800–1801 and had been released from service at the end of the Quasi-War. The secretary had offered to reinstate him in 1803, but he had declined. Yet when Chauncey needed him for duty as Sacket's Harbor, he willingly left his position at Columbia and the New York almshouse and reentered the navy. Chauncey's arguments were favorably received by the secretary, who was offended by the pretensions of Davis. It so happened that Davis had mentioned a desire for a leave of absence. The secretary reprimanded Davis for his pretensions and placed him on leave. He was destined never to be on active duty again. The departure of Davis ended any threat to Buchanan's position.[30]

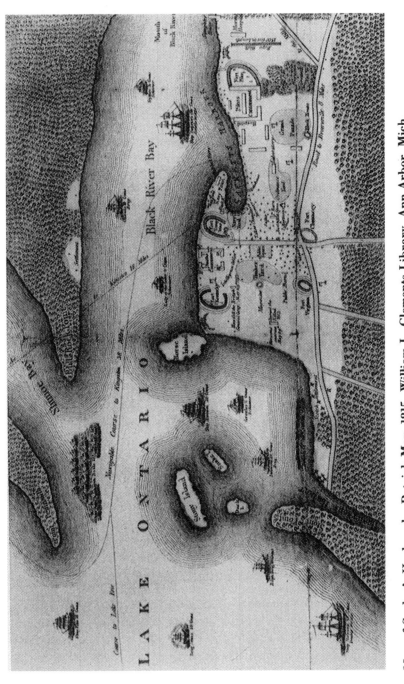

Map of Sacket's Harbor, by Patrick May, 1815. William L. Clements Library, Ann Arbor, Mich.

By this time the strengthening of British forces at Kingston, in Upper Canada, seemed to be a prelude to a more aggressive policy. Anticipating a threat in that area, in May the secretary had transferred the whole crew of the frigate *Congress* to Chauncey's command. Buchanan and his medical assistants dealt with routine cases for most of the war. Unfortunately we do not have information on the total number of men treated on that station or on the number of fatalities. We do know that it became necessary for the government to buy additional land, at Sacket's Harbor, on which a new hospital was erected in 1814. It was a two-story wooden structure that rested on supports and had no cellar. It seems likely that the floor closest to the ground was cold during the winter months.[31]

Veteran British troops arrived from Europe in the summer of 1814, and his superiors wanted Lieutenant General Sir George Prevost to attack both Sacket's Harbor and Plattsburg, on Lake Champlain. Prevost argued that he did not have the strength to do both, so he decided on Plattsburg. Up to this time there had been little activity on the Lake Champlain front. A British squadron was built on the lake and place under the command of Captain George Downie of the Royal Navy. It consisted of his flagship, the frigate *Confiance*, 38 guns, the brig *Linnet*, 16 guns, the sloops *Chubb*, 11 guns, and *Finch*, 10 guns, and 12 gunboats or row gallies. When Prevost's army moved down the west or Vermont side of the lake, Downie's ships accompanied it.

In Plattsburg Bay they found the U.S. squadron under Commodore Thomas Macdonough anchored in a north-south line that ran parallel to the army's defensive position below Plattsburg. Macdonough's force consisted of his flagship, the *Saratoga*, 26 guns, the brig *Eagle*, 20 guns, the schooner *Ticonderoga*, 17 guns, the sloop *Preble*, 7 guns, and 10 gunboats mounting a total of 16 guns. Sir George Prevost ordered a joint attack on the Americans: the British army was to ford the Saranac River and attack the American troops from the front and rear while Downie's squadron moved against Macdonough.

As Downie moved up Plattsburg Bay, the wind changed and he could not align his ships as planned. Instead the *Confiance* anchored some 300 yards from Macdonough's line and fired a broadside into the *Saratoga* which killed or wounded approximately one-fifth of the crew. Shortly thereafter a shot from the *Saratoga* killed Downie. The *Linnet* anchored and, assisted by the *Chubb*, attacked the *Eagle*. The *Finch* and most of the British gunboats engaged the *Ticonderoga* and the *Preble*. As the morning wore on, the *Finch* was disabled, drifted to Crab Island, in the bay, and was attacked and forced to surrender by a battery manned by the U.S. sick. The *Chubb* drifted out of control. Under fire from British gunboats, the *Preble*

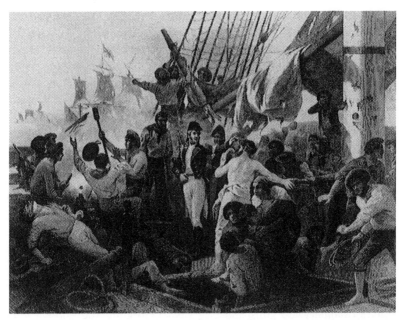

Battle of Lake Champlain. Library of Congress, Washington, D.C.

drifted ashore. The *Eagle* moved and anchored between the *Confiance* and *Ticonderoga*. During this time, Macdonough's ship had been badly battered, but he managed to turn it and bring his port guns against the *Confiance*. This, together with fire from the *Eagle*, forced the British ship to strike its colors. The *Saratoga* then turned its attention to the *Linnet*, and within 15 minutes it surrendered. The British gunboats fled. Macdonough's victory forced Prevost to break off his attack on the U.S. army and retreat to Canada with his forces.

The victory cost Macdonough 52 killed and 58 wounded; British losses were over 80 killed and 100 wounded. Macdonough was very short of medical assistance for his squadron. The *Saratoga's* surgeon was Dr. John P. Briggs of the army's Thirty-Third Infantry regiment. Because of the way in which the *Saratoga* was constructed, Briggs had to place the wounded on the berth deck, abreast of the mainmast, where he and they were exposed to shot. While he and his assistant, John Smart, were lifting a wounded man, Smart was killed by a round and Briggs was wounded by a splinter in his left leg and ankle. Nevertheless he continued to treat the wounded and did not report his wound after the battle because he thought it of no consequence. But attending the wounded kept him continually on his feet, and shortly after the battle he became lame and was subsequently permanently disabled by his wound. Dr. Briggs's diligence won the praise of Macdonough, who stated that the doctor's scientific knowledge saved the lives of a number of men. Also mentioned in Macdonough's report for their unremitting attention to the wounded were Surgeon's Mate Gustavus R. Brown of the navy and Dr. Stoddard of the army. Since he was close to shore facilities, Macdonough had no difficulty in transferring his wounded to more comfortable quarters on shore. All of the British wounded were assembled and taken across the Canadian border to the Isle aux Noix in the Richelieu River, where they could receive proper medical treatment.[32]

The British government had anticipated that their campaigns in 1814 would result in victory and would make it necessary for the Americans to accept peace terms that would involve the loss of territory and restrictions on commercial activity. Instead the reverses at Baltimore and Lake Champlain and the inconclusive results on the Niagara frontier, coupled with political and military problems in Europe, made the British agree to a peace that was very favorable to the Americans. The Treaty of Ghent was signed on Christmas Eve, 1814, but the news did not reach the United States until February 1815. It took many months for the war to wind down in all areas and for the return of prisoners. The United States narrowly avoided losing the war, but the favorable peace terms, together with the news of Jackson's victory at the Battle of New Orleans, gave rise to popular feelings that the war had been waged successfully. On the whole, the navy emerged with an enhanced reputation. No longer was there any doubt about is continued existence.

Cartel Ships

Medical officers also served on the cartel ships used to exchange prisoners of war. The treatment of the sick was stipulated in article 4 of the cartel agreement of 1813 between the United States and Great Britain. All paroled prisoners who were sick were to receive double their monetary allowance for subsistence as long as "the surgeon shall certify the continuance of such sickness." If the prisoner was suffering from an extreme illness, the attendance of a nurse was allowed. Other than that article, there were no specific provisions for the care of the sick and wounded during the transfer process. When the British prisoners were being moved from a place of confinement to a cartel ship, they were first placed in the custody of a U.S. marshal or his deputy. Those officers drew upon local physicians as needed, and they treated men in prisons, or when necessary, in local hospitals or private homes. The New York City Hospital, the Charleston Marine Hospital and the Savannah poorhouse provided such care.[33]

Upon receiving instructions from the Department of State, the Navy Department purchased the first cartel ship in December 1812. This was the brig *Analostan,* built in Talbot County, Maryland, in 1810, and measuring 94½' long, with a breadth of 24' 2" and a depth of 10' 1". It had one deck, two masts, and a square stern and could carry 200 tons of cargo. Its configuration did not allow for much movement of many humans, but the anticipated voyages would be short. A commissioned navy officer, Master William F. Smith, was placed in charge of it. The following spring a second cartel ship, the *Perseverance,* of 315 tons, was purchased and placed in service. Built in Philadelphia in 1791, it had two decks, three masts, and a square stern and was 93½' long, with a breadth of 28' and and a depth of 14'. Although similar in size to the *Analostan,* the *Perseverance* had a second deck that offered additional protection in times of bad weather. Its command was given to Master Joseph H. Dill. Both Smith and Dill had been taken prisoner early in the war and thus had personal experience of the plight of the captives. Though both captains were naval officers, they were under the authority of the Commissary General of Prisoners. The same was true of other officers assigned to the ships, including the surgeon's mates.

After an exchange of prisoners had been negotiated, the Commissary General would notify the appropriate captain of the cartel ship of the port at which the prisoners would board, the planned date of departure, and the destination. The captain would then begin the task of manning the vessel. Men were enlisted for the regular naval service but were discharged after the completion of each exchange. This practice saved money between exchanges, but it became increasingly difficult to get crews as the war went on. Additional pay for cartel duty was one attempt to resolve the problem. Before sailing, the cartel ship had to take on provisions, clothing, water, hospital stores, and a medical chest. In April 1813, Surgeon's Mate Leonard Osborne was ordered to the *Analostan,* and his colleague of the same rank, William C. Whittelsey, to the *Perseverance.*[34]

When he reported, Whittelsey learned that the ship would depart with 200–300 British prisoners and return with 400–500 Americans. The latter were coming from what Whittelsey considered "an unhealthy climate" where they were confined and constricted, and there were probably numerous invalids, who would be traveling on the ship in an inclement season. Whittelsey argued that he needed a surgeon or another assistant for this duty, which was equal to or greater than that performed by a surgeon and two mates in a frigate. If he was to act as a surgeon, he thought he should be paid as one. The secretary informed the doctor that the Commissary General of Prisons would give him such extra compensation as his duties entitled him to.[35]

When he completed the exchange, Whittelsey again wrote to the secretary about the cartel duty. He was pleased to report that most of the prisoners were healthy and that he had not lost a patient, but he doubted that he would be so lucky in the future. Whittelsey asked to be relieved of this duty. "I do not consider my age (which is but 20) or experience authorizes me to continue [in] a station where I must necessarily have charge of such a number of men laboring under the most inclement diseases—When I entered the navy I had not an idea that a Surgeon's Mate was expected to do the duty of a Surgeon." He went on to say that he got his commission immediately after he received his medical diploma, and his duties at the Philadelphia Navy Yard and in gunboats in the Delaware gave him very limited experience. The doctor's words brought a quick response. He was relieved of his cartel duties and transferred to the Washington Navy Yard, where he worked with Surgeon's Mate John Harrison and was once again under Cutbush's authority.[36]

Leonard Osborne, the surgeon's mate attached to the cartel ship *Analostan,* was a little older and had more experience than Whittelsey. He had served as a mate under Surgeon Bailey Washington in the frigate *Congress.* Whether he shared Whittelsey's apprehension about his assignment is unknown, but he was confronted with a serious health problem in the fall of 1814. At that time the *Analostan* had gone to Jamaica to pick up 170 Americans, who were delivered to Savannah. There the ship was cleaned, fresh provisions were taken on board, and preparations were made to carry British prisoners to Halifax. But before this could be done, the "sickly season" began in Savannah and some of the British prisoners died. Fearful for the health of his crew and believing that the recent British attack on Washington might cause delays in getting a passport for his next voyage, Captain Smith wanted to expedite plans. The local marshal was afraid that after burning Washington, the British might attack Savannah and was anxious to be rid of the British prisoners. Therefore 104 prisoners and 6 noncombatants were placed on the *Analostan,* and the ship sailed on September 8, 1814.

The next day, Surgeon's Mate Osborne, four of the crew, and several of the prisoners were reported to be sick. Three days later the captain had the berth deck and the hold cleaned and sprinkled with vinegar as a precautionary measure. A close watch was kept over the sick. A day out of Halifax, one of the crew died of what was described as "Savannah fever." The following day the prisoners and noncombatants were landed at Halifax. Seven members of the crew and one of the guards were now sick with fever. A second crew member died on September 24, and a third the next day. On September 27, the *Analostan* sailed from Halifax. A fourth died on the 30th, but the rest of the sick seemed to be recovering. A fifth crew member died on October 5. These deaths were making serious inroads into the strength of the small crew, so on October 10 the captain dropped anchor off Providence, and the ship was placed in quarantine. Later, after the war, the *Analostan* made another trip to Halifax to return British prisoners and one to England to repatriate American prisoners from there.[36]

In conclusion, it should be noted that though Osborne's experiences were unusual, cartel duty had its own share of problems, and the doctors assigned to it were often overworked.

Medical Statistics

At the end of the war, there were 53 surgeons and 75 surgeon's mates on the rolls of the navy. Of this number, 14 surgeons and 68 mates were appointed during the war. The largest increase came in July 1813, when 22 were commissioned and 8 promoted. Of the 82 medical men commissioned during the war, the state or district of origin has been established for 80. These are: New York, 18; Maryland, 13; Massachusetts, 12; Virginia, 8; Pennsylvania and South Carolina, 5 each; Connecticut, 4; the District of Columbia, New Hampshire, and Kentucky, 3 each; New Jersey, 2; and Georgia, Louisiana, North Carolina, and Delaware, 1 each. Demands for experienced medical men resulted in the promotion of 18 surgeon's mates to surgeon in the course of the conflict. During the war 6 surgeons and 2 mates died, but none as the result of enemy action. Despite the wartime situation and occasional shortages of medical men at various stations, the secretary accepted the resignations of 2 surgeons and 6 mates.

In his study of navy casualties, Louis Roddis estimated that 265 navy men and 45 marines were killed and 439 navy and 66 marines were wounded during the War of 1812. Records of the marine corps show that 6 officers and 335 enlisted men died during the War of 1812. Three of the officers and 39 of the men were killed in action; 4 died of wounds; 16 were missing in action; and another 16 were lost in ship disasters. Eleven of the enlisted men were drowned; 2 were executed following the sentences of courts-martial. This leaves 247 unexplained deaths, and of that total, 28 died at Sacket's Harbor, probably of disease.[37] It now seems likely that there were at least 300 combat related deaths. Accidents probably accounted for at least another 100 diseases of all kinds for as many as 300. In this as in other early U.S. wars, there were undoubtedly many who died of the effects of wounds who are not recorded in pension records.

Chapter 12

Toward a More
Professional Service

The navy emerged from the War of 1812 with a greatly enhanced reputation. Wartime frigate duels had captured the public's imagination and raised its morale. While such victories did not change the strategic balance or end the blockade, they offered a sharp contrast to apparent lack of progress by most of the army. At the end of the war, there was no longer any danger that the navy would be abolished. Under William Jones much had been done to make the operations of the Navy Department more efficient, and Congress had granted Jones's request to create a body of professional advisors to the secretary. The Board of Navy Commissioners was established in February 1815 consisting of three navy captains who, upon request, would provide specialized knowledge and recommendations to the secretary. Very early in the relationship, the secretary established that he would control the movement of ships and matters relating to the appointment, assignment, and promotion of individuals.[1] On matters pertaining to medicine and health, it was the normal practice to refer to Surgeon Edward Cutbush at the Washington Navy Yard for his recommendations. If necessary or desirable, the views of senior surgeons at other stations might be solicited.

Postwar demands on the navy meant that the members of the board had to address a number of questions. Operations against the British had scarcely been completed when it became necessary to send a naval force against Algiers to put a stop to the plundering of U.S. ships which began during the War of 1812. Captain Stephen Decatur departed from New York with 10 ships in May 1815, captured 2 Algerian warships, and sailed into the harbor of Algiers, where he forced the dey to renounce further molestation of U.S. commerce. All U.S. prisoners were released without the payment of ransom. When his work was completed in Algiers, Decatur extracted similar guarantees from Tunis and Tripoli. Thereafter the United States maintained a naval presence in the Mediterranean to protect its commerce and offer support to its diplomats and consuls when necessary.[2]

To strengthen this ability to protect commerce and to meet any potential foreign threats to the nation, Congress passed a law in 1816 for the gradual increase of the navy. Over a six-year period, nine 74-gun ships of the line, twelve 44-gun frigates, and three steam-propelled floating batteries for harbor defense would be built. It looked as though there would be many opportunities for all grades of officers to enjoy peacetime service in large ships.[3]

This optimistic outlook was undermined in part by the results of a financial depression known as the Panic of 1819. Several factors brought on the depression, including speculation in western lands, the mismanagement of the Second Bank of the United States, overextended investments in manufacturing, the collapse of foreign markets for U.S. goods as British trade recovered from the Napoleonic Wars, and the contraction of credit. The development of the American West following the War of 1812 led to an increased demand for federal services including roads, military posts for defense, and mail services. Also, the desire of Missouri to enter the Union in 1819 raised the question in the Senate of the sectional balance between free and slave states and the wider matter of the expansion of slave states. The result was the political solution known as the Missouri Compromise, which maintained the balance in the Senate by admitting Maine as a free state along with Missouri, where slavery was legal. A line was drawn at 367 30': all future states created north of it would be free; slavery would be permitted south it. In fact, the demands of the West and South worked against the idea of building a large peacetime navy. Beginning in 1821, the appropriations for the navy were steadily reduced. Postwar naval operations also tended to undermine the argument in favor of large ships, for new threats to the nation's maritime commerce came not from Europe but from the Far East and the West Indies.[4]

The search for markets led American merchants to the Orient, and the navy followed. In 1818 the small frigate *Macedonian* sailed from Boston to protect U.S. interests in the Pacific. It stopped in Valpariso and other Chilean ports, and in Peru before being relieved by the *Constellation*. The cruise of the *Macedonian* marked the beginning of the U.S. Navy's Pacific Station, and in 1821 the ships assigned to that region became known as the Pacific Squadron. When the *Macedonian* reached Boston in June 1821 after a cruise of two and one-half years, it had lost 26 of its original force of slightly more than 400 officers and men. Four had been lost overboard, 19 had died of various ailments, 1 was killed in a duel, 2 were killed and 5 wounded when Spanish troops fired on a market boat that was unwisely sent ashore during clashes between Peruvian patriots and the Spanish during Peru's struggle for independence.[5]

As part of the independence movement in Latin America, patriot leaders commissioned privateers to prey on Spanish commerce. Sometimes this degenerated into piracy, and the pirates operating in the West Indies now became the concern of the U.S. Navy. Pirates were attracted by the volume of commerce in and out of New Orleans and the growth of shipping in the Gulf of Mexico which resulted from the settlement of southern Georgia and Alabama and the acquisition of Florida by purchase from Spain in 1819. There were many prizes for those who dared seize them. Commodore Patterson's small force operating out of New Orleans did what it could, but it was clear that a larger force was needed. So in 1822 the West India Squadron was established and placed under the command of Commodore James Biddle. It consisted of two frigates, four sloops, two brigs, four schooners, and two gunboats and was based at Thompson's Island (Key West), Florida. Between 1822 and 1829 the navy was engaged in efforts to eliminate the pirates in the West Indies. This was accomplished with relatively small losses in men. Biddle learned quickly that large ships were poorly suited for this work; sloops and other craft that could operate close to shore and in shallow water were what was required. Biddle was succeeded by Commodore Lewis Warrington, who, in turn, was followed by Lieutenant John D. Sloat. Some 1,300 officers and men were involved in the campaign to end piracy and safeguard U.S. commerce.[6]

New commercial opportunities opened in Latin America when the United States recognized the independence of the former Spanish colonies. As U.S. merchants began to explore the South American markets, they looked to the navy to protect their commerce. President James Monroe's pronouncements about the Western Hemisphere in 1823, which came to be known as the Monroe Doctrine, represented an attempt to forestall any plans by European nations to restore Spanish power. The British were also opposed to any intervention, and the real strength behind the Monroe Doctrine was the Royal Navy. But the duty of protecting U.S. commerce in South American waters became the responsibility of warships that cruised off the Pacific and Atlantic coasts of that continent.[7]

Additional responsibilities were given to the navy in 1820 when Congress passed a law declaring that the foreign slave trade was piracy and those involved in it were subject to the death penalty. Beginning that year, U.S. warships returning from the Mediterranean were ordered to sail by way of the West African coast and then to the West Indies. This solution did not work, and in 1821 the schooner *Alligator* was ordered to West African waters to search for slavers flying the U.S. flag. While on that assignment, Lieutenant Commandant Robert Field Stockton, the captain of the *Alligator,* moved the colony established by the American Colonization Society for former slaves from an unhealthy site on the island of Sherbro to Cape Mesurado, where Monrovia, Liberia, is now located. Stockton's successors cruised off the west coast of Africa, but the size of the forces assigned were inadequate to accomplish the announced goal. However, these cruises did expose U.S. crews to tropical diseases.[8]

To deal with the problems and challenges of the postwar world, the Navy Department needed a strong and decisive man to manage it for a period of years. Instead it had three heads in the first eight years of the postwar period. Benjamin Crowninshield served from January 1815 to September 1818. His successor, Smith Thompson, did not assume his responsibilities until January 1, 1819. During this long interval Captain John Rodgers, the president of the Board of Navy Commissioners, acted as secretary. Although Thompson was responsible for taking action against the West Indian pirates and extended the navy's cruising grounds to the Caribbean, the coast of Africa, and South America, and while he had an interest in the education of midshipmen, his tenure was characterized by absenteeism. The administration of the Navy Department improved dramatically when Samuel Lewis Southard took over on September 16, 1823. His tenure lasted until the change in administrations on March 4, 1829. The presidency of Andrew Jackson brought new leaders, whose impact on the navy and on medicine will be treated in a subsequent chapter. It is against the background of political, economic, and naval activity during the years 1815–30 that we must now consider the efforts of navy doctors to improve their status and the state of health of the service.[9]

Rank, Pay, and Discipline

The War of 1812 on the lakes and at Washington, Baltimore, and New Orleans had given navy doctors an opportunity to observe the way in which medicine was practiced in the army. They saw a system in that service and in the British navy which had features they admired, especially in regard to rank and pay, and they began to work to improve their own service. Regulations for hospitals had been drawn up by a group of navy surgeons in 1812 and were forwarded to Congress. The subject was referred to a committee, which acted upon the suggestions and sent a bill to the House with amendments. There the matter died. Cutbush raised the issue with

Secretary Jones in February 1813, pointing out that his experience at the small temporary hospital at New Castle had confirmed for him the need for a code of rules and regulations.

It was also desirable that hospital surgeons in the navy have the same rank as their army counterparts. Army surgeons were paid more than those in the navy. In the British navy pay and responsibility increased in accordance with the number of years served and rate of the ship to which a doctor was assigned. When a man was transferred from a sloop of war to a frigate, it was considered a promotion. A surgeon ranked with a lieutenant and an army captain but was subject to the orders of a line lieutenant. There was also the matter of the public image of navy surgeons. "I can assure you," said Cutbush, "that the description of a naval surgeon, by the pen of the celebrated Dr. Smollett in his Roderick Random, has prevented many men of professional abilities from entering our service, under an idea that the surgeons and mates were considered in the same menial situation, and I must add that the pay is not a sufficient inducement. There is scarcely a village in the U.S. where a practitioner of medicine and surgery, does not received a greater compensation than a naval surgeon."[10] Despite his eloquence, Cutbush does not seem to have moved Secretary Jones. But even if Jones had been determined to act, the year 1813 was one in which the financial health of the nation reached a dangerously low point. The United States could not have afforded a pay raise then in the midst of war.

After things improved on the war and financial fronts, there were transitions in the leadership of the Navy Department. William Jones resigned as secretary in the fall of 1814 and left office on December 1. Eighteen days later Benjamin W. Crowninshield of Massachusetts succeeded him. He soon found himself caught up in problems relating to medicine in the navy.

Late in January 1815, Surgeon Cutbush sent Crowninshield a letter calling his attention to the differences between the medical departments of the army and navy. Cutbush noted that a regimental surgeon in the army received $60 a month plus three rations a day and forage for his horse. His counterpart in the navy was paid $50 a month and two rations a day. Mates were also better provided for in the army. Aside from regimental surgeons, the army service consisted of 1 surgeon and physician general, 1 apothecary general, 11 assistant apothecaries, 20 hospital surgeons, and 35 hospital mates; there was also legal authorization for stewards, matrons, ward masters, and nurses. Each regiment was authorized 1 surgeon and 2 mates, the same as a frigate. These medical men were part of a force whose authorized strength was 62,448. According to the estimates for 1815 which were presented to Congress, the naval force including marines was set at 17,293 officers and men. For this force, 50 surgeons and 80 surgeon's mates were allowed. There was no provision for any higher grades, even for those who were designated as hospital surgeons. The army made no deductions from pay for hospitals, but its sick and wounded were amply provided for there. If the authorized strength of the navy was met during the present year, wrote Cutbush, a considerable sum would be taken from the pay of navy men, but a system of naval hospitals had yet to be established.

Under the act of Congress passed in 1811, commissioners of navy hospitals were to be appointed and were to establish hospitals. While some temporary hospitals were functioning, there was no provision for appointing hospital surgeons, mates, stewards, or others. He himself, Cutbush noted, had been acting as a hospital surgeon and physician at the Washington Navy Yard, at the marine garrison, and for the ships in ordinary. He had no steward and as a result had to keep the accounts and receipts of expenditures for provisions and hospital stores. Cutbush did not believe that these were the proper duties of the physician and surgeon. In the army the person who did this work was paid $26 a month and two rations. Secretary Jones had authorized the payment of an additional $400 a year for Cutbush for superintending medical stores. The surgeon of the New York station was given $500 a year for examining and taking care of the accounts for apothecary stores.

There was also the matter of the care of pensioners. Under the act of 1811, pensioners could live at navy hospitals if they gave up their pensions. But since the maximum pension of a man was half the monthly pay while on active duty, the sums surrendered did not meet the amount spent for food. Also, there was no provision for clothing.[11]

Cutbush's effort was followed in February 1815 by one from Surgeon Samuel Marshall, who asked permission to come to Washington to discuss the hospital situation at the navy yard in New York. The Board of Navy Commissioners asked the secretary to order Marshall to Washington to consult with other surgeons, and Crowninshield complied. Similar orders went to Surgeon Heap at Philadelphia and Cutbush in Washington. When they met in Washington, the surgeons found that virtually everything that needed to be said about the need for navy hospitals had already been said. They decided that their first order of business would be to examine the quality of the medical men in the navy.

Marshall went to see Crowninshield and asked for the letters of recommendation which had been sent to the Navy Department on behalf of those who were appointed surgeons and surgeon's mates. Crowninshield turned the letters over to Marshall except in the cases of eight men, and he included the letters of recommendation for those currently seeking appointments. These letters gave the surgeons information about the professional backgrounds of their medical colleagues. The only other person who had an equivalent knowledge of both medical and line officers was Charles Goldsborough, who had served as the chief clerk in the Navy Department since Secretary Stoddert's day. Armed with details about the education, training, and experience of their colleagues, Marshall, Heap, and Cutbush were well equipped to argue the case for changes in the rank and pay of medical men in the navy. When they had completed their work, Crownin-shield ordered them back to their respective commands in mid-June. By this time the Congress had adjourned until December 1815. The arguments for an increase in the pay of the medical officers and regulations for hospitals would be needed when Congress reassembled.[12]

Cutbush was the only one of the three-man surgical board who was still on the Washington scene, and it was up to him to keep up the fight. In May 1815 he wrote to Captain John Rodgers, the president of the Board of Navy Commissioners, in response to a request from that body, and reviewed the work he had done for Secretary Hamilton on a code of rules and regulations for hospitals. Experience since then indicated that some of the rules needed to be changed. One of them dealt with the need to furnish clothing to pensioners. It was also necessary that a surgeon's mate be in residence at the marine barracks in Washington in order to take care of the sick there and at the navy yard.

Something needed to be done to place the medical department on a more respectable footing in order to attract and hold qualified applicants. "The pay of a Naval Surgeon is too small," wrote Cutbush; "the door keeper of Congress receives double the amount and there is scarcely a clerk in any public office, who does not receive more." Once doctors were in the service, some inducements to stay needed to be offered, including such positions and titles as director of a medical department, or hospital or fleet surgeon, which, if they did not greatly increase the surgeon's income, would gratify his ambition. Navy doctors "ought to have a genteel support, such, at least, as almost any small village would yield to an attentive and industrious Surgeon." Rodgers and the other navy commissioners were sympathetic to Cutbush's arguments, and their support was important not only in terms of the secretary and the Congress but within the navy.[13]

Upon hearing that the medical officers of the navy intended to send a memorandum to the secretary asking for an increase in pay, a definite ranking in the service, and the establishment of the rank of hospital surgeon, a group of seven captains and six commanders wrote to the secretary to express their support. They declared that the rank and pay of medical officers ought to be in some proportion to what men of similar professional standing could earn in civilian life. These line officers said that by their "experience, knowledge, zeal and humanity" the medical men of the navy had won the esteem and confidence of all who were associated with them. Crowninshield forwarded these letters to the Senate Committee on Naval Affairs. Nothing seems to have come of this, and the surgeons decided that they must make their own case before Congress.[14]

Early in January 1817, Congressman John C. Calhoun of South Carolina had a conversation with Surgeon Samuel R. Marshall about a memorial, or petition, that the medical officers of the navy intended to present in a few days. Marshall talked about the situation of the medical officers, and Calhoun asked him to put the facts in writing. Marshall did so. First and foremost was the matter of rank, which was not in keeping with their education, learning, and professional exertions. He argued for the establishment of the rank of hospital surgeon. Next came the matter of pay and emoluments. Marshall pointed out that after deductions for the hospital fund, the salary and the value of the rations came to $802 a year for surgeons and $502 for mates. By contrast, the pay of the army surgeon was nearly double that. Thus informed about the nature of the surgeons' complaints, Calhoun was presumably in a better position than most of his colleagues to respond, but he does not seem to have done so.[15]

The formal memorial of Cutbush and Marshall on behalf of navy surgeons was presented to the House on January 9, 1817, by James Pleasants of Virginia, and it was referred to the Committee on Naval Affairs. The chairman of the committee asked the secretary for his views, and the latter replied that the pay and emoluments sought seemed to be reasonable and consistent with what prevailed in the army. On the matter of a definite rank, he recommended that it be limited to a number of the senior surgeons in the navy who had suffered privations and hardships and who did not have opportunities for acquiring property to maintain their families.[16]

The committee also sought the views of the Board of Navy Commissioners. Captain John Rodgers, the president, replied that the board believed that navy surgeons should receive the same pay and emoluments as their colleagues in the army. It also believed that as in the army, navy surgeons should be ranked in accordance with the date of their commissions. The only point in the surgeons' petition which the board believed had no merit was that relating to the disposition of prize money. Surgeons were classed with persons with whom they could not and did not associate. Rodgers pointed out that the classification was for the distribution of various sums and had nothing to do with any necessity of association.[17]

The surgeons' petition came up in committee on January 20, 1817, and the matter was suspended. The reasons are not known.

Whatever interest John C. Calhoun had in the matter apparently lapsed when he resigned his seat on November 3, 1817, and was appointed secretary of war less than a month later. Additional pleas for reform on the matters of entrance qualifications, pay, promotion, rank, prize money, and hospitals were made by Surgeon Thomas Chidester in letters to Representative Albion Parris of Massachusetts in November and December 1817 and January 1818. Chidester argued that no one should be allowed to enter the medical service of the navy unless he had a degree from a respectable medical institution and had received a certificate to practice medicine. No one should receive a commission as a surgeon unless he had served three years as a surgeon's mate. The pay and rations of surgeons and mates should increase by a prescribed formula in accordance with their years of service. Surgeons should have a share of prize money in their own right and not be classified with lieutenants for that purpose. All hospitals on shore for the navy or the merchant service should be open to the sick and wounded of the other service. The responsibility for navy patients would rest with the navy surgeon with the oldest commission and at least a year's service at sea.

Though some of these issues had been raised before, Chidester presented points in an organized fashion. One of his arguments was that navy doctors be allowed to charge men for treating them for venereal disease. These suggestions may have been forwarded to the House Committee on Naval Affairs. In the short run, however, nothing seems to have become of them for Representative Parris resigned his seat on February 3, 1818. Later that year Chidester met Representative John F. Parrott of New Hampshire at a social event in Portsmouth. Parrott told the doctor that he had been appointed to the committee and that it had before it a proposal on the rank and pay of navy surgeons. Chidester wrote him and gave him his suggestions and asked that Senator Harrison Gray Otis of Massachusetts be informed of them. This was done, and the Senate committee also received copies of Chidester's letter to Parris. It is possible that the surgeon's views may have influenced the shape of subsequent legislation. But in April 1818 the House committee was discharged from any further consideration of the petition of the naval surgeons, as well as from the resolution on the rank and emoluments of surgeons. So, by the spring of 1818, it was clear that the surgeons had not succeeded in convincing the Congress of the merits of their case in regard to rank and pay. Chidester was no doubt disappointed by the outcome, but he did not have long to bear this. He died in August of that year.[18]

Meanwhile the naval committees of the Congress considered the hospital question briefly. In response to an inquiry from the chairman of the

Senate committee, Crowninshield reported that the sums deducted from the pay of officers and seamen for the hospital fund had been absorbed into the general expenditures of the Navy Department. This had to be reimbursed by an additional appropriation. The matter remained pending for some time.[19] Next the chairman of the House committee asked for a list of the temporary hospitals then in use, their location and the names of the surgeons in charge of them. This was delivered in February 1817.

Later that same month, Surgeon William P. C. Barton published a second edition of his book, *Treatise on Hospitals,* but it is not known whether either edition was consulted by members of the naval committees. In March 1818 the chairman of the House committee requested and received a breakdown of the estimated annual cost of each of the naval hospitals in Boston, New York, Philadelphia, Washington, Charleston, and New Orleans from January 1811 through December 1816. This showed a total annual expense of $13,783.98. The report seems to have ended for a time the discussion of the need for permanent hospitals.[20]

But on health matters there was one encouraging development in regard to regulations. Under the act of Congress of February 7, 1815, establishing the Board of Navy Commissioners, that body was authorized, with the consent of the secretary, to prepare rules and regulations for the service to be delivered to the next session of Congress. With Secretary Crowninshield urging them on, the board undertook the task, and they completed it in 1817. Congress did not act upon the matter until 1819, and in February of that year the Senate asked for a report on how the new regulations varied from the existing laws.

Smith Thompson, Crowninshield's successor as secretary of the navy, sent his reply to the Senate on January 3, 1820, early in the Sixteenth Congress. Thompson urged the creation of some additional grades for naval officers including surgeons, suggesting that surgeons be divided into classes according to the rate of the ship in which they served. It would also be beneficial, he said, to designate some officer who would be placed at the head of the medical men who would "have the immediate superintendence of this branch of the service, under regulations for that purpose to be established." Although Thompson thought that such an arrangement would contribute much for the benefit of the service, his suggestion was not acted upon. Nor were the regulations prepared by the board enacted into law, but the navy observed them anyway. Several sections in this code related to medical matters and these will be noted in chapter 13.[21]

If progress in professional matters was discouraging to the medical men of the navy, there were still young doctors who wanted to enter the service. Many wrote to the Navy Department or had someone inquire for him about the possibility of a commission. The usual answer was that there were no vacancies, but a man's name might be placed on file in case any openings occurred. Soon the accumulation of applications made it probable that most of those waiting would never get a commission. In March 1817, Secretary Crowninshield told an applicant that "no rational hope can be entertained, that the appointment you solicit will be conferred on you, at least for a considerable time." By the fall of 1818, there were more than 200 applications in the pending file.[22]

Despite this gloomy outlook, political connections could do wonderful things. When Henry Clay, the speaker of the House of Representatives, recommended Dr. Samuel C. Smith as a surgeon in 1818, he was told that the entry level was at the rank of surgeon's mate. If Dr. Smith applied himself, he would probably be promoted. This message was passed on to the candidate, and he was assured that his name would be presented to the Senate for confirmation. Unfortunately, Congress did not confirm Smith formally until March 1820. The path to promotion was evidently too slow for him, and he resigned two years later.[23]

Timing and excellent endorsements worked to the advantage of Dr. Mordecai Morgan of Philadelphia. Despite the list of people who had applied ahead of him, his name was sent to the Senate three months after his initial inquiry. He was commissioned as a surgeon's mate in December 1818.[24] Morgan was obviously hopeful about the future despite the problems of pay, rank, and the care of the sick that faced the medical men of the navy.

By 1818 matters relating to the pay of medical officers had become a part of a larger discussion on the size, role, and mission of the navy. Only one of the ships authorized in 1816 had been launched. Members of Congress began to question the wisdom of building large ships when experience had shown that smaller ones were in demand. Economy and adaptability were necessary. The yearly average of naval appropriations declined from $3,700,000 during the years 1817–21 to $2,900,000 for 1821–25. These cuts were reflected in shipbuilding and the reduction of personnel on active duty. When President Monroe sent a plan for the naval peace establishment to Congress in 1823, it was referred to the House Committee on Naval Affairs for its recommendations.[25]

Meanwhile the House approved a resolution requesting the secretary to furnish it with the names of the surgeons and surgeon's mates on duty, together with their stations and the amounts of their compensation. Secretary Thompson replied promptly and included with the information a cover letter pointing out that in two or three instances, surgeons acted as purveyors and superintendents of medicines, hospital stores, and surgical instruments, and it was believed that the interest of the nation as well as of economy had been promoted by these arrangements. Thompson's reply was read and laid on the table the day it was received. A week later the House took up the report of the Naval Affairs Committee.

After examining the information available to it on the medical department of the navy, the committee concluded that "appointments in that branch of service have hitherto been made with too little discrimination, and that many have entered it, who, on due examination of their competency, would have been rejected." While the pay might be "sufficient to induce young practitioners to engage for a few years, with a view to avail themselves of the superior practical advantages to be found in the service," it was not enough to hold the most able and the most faithful. The committee recommended the adoption of those portions of Monroe's bill which would put the medical corps on "such a basis as comports with the true interests of the service."[26]

Before such a bill was adopted, the secretary received an intriguing proposal from Surgeon Thomas Harris in Philadelphia. Some of the younger surgeons and surgeon's mates there had expressed to him their anxieties about improving themselves professionally. Their modest pay prevented them from doing anything about it through a medical school. What was needed was a refresher course to prepare surgeon's mates for promotion. This meant lectures that were focused on navy medicine and surgery or on practical information that had an immediate application to their duties on ships and shore stations. Surgeons needed to acquire skill and proficiency in operations, as well as a better knowledge of anatomy, knowledge best acquired by working on cadavers. Harris knew that there were naval institutions in Europe which offered that kind of training, but there was nothing equivalent in the United States. The young navy doctors asked Harris to give a course of lectures along the lines described. He explored the idea with Thomas Hewson, a professor of comparative anatomy at the University of Pennsylvania, and other medical colleagues. He then wrote to the secretary of the navy requesting that he be authorized to give a series of lectures on nautical medicine, anatomy, and dissection. Harris would superintend all the work and furnish medical books and journals from his private library. Philadelphia would be an ideal location because of the medical school at the University of Pennsylvania, which would be a source of cadavers to be used for practicing surgery. Also, the navy students would have the privilege of attending some lectures at the medical school. Along with this proposal, Harris sent letters of recommendation for himself and the proposed lectures by Dr. Hewson, Dr. Nathaniel Chapman, professor of practical medicine, Dr. Samuel Jackson, professor of pharmacy, and

William Gibson, professor of surgery, all at the University of Pennsylvania, as well as letters from Surgeon Bailey Washington and Commodore William Bainbridge of the navy. Harris also enclosed a letter signed by three surgeons and two surgeon's mates urging him to institute such a course of lectures.[27]

Secretary Thompson thought Harris's idea had merit, and he gave it his approval and a grant of $400 to help get the school established. Harris searched for an appropriate house in which to conduct classes and found one in the central part of the city which rented for $250 a year. The doctor wanted make some alterations, but the landlord would not agree without a five-year lease. Harris estimated that if he had the work done at his own expense, it would cost about $100. Given the moderate rent, Harris asked for permission to rent it for five years. His letter reached the Navy Department when the secretary was away, and Captain John Rodgers, the acting secretary, replied that he did not feel that he could authorize any expenditures beyond the sum already approved.[28]

The school opened in 1823. Word about its program gradually spread, and surgeon's mates began to request leave to attend. One example of this trend was the case of Benajah Ticknor, who was attached to the frigate *Congress*, then at Norfolk. Ticknor asked his superior, Captain James Biddle, for permission to apply to the school. Biddle did not want him to leave the ship but consented to the course of lectures if the Navy Department would sent him another surgeon's mate. This was done, Ticknor attended the school, and he later went on to an honorable career in the navy. Within two years it was clear that the school was doing a great deal of good with a small amount of money.[29]

Before the value of the enterprise could be assessed, however, the Eighteenth Congress assembled for its first session in December 1823. The members heard President Monroe's message that set forth U.S. policy in regard to the Western Hemisphere, the Monroe Doctrine. Afterward the Congress considered various measures, one of which was a resolution introduced by John F. Parrott of New Hampshire instructing the Committee on Naval Affairs to look into the expediency of building an additional number of sloops of war for the navy. Subsequently the secretary of the navy reported that 10 new sloops were needed.

Another matter for the committee was the motion of Representative Charles F. Mercer of Virginia to inquire into the expediency of apportioning the pay of surgeons and surgeon's mates in the navy to the time of their actual service. Mercer also suggested that the same inquiry look into the matter of "requiring an examination by a board of Physicians of all persons for admission therein." The motion was referred to the House Committee

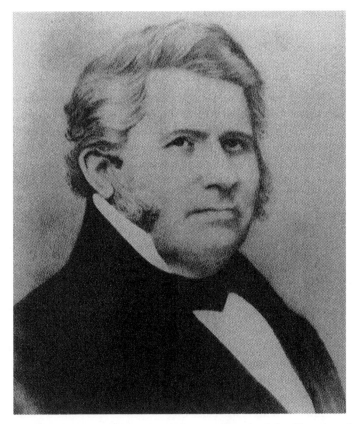

Surgeon Thomas Harris. Courtesy *Journal of the History of Medicine and Allied Sciences.*

on Naval Affairs, which was now chaired by Benjamin Crowninshield, a former secretary of the navy. Crowninshield sent to Southard, the secretary, the texts of the various resolutions that had been referred to his committee, briefly noted the intentions of this body, and asked for Southard's views on the propositions under consideration. On the matters of the pay and examination of doctors, Crowninshield said that "all that is necessary, [it] seems to me, can be said on this resolution, on the bill organizing anew the Naval Establishment." This was an accurate assessment. Nothing could be done for the doctors except in the context of a law reorganizing the navy.[30]

The larger question of the size and duties of the navy was addressed by the House on December 15, when it passed a resolution calling on the president to send it a plan for the naval establishment in peacetime.

Monroe referred the matter to Southard, who forwarded a plan to the House on January 30, 1824, along with the president's recommendations. Southard's plan emphasized the need to reorganize the navy. Discipline must be improved through the adoption of a new code of regulations. The number and grades of the officers must be limited to the number of positions available at navy yards, stations, and depots. He recommended that the bases at Erie and Whitehall be closed and that the one at Sacket's Harbor be greatly reduced. Southard wanted a force large enough to maintain an active presence in the Mediterranean, the Atlantic, the West Indies, and the Gulf of Mexico, off the west coast of Africa, and in the Pacific. He argued for higher ranks for the officers, with pay to be apportioned in accordance with the amount and importance of the service performed. Three pay scales were proposed, one for those on active service, one for those holding themselves ready for active service or who were on leave in the merchant marine, and one for those on furlough.

When discussing the medical side of the navy, Southard wrote, "No portion of the present system requires more amendment than the surgical department, in reference as well to the manner of admission into it as the government and payment of it. No one ought to be appointed surgeon's mate until after a satisfactory examination [and] proved that he is worthy of promotion." These matters were a part of a code of regulations that had already been prepared. As for pay, Southard would leave the entry salary of the surgeon's mates where it was. But after two years of service, a surgeon's mate would take an examination for surgeon; if he passed, he would receive a moderate increase in pay. The compensation of the surgeons would be the same for their first two years. It would then increase at two-year intervals during active service until it reached the maximum of $75 a month and eight rations per day. By the time the surgeon was rewarded with a permanent station at a navy yard or hospital, he would then have a fixed and adequate salary. Southard also believed that great savings could be made if "one or more intelligent surgeons" were ordered "to purchase the medical stores and supplies" for a ship.[31]

The secretary's insistence that no one be promoted to surgeon who had not passed an examination for that rank caused some problems for a veteran such as William Belt, who had been in the navy since the fall of 1811 and had performed honorable service on Lake Ontario during the War of 1812. Now he objected to orders that would sent him on a cruise as a junior medical officer on his ship. Southard agreed that he could sail in another ship as acting surgeon, but he would not be promoted until he passed an examination. Somehow Belt had got the idea that since he was among the oldest of the surgeon's mates, he would not have to take an examination, but Southard told him he was mistaken, and Belt felt aggrieved.[32]

More serious problems confronted Southard in relation to officer discipline, one of the first when he assumed office being the case of Surgeon Manuel Phillips. On September 16, 1823, Southard had to order a surgeon's mate to the frigate *Cyane,* which was due to sail to the Mediterranean, and he chose the second ranking surgeon's mate on the navy register, Dr. Manuel Phillips, who had not been to sea since 1812. This proved to be a troublesome selection.

Phillips did not go to the ship or send a letter of acknowledgment to the secretary. In late October, while Southard was recuperating from an illness at his home in Trenton, New Jersey, Phillips called on him and explained why he had not complied with the order: when he was appointed in July 1809, it was on the understanding that he would be promoted to surgeon at the first opportunity and that he would not be obliged to serve as a mate. Nevertheless, he did serve briefly as a mate on a cartel ship during the War of 1812, and while attached to the naval rendezvous at Philadelphia for two or three years. Otherwise he had been ashore or on leave for most of his time in service. During his stay in Philadelphia he had opened an apothecary shop and pursued private practice, which, Southard understood, had been profitable. As for the navy, Phillips said that he had never been promoted as promised, and he was now at the stage of life where he had achieved a respectable standing in his Philadelphia community. He did not think that he should be compelled to associate with junior officers, who were generally young men and boys whose habits and manners did not coincide with his own. Phillips brought with him letters from friends and showed them to Southard in an effort to persuade the secretary to relieve him of sea duty. The most influential of his supporters was his nephew, Mordecai Noah, the publisher of the *National Advocate,* a newspaper that advanced the ideas of Tammany Hall politicians and their followers.

Southard was not impressed by the letters or by Phillips's excuses. He observed that it was very strange that Phillips was appointed with the idea that he would not have to do his duty and that he had not been promoted for fourteen years, especially during the war, when men were advanced rapidly. Furthermore, it was the president who promoted officers, not the secretary; perhaps the president would give him an acting appointment. If so, confirmation by the Senate would be necessary for a permanent promotion, but it would not meet for a while and there were others already ahead of Phillips on the waiting list for promotion. The immediate need was for a surgeon's mate in the *Cyane.* When he finished talking, Southard was under the impression that Phillips might go to sea as an acting surgeon in the hope of getting a promotion. Phillips asked for permission to return to Philadelphia to arrange his affairs, and Southard granted it.

A few days later, Phillips returned and told Southard that charges had been filed against him for appropriating hospital property for his own use. The apothecary shop that Phillips owned apparently sold medicines to the naval commander of the New York naval station. He explained the facts of the case and asked for a public inquiry. Southard said he could not judge the propriety of requesting a hearing until he saw the charges. In the next day's mail he received a letter from the commander of the New York station which set forth the charges against Phillips, which were supported by the sworn statements of several witnesses. Recognizing the serious nature of the charges, Southard ordered a naval court then meeting in Philadelphia to determine the facts. Meanwhile Phillips was detached from the *Cyane*. Subsequently the naval court of inquiry acquitted Phillips of intentional impropriety in regard to the hospital stores, but some doubt remained. Southard chose not to pursue the matter and again ordered Phillips to duty under Captain John O. Creighton in the *Cyane*.

Creighton later notified the secretary that Phillips had not reported for duty, and Southard at once filed charges of disobedience against Phillips. The doctor immediately came to Washington to see the secretary. He told Southard that it was not his intention to go to sea, and the secretary replied that if he refused an order, he would ask the president to dismiss him from the service. Phillips then called on President James Monroe and presented his case. Monroe asked for it in writing. The doctor sent a petition to Monroe presenting his side of the story. Southard then ordered Phillips to call at the Navy Department for a copy of the charges against him. When Phillips did so, he was informed that he would be tried in Norfolk or Annapolis, which surprised him, for he expected to be tried in New York, where he had friends. Southard told Phillips that he would pay to have the doctor's witnesses travel to wherever the trial took place. At this announcement, Phillips asked if he could resign, and Southard said that the doctor would have to give his resignation to the president. Phillips did so, and formally resigned on February 19, 1824. Subsequently Noah's *National Advocate* published an article on the case which prompted an inquiry from Monroe to Southard. In response, Southard wrote that "to the very last Dr. Phillips calculated on my yielding under an apprehension of the vengeance of his friends." But Southard did not flinch from his duty; he had firm views on the necessity of prompt obedience of orders.[33]

In December 1823, Southard issued an order to all surgeons and surgeon's mates informing them that in view of the difficulties in recruiting medical men for duty on ships, in future everyone "must hold himself in readiness to obey every order for every kind of service which may be given by this Department." He added that except in extraordinary cases, medical men would not remain at any station for more than two or three years.[34]

Within two weeks, Southard accepted the resignations of Surgeons William J. Barnwell Jr. and George F. Kennon. Charges of disobedience of orders were pending against Surgeon's Mate Francis L. Beattie, but he was allowed to resign instead of facing a trial. Southard also ordered a court of inquiry into the charges brought by Surgeon Samuel R. Marshall against Surgeon Elnathan Judson. Marshall accused Judson of making improper and inaccurate remarks about a fellow medical officer. The court found Judson innocent, and Southard restored him to duty.[35]

Raising Professional Standards

Southard was also doing what he could to raise the professional standards of the navy. At the end of May 1824, he notified Surgeons Cutbush, Marshall, Barton, Harris, and Washington that they had been appointed to a board for the examination of surgeon's mates seeking promotion to the rank of surgeon. While they were so engaged, if any person appeared who wished to enter the navy as a surgeon's mate, he also should be examined on his medical knowledge. Any four of the five named surgeons would constitute the board for purposes of the testing. Examinations were to take place in Philadelphia beginning on June 14 and would continue as long as necessary to complete the tasks assigned. "Your attention will be directed to the moral character and scientific and professional attainments, and you will consider it your duty to make the examination full, minute, and rigid." He did not say so, but it is clear that this was to be an oral examination, with approaches to problems probably described rather than demonstrated. The board was to keep a record of its proceedings and send it to the secretary along with its opinions of the persons examined.[36] Notices of the forthcoming meeting of the board were placed in newspapers, and the designated surgeons met at the Mansion House in Philadelphia on June 14. Cutbush was chosen as president and Bailey Washington as secretary. A day after the first meeting, a letter was received from Surgeon Samuel Marshall asking to be excused from the deliberations because of his health and the fatigue of traveling. Southard accepted this excuse.[37]

The first matter that came to the board's attention was a letter from Surgeon's Mate Thomas Wiesenthal stating that he was attached to the brig *Hornet* as an acting surgeon and that the ship was about to sail. He asked for permission to submit his diploma in lieu of an examination. Cutbush replied that the board could not accept this, whereupon Wiesenthal appeared and was examined. When the votes of the board members were counted, the candidate did not have enough votes to recommend him for promotion, but he was not told this. Before sailing, Wiesenthal wrote to Cutbush to ask if he had hope of a favorable report. Cutbush replied that the board believed that it was not at liberty to give the information requested but would ask the secretary for an opinion; if he agreed, Wiesenthal would be given the information. In the meantime, Cutbush pointed out that the board's decision would have no effect on Wiesenthal's present commission as a surgeon's mate. A little later, as expected, Southard declined to release the information; he himself would notify the candidates of their standing. While this was understandable, it left poor Wiesenthal in a state of suspense for some time.[38]

The board's second case involved Surgeon's Mate William D. Conway, who had held that rank since December 1814. During the past five years, he had applied to the Navy Department for promotion and had been turned down. More recently he had been informed of the existence of the board and the need for candidates for promotion to appear before it. Writing from Baltimore, Conway said that he had received his degree from the medical school of the University of Maryland eight years ago. Before receiving it he had to undergo public examinations before a body of "learned and respectable citizens" in "all branches of the healing art." In view of the high standing of his medical school and his own self respect, he could not submit to any subsequent examination of his competency, which the regents of his university had already accepted. He hoped that his failure to appear before the board would not be considered a want of respect for its members, both individually and collectively, or for the secretary. Conway felt that the manner in which he performed his duties should be known to the secretary from the documents on file in the Navy Department. Cutbush replied that the board had no power to excuse candidates; one with a degree from a respectable university had already appeared before the board, and the examination of others was pending. Conway held his ground and corresponded with Southard, but the latter was firm in his decision. The upshot was that Conway resigned his commission on April 11, 1825.

Meanwhile on June 16, 1824, four doctors presented themselves to the board. Two, DeWitt Birch and Madison Lawrence, both from New York State, sought to enter the navy as surgeon's mates. The two others, Surgeon's Mates J. T. Armstrong and John W. Peaco, sought promotion. The two navy doctors were examined first. Armstrong failed to receive enough votes and was not recommended for promotion; here was another case of a doctor who had been serving since May 1812 but who could not be advanced. Peaco had been in the navy since June 1814, but he did better in his examination, and his promotion was endorsed. He was promoted in July 1824, but he enjoyed his new status less than three years and then died.

On June 17 the board examined two more candidates for promotion. These were Benajah Ticknor, who was found qualified to be a surgeon, and Charles Chase who was not. The next day two New Yorkers, Augustus A. Adee and DeWitt Birch, were approved for the rank of surgeon's mate. English-born William Birchmore, who had been serving as a surgeon's mate since January 1815, was found to be qualified for promotion. In succeeding days the board examined Surgeon's Mate Mordecai Morgan, who passed, and John S. Wiley, who failed. For the entry-level exams there were two candidates, Madison Lawrence of New York, who failed, and Benjamin F. Bache of Pennsylvania, who passed. No candidates appeared on June 22, and the board placed a notice in the Philadelphia newspapers that it would adjourn the following Thursday if no additional candidates appeared.

The next day, June 23, the board received a letter from Surgeon's Mate Wilmot F. Rogers, who had been in the navy since July 1813, asking it to consider his situation. During his time in service, he had not had the advantage of a library or the time to study and as a result was not as well prepared as other candidates. If he appeared before the board and just passed his exam, it would be a reproach. On the other hand, if he failed, it would be a source of mortification to his family and friends. He wanted a leave of absence to prepare for the next examination period. A postponement and a leave of absence were matters that the secretary must decide, Rogers was informed. When the matter came to Southard's attention he apparently granted the reprieve. Rogers never took his examination, for he died in August 1824. In the meantime on June 23, 1824, the board approved Thomas F. Boyd for promotion and found Robert P. Macomber of New York qualified for entry as a surgeon's mate. The next day, Jonathan R. Gilliam of Virginia presented himself for the examination for the entry-level grade and was found not qualified. Samuel Biddle and C. B. Jaudon, both of Philadelphia, passed the examination for surgeon's mate.

No other candidates appeared on June 26, so examinations were closed. The board then ranked the successful candidates for promotion in terms of professional merit. Its choice for first place was Benajah Ticknor, followed by Mordecai Morgan, Thomas J. Boyd, John W. Peaco, and William Birchmore. The ranking of the candidates for commissions as surgeon's mates was Benjamin F. Bache, Charles Biddle, C. B. Jaudon, Robert P. Macomber, DeWitt Birch, and Augustus A. Adee.

The board then made inquiries into the moral character of the doctors who had been selected, presumably by writing to prominent doctors in New York, Philadelphia, and other cities. Whatever the method used, the board decided that the moral character of all the men it had selected was "correct and honourable."

Also of correct moral character were the doctors who did not pass the examinations. The board recommended to Southard that they be given an opportunity to improve themselves professionally by attending a course of lectures and by taking the examination another time. On June 28, the board met for the last time during this first examination period in order to read and approve the record of their work before forwarding it to the secretary. Members then returned to their respective stations.[39]

Southard carefully considered the board's report and acted quickly. On July 10 the Senate confirmed the promotion to the rank of surgeon of Ticknor of Vermont, Morgan and Birchmore of Pennsylvania, Boyd of Delaware, and Peaco of Maryland. Following the advice of the board, Southard dated their commissions so that they would rank as recommended, with Bache first and Birch fifth. But a new name, John R. Chandler of the District of Columbia was added before that of Augustus A. Adee. The new commissions were forwarded to the appropriate commanding officers for distribution to the doctors.[40]

How did Chandler make the final selection? Appointed as a surgeon's mate on November 14, 1824, Chandler saw brief service on the schooner *Shark* before being assigned duties ashore. The appearance of his name on the list of commissioned officers raised questions in the mind of Surgeon's Mate August P. Beers, who received his commission on November 16, 1824. Beers wondered if his commission had been properly dated, and he wrote to Southard about it. Southard replied that Chandler was appointed some months before the examination and before it was expected that one would take place. When he received his commission he was told that if he passed his examination he would be confirmed by the Senate. Therefore Beers' commission was dated as it should be.[41]

It was Southard's intention to announce that the next examination would be held in the fall, but Surgeon Harris suggested to him that it be held in February. Such an early announcement would stimulate navy doctors to study and would allow candidates "to pursue a course of dissections." He left unsaid the fact that he was running a school designed to meet the needs of such officers. Southard went forward with his plans for a fall examination.[42]

In November 1824 the Navy Department announced that the board of navy surgeons would meet in Gadsby's Hotel in Washington to examine surgeon's mates for promotion. The board consisted of Cutbush, Barton,

Harris, and Washington. One of those advised about the examination was Dr. John H. Imlay of Allentown, New Jersey, who had just been appointed an acting surgeon's mate. Southard wrote him that he was receiving a commission on condition he present himself before the board of surgeons. If he passed that examination, his appointment would be confirmed; if he failed, the appointment would be considered revoked. The board met, but no record survives of how many candidates it examined. Possibly an oral report was given to the secretary. Harris did write to Southard about Dr. Imlay, who had failed the examination. This created some difficulties for the secretary, for Imlay had studied under a doctor who was a friend of Southard's. Harris worked with Imlay to help him prepare for another try. In 1826 he made another unsuccessful attempt to pass the examination. The matter was still unresolved when Southard left office on March 3, 1829. The new administration may have had someone suggest to Dr. Imlay that he was wasting his time, or he may have reached that conclusion himself. Whatever the situation, Imlay resigned from the navy in September 1831.[43]

Meanwhile, in January 1825, as the time for the winter examination approached, Harris wrote to Southard about changes in the membership of the board. It seemed likely to Harris that Surgeon Marshall would continue to be indisposed, and it was known that Surgeon Washington was about to begin a cruise. If one of these officers could not attend the meetings of the board, Harris suggested that Surgeons Robert K. Hoffman or John H. Gordon would be qualified substitutes. Both were graduates of medical schools, and both had improved themselves in their profession. Harris observed that the next board would probably have to reject more candidates than at the previous meeting, and it was therefore important that it be composed "of proper persons." He went on to say that most of the officers attending his medical lectures were "attentive and studious," especially Surgeon's Mate Charles Chase. Harris thought it likely that Chase would "retrieve the character which he lost in the last examination." Southard saw fit not to reply to this letter, probably because he was now busy with other matters. As a result, he did not announce the date for the winter examination, causing some anguish among the surgeon's mates who had been busy preparing themselves.[44]

Surgeon's Mate Charles Chase wrote to Representative John Parrott about the matter in mid-February 1825. He pointed out that he had been in Philadelphia since the previous November preparing himself for an examination that he expected to take place in early February. Feeling himself qualified to pass, and wishing for a promotion before the end of the present session of Congress, he asked Parrott to use his influence with the secretary to find out what had happened. Parrott sent the letter to the secretary. Chase sent a similar letter to Southard asking if, with the press of business, the secretary had forgotten about the examination and the men waiting to take it. A letter with the same query was received from Surgeon's Mate James Cornick. Southard's response was that they had not been forgotten; examinations were held at the convenience of the Navy Department, not of individual officers. The next examination did not take place until April 15, 1825. This time the group that met in Philadelphia consisted of Cutbush, Barton, Harris, and two new members, Surgeons Richard Hoffman and John H. Gordon. Both Chase and Cornick passed their examinations and got their promotions within a few months. Thereafter examinations were held whenever they were needed, normally in Philadelphia but occasionally in Washington.[45]

While Southard and others were doing what they could to improve the professional environment of the service, there was concern among medical men about how they would fare under the act for the gradual improvement of the navy then pending in Congress. An expression of this sentiment was published in an article on "The Navy" in the *National Gazette and Literary Register* of Philadelphia in March 1826. Signing himself *Fiat Justitia*, the author said that in anticipation of congressional approval of a pay raise, "many of the most respectable young medical gentlemen in the country applied for commissions, and those that were already in the service, devoted themselves to their profession, with a degree of zeal before unknown in the service." This great influx of talent into the medical department was such "that there was every prospect of as great a revolution being effected, in the service," as had taken place in the Royal Navy during the administration of Melville. But instead of passing this popular bill, the naval committee of the House reported a substitute measure that was inadequate. The proposed bill would give to assistant surgeons, a rank being substituted for that of surgeon's mate, the pay of $40 a month and one ration a day which was valued at 25¢. After he passed his examination for surgeon, he would receive $50 a month and the single ration. When the medical officer was promoted to surgeon his pay would increase to $60 a month, but there was no change in the ration allowed. After that he would receive $10 extra a month for each additional five years of service up to the limit of $100 a month, but still only one ration a day.

Under this formula, wrote the columnist, a doctor who entered the navy at the age of 21 and served 30 years would receive as an annual pay, counting the value of his rations, $1,299. This sum was less "than is frequently given to a third rate clerk in one of our departments." He asked if this "paltry consideration" was "likely to secure the services of ambitious men, for, it should be recollected that men of talents are always ambitious." Likewise, a surgeon of a fleet, who had great responsibilities and whose talents should make him "one of the first men in the nation," would receive only $20 a month extra or $240 a year for this important duty. Nor did the pending law contain any provision for hospital surgeons to retire on a reduced pay after 20 or 30 years of service, as was the case in the British and French navies. *Fiat Justitia* listed the sums paid to British navy and army surgeons who held various posts. He went on to note that the Mexican government paid its full surgeons the equivalent of $135 a month. Medical men of the next lowest rank, or assistant surgeons, were given compensation in proportion to this sum. Surgeons of hospitals were paid liberally. He urged the naval committee to compare these rates of compensation with those proposed for the medical men of the U.S. Navy. "In short, there is no naval service in the world which does not offer more lucrative positions than that of this country."

In publishing the criticisms of *Fiat Justitia,* the editor of the *National Gazette* expressed the hope that they would be considered by those to whom they were addressed.[46] Whether on not this was the case is not known. It seems likely that the arguments would have been brought to the attention of the House committee. Certainly some of the provisions of the original act were changed. Congress did not pass an act for the gradual improvement of the navy until March 3, 1827. This authorized the procurement of timber for ships and steam batteries so that it could be seasoned and made available for immediate use, if necessary; the building of two dry docks and improving the preservation of property in the navy yards. The president was authorized to preserve live oak timber on U.S.-owned lands and to investigate the expediency and practicability of a marine railroad at Pensacola. Finally, it was stated that the $500,000 for six years that was appropriated to carry this law into effect could not be transferred to other purposes.[47] This law was a far cry from the comprehensive legislation that Southard had initially looked for. When it became apparent that the pending legislation did not address the longstanding questions of the rank and pay of medical men and other officers, Southard and others sought to deal with these matters by means of specific legislation.

Meanwhile another article on the pay of naval medical officers was published in Baltimore in *Niles Weekly Register.* Unsigned, it said that the present secretary had introduced regulations "which are calculated to give medical officers a professional standing, not exceeded in respectability by any establishment of the kind in any country." These regulations made it "impossible for any to become surgeons and surgeons' mates but those eminently qualified." The secretary "encourages the cultivation of medical knowledge, by affording the members of the profession every facility in the prosecution of their researches, compatible with the interests of the service." But the inadequate pay they received made it difficult for navy medical men to support their families and themselves or to pursue "those inquiries in foreign countries which would enlarge the sphere of their knowledge and usefulness, and extend the boundaries of science." Because of the poor compensation, 12 out of 40 able surgeons had resigned in the last four years. Naval surgeons received $30 a month less pay than an assistant surgeon in the army but did not endure fewer privations or less exposure. The anonymous author concluded with the assurance that in the next session of Congress, the claims of naval medical officers would be addressed. In presenting these arguments of "an esteemed friend in the medical department of the navy," the editor of *Niles Weekly Register* said that it was right and proper that naval medical officers should be paid so that they could live decently. Otherwise valuable men would continue to leave the service, and the health and lives of seamen would be in the hands of less experienced medical officers.[48]

A petition to Congress calling for an increase in pay, signed by four surgeons and five surgeon's mates, was referred to the House Committee on Naval Affairs on January 14, 1828. Eleven days later a similar appeal came from navy lieutenants. On February 12 the committee reported a bill on these subjects. Through Southard's close association with Robert Y. Hayne, the chairman of the Senate Committee on Naval Affairs, a bill was introduced there to increase the pay of surgeons, surgeon's mates, lieutenants, and midshipmen. It did not get very far, but in the next Congress the lieutenants and the medical men got pay raises in separate laws.

Under the act of May 24, 1828, entry-level medical officers would henceforth be known as assistant surgeons. This was regarded as a more dignified title than that of surgeon's mate. No one could enter the naval service unless he was examined by a board of navy surgeons appointed by the secretary. No one could be appointed as a surgeon until he had served at least two years as an assistant surgeon in a public vessel of the United States at sea, and after he had been examined and passed by a board of surgeons. The law also authorized the president to appoint "an experienced and intelligent" navy surgeon in every fleet or squadron as "surgeon of the fleet," who would be the surgeon of the flagship and in addition to his regular medical duties, would inspect the quality and examine and approve all the requisitions for the medical and hospital stores of the fleet. In difficult medical cases, he would consult with the surgeons on the other ships of the fleet or squadron and keep records on the character and treatment of diseases, which would later be sent to the Navy Department.

For these additional duties the surgeon of the fleet would be allowed double rations.[49]

On the matter of pay, the law provided that every surgeon would receive $50 a month and two rations a day. After 5 years of service, this would be raised to $55 a month and three rations; after 10 additional years, $60 a month and four rations; after 20 years of service, $70 a month and four rations. An assistant surgeons with less than 5 years' service would receive $30 a month and two rations a day. After 5 years he would be examined by a board of naval surgeons, and if he passed, he would receive and additional $5 a month and one ration; after 10 years of service, another $5 a month and one ration per day. While at sea, the assistant surgeon with 2 years of service would receive double rations and $5 a month in addition to his normal pay. Surgeons on sea duty would get $10 a month and double rations as well as their usual compensation.[50]

In passing this legislation the Congress gave hope to the medical officers of the navy except for a few surgeons. As they read the law, they would not receive a pay raise because they had not been examined and they already held the rank of surgeon. To meet this situation, an amendment was passed on January 21, 1829, giving such men additional pay and rations according to their length of service despite the fact that they had not been examined.[51]

With the passage of these laws, the morale of the medical men of the navy rose. Conditions had improved enough for men to be able to make a career of the public service. Many of the medical officers who began their careers immediately before and after the passage of the first law served for a number of years and became the transmitters of a newer and more professional tradition.

Chapter 13

Health Care
and Hospitals,
1816–1829

Immediately after the War of 1812, the navy again turned its attention to Algiers, which had resumed attacks on U.S. commerce. Squadrons under Captains Stephen Decatur and William Bainbridge were sent to the Mediterranean. Decatur arrived first and forced the Algerians to cease their attacks. War had been averted, but there was no assurance that a new threat would not develop, and the United States was determined to maintain a naval presence in the area. Bainbridge and Decatur went home, and Commodore Isaac Chauncey was placed in command of the Mediterranean Squadron.[1]

It was the intention of Secretary Crowninshield that a supply depot and a hospital be established in the Mediterranean, and he suggested the port of Cagliari, on the island of Sardinia, as a convenient location. He appointed Dr. John D. McReynolds as the surgeon of the Mediterranean hospital and assigned Surgeon's Mates Thomas G. Peachy and George P. Doane to assist him. Chauncey examined the situation at Cagliari but rejected the site because it did not have a sheltered harbor for his ships. He now had to find a base for ship repairs which would also be suitable for rest and recreation for crews, provide a safe haven during winter months, and be an appropriate site for a hospital. After investigating several ports, Chauncey thought that Port Mahon, on Spain's island of Minorca, was an ideal spot: it was close to North Africa, yet near the French port of Marseilles; it had an excellent harbor, a good climate, and friendly people; the squadron had spent the winter of 1816–17 there; and a naval hospital of sorts was established on shore. The Spanish government was not receptive to U.S. overtures for long-term base rights, so in January 1817, Chauncey

267

ordered all the invalids in the squadron to be sent home and discharged. He closed the hospital and gave Surgeon McReynolds permission to return to the United States.[2]

About the time the squadron was ready to sail, the frigate *United States* had an outbreak of smallpox. Chauncey asked the governor of Minorca for permission to land the sick at the quarantine station at Port Mahon. The governor consented. Chauncey's squadron sailed as planned, but the *United States* under Captain John Shaw was left behind at Mahon until the men recovered. While Shaw was waiting, he apparently requested and was granted permission to unload his stores at the dockyard while he cleaned his ship. In gratitude, Shaw evidently assisted the Spaniards to refit an old warship. When Shaw's men recovered, they returned to their ship, and the *United States* sailed to rejoin the rest of the squadron. Throughout the period of illness, the Spaniards were accommodating, but they did not change their mind about a U.S. base at Minorca.[3]

Spain had a weak government and was faced with the threat of a revolt. It had not acknowledged the validity of the Louisiana Purchase, and it was worried about U.S. intentions in regard to Florida and toward Spain's former colonies in Latin America, which were struggling to maintain their independence. Adding to these problems was the fact that a Spanish warship that the Americans had helped to refit, and to which they had lent some seamen for a voyage to Cartagena, had foundered en route. There were suspicions among some Spaniards that foul play might be responsible for the loss of the ship. Closer to home, a riot had taken place in a Port Mahon tavern between 125 Americans and some 300 soldiers of the local garrison, and one U.S. midshipman was killed. After considering these incidents the Spanish government saw no reason to grant the U.S. request for base rights.[4]

Faced with this decision, the Americans had to make arrangements to deposit their stores at Gibraltar and to have the ships of the squadron visit various Mediterranean ports. When the *Franklin* reached Naples in May 1819, Commodore Stewart paid a visit to Francis I, the emperor of Austria, who was attending a ball at a villa in the country. A number of Italian states were then ruled by dukes loyal to Austria, and the wife of King Ferdinand I of Naples was the daughter of Maria Teresa, the late empress of Austria. After being presented to the emperor, Stewart invited the monarch to visit his ship, and he promised to do so on the same day that he was scheduled to visit the ship of a British admiral. On the appointed day the royal party visited the *Franklin*, where they were received with appropriate honors and toured the ship. When they were preparing to depart, the nearsighted grand master of the empress fell down the hatch and into the cockpit. The accident was the cause of much distress to the royal party, for it was feared that the court official might die. Surgeon Thomas Salter examined him and found that he had only broken a leg, which he immediately set. The empress was very relieved to learn that the grand master was only slightly injured, and in gratitude the emperor presented Dr. Salter with a large purse filled with gold pieces. With great delicacy and propriety, Salter declined the gift. A few days later the queen of Naples visited the *Franklin* and told Stewart that the emperor had been highly gratified by his tour of the vessel and that since that time little else had been discussed at court.[5]

The *Franklin* sailed shortly after this, but Dr. Salter's quick action may have influenced the royal decision to allow the navy to establish a hospital at Pisa, on the Arno River, in the Italian province of Tuscany. We know very little about this arrangement. It would seem that space for sick U.S. seamen was acquired in an existing hospital. Surgeon Salter was placed in charge and was assigned two surgeon's mates to assist him. Apparently the hospital turned out to be entirely unsatisfactory from the point of view of the officers of the Mediterranean Squadron. It was distant from the normal cruising areas of the squadron, and it took time to get the sick to the hospital. Quarantine laws at Naples were so strict that ships had to wait 20–40 days before any of the sick and disabled could be landed. Once on shore, they were subject to many local restrictions. When their journey to Pisa could be resumed, they had to travel up a canal for about 15 miles. Neither the nature of the accommodations at Pisa nor the number of patients treated there has been ascertained. It soon became apparent to a few line officers, at least, that more suitable arrangements would have to be made.

Late in 1821, Captain Jacob Jones, who had a medical background, informed Secretary Thompson that the hospital at Pisa was unnecessary, and Thompson ordered him to close it. Responding to this order, Jones found that the hospital had been abandoned for a year or more. Surgeon Heap, who had previously been in charge of it, was now in Florence. Reporting to the secretary, Jones promised to visit Pisa to remove any hospital stores that remained and send home in the first available naval vessel any officers who were still attached to the hospital. When Jones reached Pisa, he found that there was nothing for him to do. Hospital arrangements for Americans there had been discontinued.[6]

By 1821, U.S. relations with Spain had improved. The United States purchased Florida in 1819, and a boundary line between Spanish and U.S. territories west of the Mississippi River was established by a treaty. In August 1820 the captain of the U.S. brig *Spark* asked the authorities at Port Mahon if he could use the navy yard there in case of need, and the authorities agreed. At Madrid the U.S. minister twice raised with the king the question of granting the privilege of depositing stores duty free at Port Mahon. The king consented to a six-month period with the possibility of a renewal.

Thinking positively, the Americans quickly moved their stores from Gibraltar to Minorca. The naval hospital at Pisa was deactivated and a new one established at Port Mahon with Surgeon John D. McReynolds in charge. It was hoped that this large-scale build-up would make it difficult for Spain to refuse to renew the lease, but this proved not to be the case. Spain was again irritated by the U.S. recognition of the independence of the former Spanish colonies in Latin America, and in May 1822 it refused to renew the U.S. rights at Port Mahon. Once again Americans moved their supplies to Gibraltar, and the squadron was without a permanent base. But a year later the Spanish consented to the repair of two U.S. warships at Port Mahon. Then in 1825, through the efforts of Commodore Rodgers and the U.S. minister at Madrid, the king approved the duty-free deposit of supplies and the establishment of U.S. naval base. This was the first long-term overseas naval base in U.S. history, and the arrangement lasted nearly 20 years.[7]

When entering the harbor of Port Mahon, a ship first passed a large diamond-shaped island that was the site of the lazaretto. It was large, clean, and airy and was regarded as one of the finest in Europe. Among other accommodations it had two infirmaries. Next was a small island opposite the city of Georgetown which was known as Quarantine Island. Here ships and crews were held for various periods to determine whether there were any diseases on board. The location facilitated communication between the authorities on shore and the ships in quarantine, as well as among the ships being held there. On this island the Americans again established the hospital. Moving up the channel, just above Georgetown and below the city of Mahon, was another small island known as Hospital Island, the site of a military hospital. The quarters for the sick were numerous, clean, and well aired, and the hospital had an excellent supply of water from a well. A Spanish surgeon and a chaplain were regularly stationed there.[8]

At the U.S. hospital a navy surgeon was assigned to treat the sick transferred from the squadron. Bruises and knife wounds inflicted on U.S. sailors as a result of fights on shore were usually treated on board the ship to which the man belonged by its medical officer. There is little in the surviving records to tell us much about the number of men treated at the hospital and the nature of their ailments. The evidence suggests that there were few deaths.

Valuable information on the state of health in the frigate assigned to the Mediterranean survives in the records kept by Surgeon Usher Parsons in the *Java*. When he reported to that ship at Baltimore early in 1815, he first prepared a list of the medical and hospital stores needed for the voyage. On July 1, he saw his first patients; among the ailments he encountered on this first day were pleurisy, venereal diseases, fever, dysentery, contusions, and a fractured foot. The ship went to Norfolk for additional supplies, and while there both officers and men enjoyed shore leave, which resulted in 12 cases of venereal disease. About this time, Captain Oliver Hazard Perry complained of a swelling in a knee joint. Parsons said that such swellings were sometimes caused by mercury, a common treatment for both gonorrhea and syphilis. Perry replied that he had never been treated with mercury, nor had he ever had a disease that required it.

From Norfolk the *Java* went to New York, where on December 16, Perry was ordered to prepare his ship for duty in the Mediterranean. Through windy and stormy weather the *Java* made its way across the Atlantic. In his diary, Parsons observed that the dampness had caused much sickness, such as dyspepsia and slight fevers, but of the 30 men on the sick list, probably 20 had lacerations, contusions, and sprains due to the pitching of the ship.

Off Cape St. Vincent, Portugal, a dry, rotted main-topmast broke off and in falling, tore loose a part of another mast and some spars. Ten men were aloft furling a sail when the accident happened. One dropped on the muzzle of a cannon, fell overboard, and was lost; three others died in falls; one struck the bottom of an upturned boat and fractured his skull; some were crushed under the rigging and spars that fell to the deck and were screaming in pain; others managed to hang on to yards, crosstrees, and rigging and were yelling for help. Surgeon Parsons rushed to the aid of the injured. While helping to move them, he was hurled between decks and fractured his kneecap. Unmindful of his own injury, Parsons quickly set up a temporary cockpit on the aft part of the main deck and began to treat the injured. The sailor who split his skull was trephined but later died. The next morning, four of the dead were buried. The weather improved greatly and the ship reached Gibraltar safely. After a brief stop there and at Malaga, it headed for Port Mahon.

The surgeon in charge of the U.S. hospital on Quarantine Island was Dr. McReynolds, an old friend from the War of 1812, and to his care Parsons transferred his injured patients. While the ship was being repaired, Parsons went to the hospital several times to transfer patients and to see McReynolds. In a letter to his family on March 12, Parsons said he had three cases of pleurisy. "This is an epidemic peculiar to this island at this

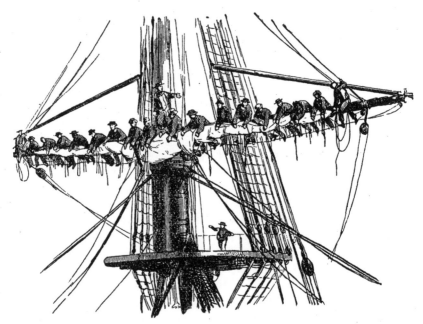

Sailors Furling Sails, circa 1840. Smithsonian Institution, Washington, D.C.

season, & it is to be feared it will take off a great many of our sailors." The local response to the disease was to bleed the patient extensively during the first two days until the pain was relieved, a treatment introduced by a British army surgeon, George Cleghorn, during his country's occupation of the island.

The *Java* left Port Mahon in late March for Algiers, then went on to visit Tunis, Tripoli, Syracuse, Messina, Palermo, Gibraltar, and Naples before returning to Mahon for winter. In January 1827 it was one of two ships selected to carry separate copies of the newly negotiated treaty with Algiers to the United States. Prior to its departure from the Mediterranean, Surgeon Parsons prepared a medical report covering the duty of his ship there: the total number of cases treated was 8,142, or an average of 22 patients a day; and there had been only one death, that of a man in the advanced stages of consumption.

Eleven days after the ship left Port Mahon, a seaman was stricken with a severe case of smallpox. His enlistment term was nearly up, and he had been transferred into the ship for the voyage home. The rest of the crew was mustered, and it was discovered that 18 men had never had smallpox or cowpox, whereupon Captain Perry ordered them to be vaccinated.

Unfortunately the vaccine that Parsons had was a year old and was believed to be ineffective. In case it failed, he inoculated the men and then paid strict attention to their diet and regimen. All those vaccinated came down with a mild form of smallpox, and all recovered in two or three days. Eighteen others who failed to report for vaccination were stricken and 4 of them died. The other 14 had a difficult time but gradually recovered. By the time the ship reached the United States, there were only 6 remaining smallpox patients. During the passage home there were also three deaths due to "pulmonary consumption." In his report to the secretary, Parsons said that while the total number of seven deaths from all causes was "unusual" for one ship, it should be borne in mind that the *Java* was taking home 40 or 50 of the incurable cases from the squadron and hospital during a long winter passage. In light of these circumstances "the number of deaths will seem as moderate as could have been expected." When the ship arrived off Newport, Rhode Island, 5 cases of smallpox were transferred to a hospital on shore.[9]

Some indications of the state of health of men in the frigate *Constitution,* who were in the Mediterranean during 1824–25 and spent a part of that time at Port Mahon, can be gleaned from the journal of Midshipman Andrew Harwood. The ship sailed from New York on October 29, 1824, under the command of Captain Thomas MacDonough. The first death took place at Gibraltar on December 19, but the man had suffered from consumption since the ship left New York. February 1825 saw a duel between two midshipmen in which one received a severe wound in the arm. MacDonough issued an order forbidding duels. April brought the death of Marine Lieutenant Henry W. Gardner from constipation. Harwood says that the short illness of the lieutenant "baffled the united efforts of the Surgeons of the squadron, who resorted to every remedy in vain to save him." Gardner was buried in the English Protestant cemetery in Messina, Sicily. Other deaths recorded at this time by Harwood were those of a seaman who drowned while trying to swim ashore "for a frolic," an old and enfeebled seaman who fell off the foreyard and was killed when he struck the deck, and a boy who died because he let his fever go too long before he reported it to the surgeon. Harwood noted, "The weather is very unhealthy at this season of the year particularly for persons predisposed to pulmonary complaints, and indeed few or none of us escape an almost perpetual cold."

Midshipman Harwood compiled his own statistics on the sick of the *Constitution* between March 21, 1826, and June 10, 1827, his numbers taken from the surgeon's daily report. While Harwood's record does not include names, illnesses, or the length of stay of patients, it does provide at least some insights into the health of the ship. Of the 440 days covered by his entries, there are 116 for which there are no notations. For many of these days the context suggests that there was little or no change from the day preceding. On the other hand, 3 or 4 consecutive days without entries may mean that there were no men on the sick list. The number reported sick on a single day ranged from 1 to 26 out of a total of 738 men assigned to the ship during the time span of the journal. From September 18, 1826, to March 10, 1827, the *Constitution* was in Port Mahon, including 18 days in quarantine. During this period the daily average number of men on the sick list was 15. Harwood's journal does note any transfers to the hospital on shore, so we must assume that most of these illnesses were not serious and fairly routine for a ship of that size.[10]

A much more serious situation confronted the captain of the frigate *North Carolina* in 1827. After having touched at Toulon and Tunis, it entered the harbor of Malta and transferred 90 smallpox cases to the lazaretto. But to the surprise of the Maltese, only 4 men were reported to have died out of a crew of about 900. Upon investigation it was discovered that during the previous two years, many of the crew had been vaccinated three times. The low death rate among so many men was regarded in Malta as a proof of the protection afforded by vaccination.[11]

Closer to home the deployment of a naval force to fight the pirates in the West Indies led to serious health problems. In 1822, Captain James Biddle was given the command of the squadron that was to suppress piracy. To carry out that mission he was first to go to Havana and cultivate the friendship of the Cuban officials. Then he should proceed to Port-au-Prince to seek the cooperation of the Haitian authorities. Biddle set sail in the frigate *Macedonian* accompanied by the *Hornet, Spark, Enterprise,* and four schooners. While he was in Havana, yellow fever struck the crew of the *Macedonian* and seven men died. Biddle broke off his negotiations and sailed for Haiti. The fever continued. Believing that offensive and impure air from the ship's hold was the cause, Biddle ordered a series of measures to try to purify the environment. Ventilation, whitewashing, letting fresh water into the hold, fumigating, and starting fires to dry timbers were all tried, but the fever continued. By July 24, or 20 days after he left Havana, 80 men were on the sick list and 9 had died out of a crew of 376. Biddle decided to head for home.

Writing to Secretary Southard about his decision, Biddle charged that the sickness and death were due in a large degree to "the negligence of the Officers of the United States Navy Yard in Charlestown, Massachusetts in omitting to cleanse sufficiently the Hold of the ship" before the last voyage. By the time the *Macedonian* reached Gosport, Virginia, in July 1822, it was in a deplorable state: 77 men had died of yellow fever, and another 52 were ill with it. When the news of this disaster reached the Navy Department, it caused much anguish. Surgeon Cutbush was sent from the Washington Navy Yard to Norfolk to bring his expertise to bear on the problem.

At Norfolk the ship was moored off Craney Island to keep the diseased men away from the rest of the base. Medical men from the hospital, the Norfolk Navy Yard, and other ships lent a hand in caring for the patients. By the time the disease abated, 100 officers and men had died.[12]

In the meantime, Biddle's charges had been brought to the attention of President Monroe, who instructed Secretary Thompson to look into the allegations. Thompson ordered Captains John Rodgers, Isaac Chauncey, and Charles Morris to investigate the charges against Captain Isaac Hull, the commandant of the Charlestown Navy Yard. To defend himself, Hull relied on his counsel, Samuel Hubbard, as well as on Daniel Webster, a former member of the House of Representatives from New Hampshire, who was now running for Congress from Massachusetts. Using the journal of the navy yard and the testimony of officers and workmen, Hull's defense was able to show that the ship had been cleaned, pumped, and whitewashed and everything stowed properly before it sailed. Medical testimony was introduced to show that the disease was brought on by a number of factors including the sudden transition from a cold to a warm climate, dampness, the lack of proper clothing, the lack of tea, sugar, and other extras, sleeping on the deck, fatigue brought on by the frequent exercise of the guns, letting water into the hold at Havana, errors in the treatment of the sick after the death of the surgeon, and a feeling of despondency after Biddle made a speech to the crew in which he blamed the navy yard for their sickness. Much to Biddle's chagrin, the court found Hull not guilty.[13] Secretary Thompson now declared that the *Macedonian*'s casualties were caused by the climate, and a general order was issued temporarily forbidding any naval vessel from entering the harbor of Havana.

The secretary tried to seek out and change any other situation that was regarded as a threat to the health of navy men. Earlier Porter, who succeeded Biddle as the commander of the naval force in the West Indies, had complained about the decision of the secretary to locate a navy base at Key West, then called Thompson's Island. Porter objected to the climate, the sandflies, and the mosquitoes there and recommended that it not become a permanent base. He was overruled, and as a part of the base, a hospital was established with Surgeon Thomas Williamson in charge. In August 1823 there was an outbreak of yellow fever at the site which prostrated large numbers of officers and men. Of the 25 officers stricken, 23 died. Porter himself became ill and narrowly escaped death. While he was sick, an attending navy surgeon noted that an old wound in the arm which Porter had received during the Quasi-War, was affected. His left clavicle began to separate and pieces of bone came off in layers. The doctor believed that the fever was the cause of the exfoliation. As soon as he recovered sufficiently, Porter was advised to leave the area. He complied, and he reached Washington on October 26.[14]

In the meantime, Secretary Southard had become concerned about Porter's health and the reports from Thompson's Island. He decided to send Commodore Rodgers and three experienced surgeons to investigate the causes of the disease. Doctors Harris, Washington, and Hoffman made a rough passage with Rodgers in the schooner *Shark* and reached the base on October 23, 1823. Porter having already departed for Hampton Roads, Rodgers assumed command of the station. By this time the yellow fever had abated, but there were still 59 men on the sick list. These were moved to the *Hero* and the *Harmony* and taken to the hospital at Gosport. The surgeons then began to look into the health problems of the station. They decided that the outbreak of the fever was caused by miasma and the hardships of service in a tropical climate, two of which were mosquitoes and sandflies.[15] Rodgers and the surgeons returned to Washington in late November.

The navy continued to use Thompson's Island as the site for a hospital and base but was looking to Pensacola as a better location. The area had become a part of the United States as a result of a treaty with Spain in 1819, by which Florida was purchased and the boundaries between Spanish and U.S. territories in the west were defined. It was not until July 1821, however, that Pensacola formally became a part of the Union. On February 2, 1825, a bill was introduced in Congress authorizing the president to select and purchase a site for a navy yard on the coast of Florida and the Gulf of Mexico. Buildings and improvements to accommodate and supply the ships of the navy in that quarter were also authorized. Congress gave its final approval to the bill on March 3, 1825. In October of that year, a three-man naval commission went to Pensacola to select the site of the navy yard. They chose Tartar Point, on the west side of Pensacola Bay, and Southard forwarded their recommendations to President Adams on December 2. Adams approved the report the next day, and on February 26, 1826, the construction of the navy yard began. Despite this promising beginning, shortages of food, labor, and building supplies delayed its completion for many years.[16]

The same problems that made it difficult to finish the yard also affected the building of a suitable hospital. As a result, there were delays in closing down the one at Thompson's Island. While it was still serving the sick, a young surgeon's mate named Samuel Biddle, who was attached to the hospital, came down with a fever. He continued to work and was treating himself with a mixture that included acetate of ammonia. His steward was to bring him the mixture, but instead he gave him a quantity of the black drops. When the doctor felt the effects, he knew what had happened and tried to induce vomiting. Unfortunately only a part of his stomach was emptied, and he died shortly afterward. The death of this skillful surgeon and benevolent man again focused attention on Thompson's Island.[17] In a letter to Mordecai Noah's newspaper, the *New York National Advocate,* a person who was presumably stationed at Thompson's Island and who signed himself with the pen name Coram charged that Southard continued to use the locale even though he knew it was unhealthful. Evidently the writer was not familiar with the problems at Pensacola. There things were slowly changing. In 1826, Surgeon Isaac Hulse was assigned to the base to take charge of the temporary hospital, and the sick were transferred from the squadron. Additional space was needed in the fall of 1827, and an investigation showed that the only suitable structure in the vicinity of the yard which could absorb the overflow of patients was a house outside the yard near Ft. Barrancas. This house had formerly been occupied by the officers from the yard while that facility was being built.

If space could be found for the sick, there was still the need for additional medical help. The commandant of the yard told Secretary Southard in September 1828 that the duties of Dr. Hulse were very arduous. He had no permanent assistant, and at that time he was treating a total of 23 patients in the two locations. More sick men were expected soon. Southard assigned additional doctors to the base. As for the yard itself, a decade after it was established, it still lacked the facilities that were associated with a first-class naval installation.[18]

Ventilating Ships

A significant effort to improve the health of sailors in ships was made by Commodore James Barron with his invention of a ventilating bellows. The device consisted in part of cast iron pipes that were readily available in any hardware store and could easily be installed by a ship's armorer. The device was installed in the *Hornet* as an experiment during its operations in the West Indies. In his report on the experiment in November 1824, Commander Edmund P. Kennedy noted that on two previous cruises the *Hornet* was considered a very sickly ship, and yellow fever had played havoc among the officers and crew. On the most recent cruise, the bellows was put in operation for 15 minutes of every hour. Generally it took about that amount of time to expel all the foul air. With the exception of the sail-maker, who had come down with "the bilious intermitting fever," which he contracted in Portsmouth before sailing, there were no sick on the ship during the cruise. And the sailmaker recovered shortly after the ship put to sea. Kennedy recommended the ventilating device to the Board of Navy Commissioners and Commodore David Porter, the commander of the U.S. naval force in the West Indies. Praise for the ventilating bellows also came from naval constructor Charles D. Brodie at Portsmouth. Apparently these reports were not acted upon, perhaps because of indifference or because there was no admiration for Barron among some of the senior officers of the navy. Barron had killed the popular Captain Stephen Decatur in a duel in 1820.[19]

The matter was raised again in November 1825 by Thomas V. Wiesenthal, who had served as acting surgeon of the *Hornet*. Writing to Secretary Southard about the experiment, Wiesenthal said that the *Hornet* had sailed from Norfolk in July 1824 and returned in August 1825. During the interval the ship operated principally in areas around Cuba and Key West. There was no yellow fever on board until July 1825, and although that was an epidemic, "it had very little of that malignancy which generally characterises [sic] that disease." The acting surgeon attributed this to the constant use of the bellows during the epidemic. Though about 80 men became ill with the disease, none died. In the course of the 13-month voyage, there were only four deaths, none the result of "malignant fever" and one of "an acute disease."

In his letter to Southard, Wiesenthal gave an account of an experiment he had conducted. With his thermometer he measured the temperature of the air on the main deck in September and found it to be 98 degrees. Descending to the hold of the ship, he took another reading and found the mercury at 98 ½ degrees. The heat in the hold was accompanied by an offensive smell. Leaving his thermometer in the hold, he had the bellows turned on. After two hours of operation he found that the temperature in the hold had fallen only half a degree but the offensive smell was gone. During the cruise he conducted similar experiments, with generally the same results. Wiesenthal understood that Barron intended making some modifications in his invention, and if so, he thought it would be expedient to use it on ships, especially those operating in tropical climates.[20] Despite this positive endorsement, the matter was not pursued. Barron's ventilator was removed from the *Hornet* and not reinstalled when the ship sailed.

This time the results were very different. Commander Alexander Claxton reported that the ship had 54 cases of yellow fever, 9 of them fatal. Since the ship had visited no ports and there had been no relaxation of the strict regulations regarding cleanliness, Claxton was convinced that the disease originated in the ship. He blamed the removal of the ventilator as a cause. When the disassembled device was located, it could not be reassembled. Claxton also pointed out that the *Natchez* had also suffered from yellow fever and that it had attempted to rig a bellows pump, but this was an insignificant effort in comparison to Barron's ventilator, which he called a "Barroneter." In the future, wrote Claxton, he would not willingly go to sea without one of Barron's ventilators.

As a result of this report, Barron's invention was now regularly installed in navy ships. In 1834, Barron wrote the secretary that the government should pay him for its use; Levi Woodbury replied that he could not pay him, and that Barron must present his claim to Congress. Barron did so but was unsuccessful.[21]

Smallpox

Another health problem that was a matter of concern was smallpox. In December 1824, Surgeon Mordecai Morgan reported to Southard from the frigate *Constellation* that smallpox was showing up among the men recruited in New York for duty in the West Indies. He recommended that the surgeons on duty at all the recruiting rendezvous vaccinate all incoming men who had not had smallpox before they were sent to his ship or the New York Navy Yard. It was a good suggestion, but nothing seems to have come of it.[22]

Fortunately other individuals in Congress became interested in the cause of prevention, perhaps as the result of appeals by naval medical officers or other interested parties. In 1826 the House of Representatives passed a resolution directing the secretary of the navy to inform it of any regulations that had been adopted to encourage vaccination in the navy. Southard replied that none had been adopted other than those that related to the general health of men in ships. It was the duty of the commanding officer and the surgeon to take every precaution to prevent and stop the spread of contagious diseases. He added that cases of smallpox were rare in the navy. There had been an outbreak in the *United States* the previous September in which one seaman died, but the rest of the sick had recovered.[23]

It was now clear that Congress had an interest in the subject, so Southard decided to issue a special order. On May 26, 1826, he informed the commanders of navy yards and ships:

> It is necessary that the Surgeon, attending the Recruiting rendezvous ascertain with certainty, of every recruit, whether he had had the small

pox or been vaccinated; and cause all such as have not, or about whom
there is the least doubt, to be vaccinated without delay. All the seamen
heretofore enlisted and now under your command will be treated in the
same way. You will consider it your duty to attend particularly to this
matter, and require from the Surgeons the necessary reports on the
subject.

Commanders of vessels embarking on a cruise were to see that similar
examinations and vaccinations took place.[24] This was a step forward in the
prevention of disease, but three years later a failure to implement the
order fully brought problems.

While cruising off Cuba in 1829, the crew of the schooner *Grampus* was
infected with smallpox and several men died, including the surgeon. The
captain took the ship to Pensacola to be fumigated. While there a few
officers came down with a mild form of smallpox. Surgeon James Page
faced a problem of where to put these patients. The "miserable huts" that
had previously been used as a temporary refuge for the sick were now
unhabitable in hot weather. A house in the yard which had been used as a
temporary hospital the previous summer was private property and was
now rented. There was no suitable building in or near the yard for the sick
of the *Grampus,* so they were placed in a barn that was now the designated
hospital for smallpox patients. The roof was partially blown off and a sail
was spread over it to protect the patients from sun and water. Surgeon
Page and Assistant Surgeon William Whelan of the naval station oversaw
the transfer of the sick to the makeshift hospital and then departed. One of
the patients, Lieutenant George Smith Blake, wrote: "In a few moments the
Doctors left us. Good God how wretched is this situation. We have no
attendance saving that of one of our own men who was one of the first
taken sick, & is now convalescent and an old Black woman. Every one
shuns us for the disease is contagious." Blake and his shipmates recovered.[25]

Problem Cases

With the return of peace in 1815, the duties of medical men in the navy
focused on the care of patients who suffered from an assortment of illnesses and injuries that were considered normal to the nature of seafaring
life. These included broken bones, sprains, cuts, bruises, hernias, rheumatism, various disorders of the digestive and respiratory systems, and venereal diseases. Such disorders were also to be found in men attached to navy
yards and shore installations. Amid all the more or less routine cases there
were some that the attending physicians considered unusual, and therefore
sometimes the surgeons and mates described them in more detail in their

records. In addition, the 15 years following the end of the War of 1812 brought some large and serious outbreaks of sickness, as has already been noted.

For Surgeon Amos Evans, who had treated combat casualties in the *Constitution* during the War of 1812, an assignment to the hospital in the Charlestown Navy Yard offered no great challenge to his medical skills. There was, however, a case with some unusual aspects which began on January 25, 1816, when one William Oaty, about 25 years of age, accidentally shot himself with a pistol while he was seated. The ball entered about midway between his breast and umbilicus, passing through the linea alba and moving downward and obliquely toward his left side to lodge in his pelvic cavity. Immediately afterward the surgeon found Oaty's pulse to be full and regular. There was no external hemorrhaging, but there was a constant flow of urine from the hole. Oaty complained of pains in the glans penis and in his loins to the left thigh. The patient was placed in bed with his shoulders and knees elevated. His wound was dressed with a simple "pledge" and cataplasm. At 4 P.M. that day it was noted that his pulse accelerated and became irregular.

During the next day and a half the surgeon bled Oaty three times for a total of 29 ounces. He was catheterized four times and given an enema four times, with good results for both treatments. Originally he was given a solution of "super-tart. potass in water" and an anodyne at bedtime. But it was found that he was unable to retain anything, even warm or weak wine and water. Oaty suffered greatly from thirst and vomiting, and his skin became hot and pungent. He complained of pain in the abdomen and left thigh, the latter relieved by a tight bandage. There were signs of delirium, and he slept little. The poultices on his wound became painful and were omitted, and fomentations were ordered applied during the night. In the beginning he had a full and hard pulse of 120 a minute, but it became "quiet, irregular and small." A day later it was scarcely perceptible at the wrist. At 1:00 P.M. on the second day he died.

When the body was dissected, it appeared that the ball had passed between the abdominal parietes and peritoneum without entering the abdominal cavity. On its downward course it went through the anterior fundus of the bladder and emerged just above the entrance of the urethra on the left side. It then entered the brim of the pelvis on the inside of the large blood vessels and passed through the pubis, which it fractured, and entered the pelvis through the obturator foramen, where it lodged between the rectum and the a coccyx.[26]

This turned out to be one of the few cases that intrigued Surgeon Evans. He hoped for a more challenging assignment, but this was not forthcoming. There were too few berths for surgeons in the postwar navy. At his request, Evans was given a year-long furlough in 1819 which was renewed for another year in 1820. When ordered to sea in 1821, he did not comply, and the order was revoked. He resigned his commission in 1824. With his departure the navy lost one of its best surgeons, according to Captain Isaac Hull.[27]

A case that threatened to injure the professional reputations of two surgeons grew out of the treatment of Commander Thomas Gamble of the sloop of war *Erie* in the Mediterranean in 1817. When Surgeon's Mate Alexander Montgomery joined the ship in January of that year, he learned that earlier Gamble had suffered from tumors about the abdomen and that when he had a cold, they also appeared in his groin. Gamble told Montgomery that he had never had venereal disease and that he had been told by two civilian doctors, Philip Syng Physick and John Syng Dorsey, that he suffered from scrofula. Surgeon Robert S. Kearney of the navy had also examined him and had given the same opinion. Montgomery said that he was inclined to regard the disease as such even without the testimony of those authorities. Later Montgomery noticed that when Gamble was stricken with colds, cholera morbus, and once or twice with diarrhea, a tumor appeared in the groin. The tumors on the abdomen generally enlarged about the same time as that on the groin. When Gamble recovered, the growth on the groin disappeared. This had taken place without resort to mercury.

Then in November the ship stopped in Malaga, and there, according to Montgomery, Gamble contracted a venereal disease, which manifested itself in a chancre and bubo. Montgomery treated these with mercury over a 50-day period and Gamble was considered cured. Sometime after this, Gamble came down with cholera morbus and again had a tumor on the groin that grew larger than a hen's egg. Montgomery treated Gamble's cholera morbus, by giving him two "mercurial inunctions" at the beginning but did not do anything about the tumor. It disappeared along with the cholera morbus after 10 days. About four weeks later, Gamble caught a severe cold and the tumor reappeared on the groin. It was colorless and grew slowly except in good weather, when it temporarily diminished. It caused little pain and neither it nor his cold kept Gamble from enjoying himself on shore at balls and parties. But Surgeon Heap was brought in for a consultation on the character and treatment of the tumor.

In the presence of Gamble, Dr. Montgomery told Heap that the scrofulous tumors had shown themselves on the captain's abdomen and groin long before he had any venereal infections. He repeated what he had been told by Gamble about the opinions of Drs. Physick and Dorsey. Montgomery reviewed his own experience with the tumor that appeared and disappeared. Since the chancre and bubo had been cured, Gamble had stated that he had not been exposed to venereal disease. Nevertheless, Surgeon Heap decided that the tumor was venereal and prescribed a course of treatment with mercury which Montgomery was to follow. Montgomery did as he was instructed with the result that the captain's mouth was constantly sore, the tumor grew worse, and his health was undermined. It was decided that Gamble should be sent to see Heap, accompanied by Montgomery.

According to Montgomery, at this meeting Heap told the captain that "no venereal taint" remained in his system. Gamble was happy to hear this and hoped that he would have to take no more mercury. Heap assured him that this was the case. About 10 days after this, Gamble returned to his ship, supposedly fit for duty. But Montgomery found that the captain's tumor was worse and that his mouth was still sore from the mercury. Gamble delivered a letter from Heap to the surgeon's mate informing him that Heap and Dr. Varca, an Italian physician at Pisa, had determined that Gamble's tumor was a local infection and that blisters should be applied until the tumor was ready for the lancet. Montgomery followed these orders and Gamble's condition worsened. The ship encountered stormy weather, and while dealing with this problem Gamble came down with intermittent fever. Montgomery treated this condition with customary medications, including wine and arsenic. While the ship was off Portugal, Montgomery went to see Surgeon Thomas B. Salter on an accompanying vessel and showed him Heap's letter of instruction and his own register of daily practice. Salter thought that Gamble should be returned to the hospital in Italy as soon as possible. This was done.

At the hospital in Pisa, Surgeon Heap told Montgomery that Gamble's disease was "now evidently mercurial." Montgomery agreed and said that he had so reported it. Three or four days later, Montgomery heard that Heap and Dr. Vacca had again decided that Gamble was suffering from a venereal infection and had resumed the mercury treatment. Upon hearing this, Montgomery, in the presence of other officers, said that if they did as reported, Gamble would be dead within a month. Gamble survived beyond a month, but on October 10, 1818, he died. Heap then reportedly wrote to his commanding officer that Montgomery had been responsible for Gamble's death. Montgomery reported that he carried out the orders given to him and that he had objected to the conclusion that Gamble's problem was due to venereal disease; he thought that if Gamble had never seen Heap, he would still be alive. Montgomery asked for a court-martial or court of inquiry, whichever the secretary though would be the best way for him to vindicate himself "with the least injury to the public service."[28]

Secretary Thompson evidently decided not to do anything about this case. Within a short time things were resolved at least as far as the doctors were concerned. Heap was appointed a temporary consul at Tunis in January 1824, and in December 1825 he resigned his commission to accept a diplomatic appointment. Meanwhile in May 1825, Montgomery was promoted to surgeon, and in January 1828 he died.[29]

The Naval Hospital Fund

One of the great and recurring problems of the postwar years was the state of the Naval Hospital Fund, including the lack of progress in achieving the goal of the law of 1811 of erecting permanent hospitals. Early in 1812 the Commissioners of Navy Hospitals had studied several possible locations for a hospital in Washington. An architect had been appointed and ordered to prepare a plan and estimate the cost. The outbreak of war had prevented anything more from being done. A fresh start had been made on January 1, 1815, when Benjamin H. Latrobe, the architect, wrote to Benjamin Crowninshield, the newly appointed secretary of the navy, that a new set of drawings for a marine hospital would be delivered to him the next morning. The original set had been sent to Secretary Hamilton in 1811, but they had since been lost. Also, a meeting had been scheduled at the office of Secretary of the Treasury Alexander J. Dallas which Crowninshield should attend in his capacities as secretary and as one of the Commissioners of Navy Hospitals. Presumably Crowninshield did attended. Latrobe evidently soon learned that there was little disposition to move forward on the marine hospital building. The rather grand design of the structure and the probable costs of operating it no doubt cooled whatever enthusiasm there was in Congress.[30]

The Navy Department received a resolution of the Senate asking for reports on several subjects, and it sent the answers a few days after Congress met in December 1815. One of the questions dealt with the measures that had been taken in regard to navy hospitals. Crowninshield reviewed what had been done since 1812. The Commissioners of Navy Hospitals were preparing a report on the subject. It was already clear, however, that the unexpended balance in the Marine Hospital Fund, amounting to $50,000, and the contributions of 20¢ a month by naval officers and seamen were insufficient to meet the goals envisioned by Congress. The commissioners were not estimating the amount they would need to meet public expectations. That subject was referred to the attention of Congress. But Congress had other issues on its mind. In 1815 and 1816 the commissioners met, and finding that there were no moneys at their disposal to carry out the the provisions of the law of 1811, they adjourned. They took comfort in the knowledge that medical assistance was being given to the sick at temporary hospitals, which were all that could be provided in existing circumstances. Late in 1817 the House turned its attention to the subject.[31]

In a resolution passed on December 22, 1817, the House of Representatives asked the secretary of the navy for a report on naval hospitals, the names of the surgeons in charge of them, and the Marine Hospital Fund. Crowninshield forwarded a copy of the resolution to the naval surgeons at the various navy yards with a request that they supply the hospital information requested. They reported that frame houses in or near the navy yard were being used as hospitals in Brooklyn, Philadelphia, Washington, and New Orleans. In Boston a part of the marine barracks in the Charlestown Navy Yard was also being utilized.[32]

As commissioners of navy hospitals, Secretary of War John C. Calhoun, Secretary of the Treasury William H. Crawford, and Secretary of the Navy Crowninshield sent their own unified report to Congress. They recommended that the portion of the law of 1811 separating the Navy Hospital Fund from the Marine Hospital Fund be repealed and that combined funds be placed under their direction. The existing marine hospitals and those that might be erected in the future for the navy should also be under their direction. The commissioners would make the rules and regulations for these hospitals. Appointments as surgeons, officers, attendants, and so on would be made from those associated with naval hospital establishments. Unless Congress saw fit to appropriate funds for a permanent asylum for the crippled, aged, and infirm, that portion of the law of 1811 relating to them should be repealed. These recommendations represented a substantial retreat from the ideas advanced by Secretary Hamilton in 1811. Members of Congress were apparently convinced by the arguments and began to draft legislation to make them a reality.

Along with their recommendations, the commissioners sent a report on the state of the funds, which showed that in 1809 the Navy Department paid into the Treasury the sum of $38,513.96 and that this was the only money transferred since 1799. The Treasury reported that the Marine Hospital Fund had a balance of $3,782.86 as of February 1811. The accounts of the Naval Hospital Fund were incomplete and showed only funds transferred in February 1811 and March to November 1817 which totaled $77,701.45. From the reports sent by the navy yards, it was estimated that the annual expenses for rent for hospitals, pay, rations, and quarters of surgeons and surgeon's mates at Boston (Charlestown), New York (Brooklyn), Philadelphia, Washington, and New Orleans came to a total of $13,783.98. Crowninshield sent all information to the House in January 1818, along with his own report reviewing what had happened in regard to the Marine Hospital Fund since 1811 and the actions of the commissioners in 1815 and 1816.[33]

If Crowninshield thought that Congress would be satisfied with this, he was soon to change his mind. In April 1818 the House asked both the Treasury and the Navy departments for separate reports on the number of the sick treated at each hospital each year and the expenses for them. Once again Crowninshield relied on the surgeons at the navy yards, and the information they sent provides useful glimpses of the state of navy medicine at several of the yards mainly for the years 1813–17.[34]

The report from Cutbush at the Washington Navy Yard showed a total of 375 patients or a yearly average of 75 for the period, the greatest numbers being in the war years. Baltimore's report covered July 1812–March 1817 for a total of 724 and a average of 120. New Orleans sent statistics spanning 1811–17, during which 2,334 patients, or an average of 334 per year, were treated; Surgeon Heermann reported that of the total, 2,089 were cured, 43 were relieved, 19 were incurable, and 183 died. Incomplete records permitted the surgeon at Gosport (Norfolk) to send only the figures for 1816 and 1817, for a total of 260 or a yearly average of 130. The report from Newport covered January 1815–January 1818 for a total of 219 patients and an average of 73 a year; the greatest number of these came from the Mediterranean Squadron, commanded by Commodore Bainbridge, and the frigate *Java*.[35] Surgeon Samuel R. Trevett pointed out that there was no hospital or other building in the Charlestown Navy Yard for the sick, who were generally placed in the hull of an old merchant vessel. At that time they were in the frigate *Java,* which was in ordinary. During the past three years, his sick list averaged 17 or 18, but this was not a true measure because many were treated in their own ships. An even briefer report was submitted by Surgeon Samuel R. Marshall from the Brooklyn Navy Yard. He said that the number of sick admitted annually ranged from 180 to 230. At Charleston, South Carolina, Surgeon Logan reported that the number of sick during 1814 and 1815 exceeded 62 a year. With the postwar reductions in the naval force the annual total was 17.[36]

The lack of uniformity in the reports of the sick made it impossible to break down the cost of care at each yard, for most surgeons did not include that information. Such financial information as was provided was either too skimpy or too detailed for useful comparisons to be made.

From the point of view of the Senate however, enough information was apparently available for it to proceed with a bill to create a general fund to which both merchant and naval seamen would contribute. Thirty-five cents a month would be deducted from the pay of officers, seamen, and marines and paid to the commissioners of a marine fund. When a patient was admitted to a hospital, one ration a day would be deducted from his pay and paid to the commissioners. In the case of persons on pensions, the amount of the pension accruing while the patient was in the hospital would be paid to the commissioners. Those appointed as directors of marine hospitals would receive as compensation 1 percent of their expenditures. Another part of the bill dealt with the purchase or acceptance of lands or buildings for these hospitals. After the measure passed the Senate in 1819 and was sent to the House, the chairman of the House Committee on Naval Affairs asked the Board of Navy Commissioners for its opinion of the bill.[37]

As head of the board, Captain John Rodgers was at first hesitant about expressing its opinion on a measure that had already passed the Senate. But since an opinion was requested, he responded at length. He expressed strong objections to the plan to send sick navy seamen to marine hospitals, for experience suggested that as soon as they were convalescent, they would desert. Hence captains would keep sick men on ships for longer in the hope of curing them. The current bill did not seem to afford relief to the sick and disabled seamen of the navy.

There was also the matter of the unequal contributions of navy and merchant seamen. Most merchant voyages averaged about four months, and unless he shipped out soon after completing one voyage, merchant seaman did not pay into the fund for eight months of any given year. On the other hand, the navy men never served less than two years and would be making continuous contributions to the fund during that period. In addition, the pay of the merchant seaman was generally higher than that of his navy countryman, and indeed naval pay had been reduced. Thus navy men would be contributing a higher proportion of their pay than merchant seamen. At the present time, the annual contributions of the officers, seamen, and marines amounted to $10,500. Rodgers also expressed the board's objections to the provisions of the bill in regard to pensioners and the compensation of the hospital directors.[38]

These objections evidently had the effect of eroding support for the Senate bill in the House. If merging the funds for the care of navy and merchant seamen was not the answer, there was still the need to do something soon about permanent hospital arrangements for the navy. In his annual report in December 1821 on the state of the navy, Smith Thompson referred to past reports from the Commissioners of Navy Hospitals, the body in charge of the Naval Hospital Fund. He said that while they still could not carry out the 1811 law, they had established "a separate and distinct fund for that purpose by drawing on the appropriation for the pay of the Navy such sums as may, from time to time, be spared until the amount in the Naval Hospital Fund shall be completely reimbursed." This was a start at resolving the problem, but it would take some time to correct past mistakes.[39]

Southard understood the situation and brought the problem to the attention of the fourth auditor of the Treasury Department, who supervised navy expenditures. The secretary directed that beginning on January 1, 1824, the money deducted from the pay of officers and seamen was to go into a separate naval hospital fund. He then began to urge Congress to vote the amount needed to repay the fund with interest. From the fourth auditor Southard learned that in February 1811, when the navy and merchant marine funds were separated, there was a credit of $3,782.96 in the Naval Hospital Fund. Between that date and the end of December 1823, the sum of $187,918.81 had been paid into the naval fund, bringing the total credit to $191,701.67. After deducting expenditures of $71,988.72, there was a credit of $119,712.95 which had been absorbed into the pay of the navy.[40]

While the fund was being restored, the Commissioners of Naval Hospitals purchased land in September 1823 in Chelsea, a suburb of Boston, on which to build a new hospital. In May of the next year, land was purchased in Brooklyn, New York, for the same purpose. Next came the acquisition of property in Philadelphia in June 1826 for a naval asylum. Then, in 1827, land was purchased for a hospital at Norfolk. That same year the House of Representatives asked the commissioners for a report. They replied that although the act of Congress providing hospitals and an asylum for seamen had been in effect for almost 28 years and money had been deducted from the pay of seamen during that time, not one building had been erected. "The effect upon the feelings of our officers and seamen may well be imagined. The commissioners are assured that it has been one powerful cause of the difficulties sometimes encountered in procuring seamen for public vessels." Congress took no action on the matter and addressed another inquiry to Southard in December 1828.[41] In his reply Southard pointed out that the government had kept and used the money contributed by the men of the navy and marines and said that the sum misspent should be repaid with interest. No person in the service had received any advantage from the fund. The secretary added: "The government has never given a cent to create hospital establishments in the navy. In no other country, and under no other civilized government, is this a fact."[42]

The House Committee on Naval Affairs recommended an appropriation to repay the whole amount due: $195,351.81 according to Southard; $167,759.37 according to the committee. When the matter finally came to a vote, by the act of May 24, 1828, Congress appropriated $46,217.14, which was the balance of the $50,000 presumably transferred in 1811. This was followed by an additional appropriation on March 2, 1829, of $125,000. Congress declined to appropriate funds on its own to build naval hospitals. Two days after this, Southard's term of office ended and the party of Andrew Jackson took over the government. It was not until 1830 that the first naval hospital opened in Norfolk.[43]

Chapter 14

Continuing Reform
Efforts

When Andrew Jackson became president on March 4, 1829, he chose as his secretary of the navy John Branch of North Carolina, whose earlier career had embraced service as governor of North Carolina and as a U.S. senator from that state. Most of the new administration's attention was devoted to domestic affairs. In naval matters the emphasis was on economy. This meant that the task of protecting U.S. commerce was done through the use of smaller ships, which were more economical to employ and could operate in shallower waters. It also meant that the shallower waters in southern harbors could be used more, to the economic benefit of that area. During Branch's tenure the United States had only 5 frigates, 10 sloops of war, and 4 schooners in operation. The usual practice was to use 2 or 3 of these ships on tours of two or three years on foreign stations.

While Branch was in office, congressional appropriations for the navy were approximately $3,500,000 a year. The Board of Navy Commissioners sought funds for the construction of new ships, and when these were denied, it accomplished the same goal under the guise of repairs. Branch was dissatisfied with the board and recommended to the House Committee on Naval Affairs that it be replaced with a bureau system. The committee took no action, and the matter remained pending for another 12 years.

Branch also suggested that the officer corps be pruned, that the pay of the naval officers be placed on a par with that of the army, and that the grades of vice and rear admiral be created. He urged that the marine corps be merged with the infantry or artillery of the army. The fiscal concerns of the navy were confused and unsettled and needed reforming. Nothing came of these proposals. If he had been able to serve for a full four years,

Branch might have achieved more of his goals. However, he and his wife, along with other members of the cabinet, were caught up in a dispute involving the social acceptance of the wife of the secretary of war, and Jackson forced him to resign on May 12, 1831.[1]

The new head of the navy was Levi Woodbury of New Hampshire, a former senator, who served from May 23, 1831, to June 30, 1834, when he became secretary of the Treasury, a position he held until 1841. Under Woodbury economy continued to be the watchword. Congress appropriated about $4 million annually for the navy, but he spent less than half that amount. Woodbury urged the construction of steam batteries for harbor defense, the reorganization of the Board of Navy Commissioners, higher pay for officers, and the better teaching of midshipmen. He was also interested in reducing the daily ration of whiskey and water, or grog, in the enlisted force and limitations on the practice of flogging. Some changes in the teaching of midshipmen and in relation to flogging and grog took place during his tenure.[2]

Woodbury was followed in office by Mahlon Dickerson of New Jersey, who earlier in his career had served as governor of and U.S. senator from that state. His years in the Navy Department were from July 1, 1834 to June 30, 1838. Congressional appropriations for his department were kept near $3 million, but in 1836 he requested an additional $2 million to fund an exploring expedition to the South Seas and to place more ships in operation. During Dickerson's tenure the first steel warship was built, and the ship of the line *Pennsylvania*, the largest of the sailing ships of the navy, was launched. The latter was destined to spend most of its career in port functioning as a receiving ship for recruits. Dickerson felt that the navy needed two or three steam batteries for harbor defense, but he recommended the construction of only one to Congress. During his years in office, there were more ships in commission than at any time since the War of 1812. The United States had as operational units the Mediterranean, West Indian, Pacific, Brazil, and African squadrons. Also, when the Second Seminole War began in 1835, the navy supplied a small unit to aid in the campaign against the Indians. The war in Florida continued until 1843.

Other matters of interest to Dickerson were the reform of the Board of Navy Commissioners, the placing of navy officers on a par with the army, and the creation of the grades of admiral and vice and rear admiral, but he believed that the initiative on the matter of the higher ranks should come from Congress. At the same time, a concern about the large number of foreign-born seamen in the enlisted ranks of the navy made him press successfully for an apprentice program designed to bring young, native-born American boys into the service. Public debate about their environment on shipboard also led to additional attention both in and out of the navy to the subjects of flogging and grog. It was under Dickerson that the South Seas or Wilkes Exploring Expedition finally set sail. The debate on the enterprise had gone on since Samuel Southard's term in office.

When Jackson's designated successor, Martin Van Buren, became president in March 1837, he asked Dickerson to remain in office, and the secretary did so. It was Van Buren's misfortune that the financial crisis known as the Panic of 1837 took place early in his term. The results of the panic on Dickerson's business interests, as well as his poor health, induced him to resign on June 30, 1838.[3]

Van Buren replaced him with James Kirk Paulding of New York, who had served from 1815 to 1823 as secretary of the Board of Navy Commissioners and from 1824 to 1838 as the navy agent at New York. These activities had given him financial security, so that he could devote some time to writing, and he had gained a reputation for his work in naval history, poetry, and fiction. His earlier naval associations brought him in close contact with Commodore John Rodgers, who dominated the Board of Navy Commissioners and naval affairs in general for over 20 years. From Rodgers he apparently imbibed or reinforced his dislike for the new steam technology, and he resisted its application in the navy. He did, however, try to have as large a navy as Congress would fund, and he felt that officers and men should get experience at sea. He also tried unsuccessfully to get the rank of admiral created. Among the changes he advocated were the reorganization of the Navy Department and bringing all the acts of Congress relating to ship construction under one appropriation. Near the end of his term, the movement for reform of the Board of Navy Commissioners and in ship construction reached a point where Congress finally took action. The results of these changes were not seen until the new Whig administration under President William Henry Harrison took office in March 1841.[4]

Sea Duty

Making more equitable arrangements in assignments to sea and shore duty had been a matter of interest to Southard, and the policy was applied more vigorously under Branch. When Surgeon George Logan, who had long been stationed at Charleston, was ordered to sea, he resigned.[5] Branch also turned his attention to Dr. Cutbush, who had reportedly been a strong supporter of John Quincy Adams in the election that brought the Jacksonians to power. On June 6, 1829, Cutbush was ordered to report to Commodore Barron for duty in the frigate *Constellation*. The surgeon sought to have his orders revoked. He pointed out that he was now 57 years old and suffering from diminished eyesight, and hence poorly equipped to function in the dimly lit area of the cockpit. He therefore asked for some consideration of his age and services. Branch was adamant: Cutbush must go to sea. So on June 10, Cutbush resigned, ending a distinguished career dating from 1799. The way in which Cutbush's separation from the service was handled reflected a lack of feeling and gratitude for a man who had contributed much to the advancement of medical care in the navy.[6]

Orders for sea duty were also issued to Surgeon William P. C. Barton in Philadelphia. Barton chose to go to sea on what proved to be a short cruise in the West Indies. Problems relating to the health of crews in that area and his own recent experience there had the effect of enhancing his reputation at a time when other older surgeons were no longer in service.[7]

The Liquor Ration

By the late 1820s there was a growing sentiment in the country for temperance and against the misuse of alcohol. Individuals who shared that conviction now began to present petitions to Congress urging it to act to abolish the daily ration of grog in the army and navy. Other petitioners urge that a substitute be introduced in lieu of the liquor ration. In reporting these developments, the *Sailor's Magazine,* published by the American Seamen's Friend Society of New York, suggested that the surgeons of the army undertake an inquiry as to the fitness of the liquor ration for the promotion of the physical and moral strength of soldiers.[8] A month later the same journal suggested that navy surgeons institute an inquiry into the effects of the daily ration of grog. The editor believed that it was sufficient "to create an unconquerable thirst for strong drink," make sailors prone to temptation in order to satisfy their craving and to drink to excess, thereby destroying their minds and bodies. He also questioned the utility of the continual rotation of the diet of sailors and concluded, "Men feed more uniformly when their diet is more uniform."[9]

Some of the sentiments of the editor on the matter of the liquor ration were reflected in the House of Representatives on February 25, 1829, when it passed a resolution calling upon the secretary of the navy to institute and inquiry into the effect of the grog ration on midshipmen. Branch gave this task to Surgeons Heermann, Barton, and Harris. He asked them for their individual opinions on whether the grog ration was "necessary or expedient" for midshipmen and its effect on the morals, health, discipline, and character of the navy.[10] The surgeons were careful in considering and formulating their replies. All believed that the spirit ration was unnecessary and harmful to morals and health. Heermann thought it was also subversive to discipline. Barton advocated a more wholesome ration for midshipmen and questioned the wisdom of allowing the commander of a ship to determine whether spirits should be used. He believed that an act of Congress was necessary. Harris said that the inquiry ought to be extended into the effects of grog on the young men and boys in the crews. He thought that tea and coffee should be substituted but admitted that old sailors would not submit to the abolition of grog. Branch had the replies of the three surgeons in hand in September, and he expressed his concurrence with the sentiments expressed when he forwarded the letters to the speaker of the House in January 1830. He recommended that seamen who commuted the spirit ration be paid a liberal sum of money that could be used to purchase small stores.[11]

This information was useful to Dr. Lewis Condict, a representative from New Jersey, who was already at work trying to end the liquor ration in the army. Turning his attention now to the navy, he introduced three resolutions in February 1830. One asked for an inquiry into the advisability of paying seamen and marines double the value of their discontinued whiskey ration at the end of a voyage; the second proposed the payment of a bounty in money or clothing for total abstinence from the liquor ration and good behavior; and the third hoped to hold out inducements to younger officers to embrace total abstinence. These resolutions precipitated a debate in the House on the liquor problem. The exchanges reflected the belief by some that reform must come from the individual and that abolition would be resented by sailors and would do no good. Others spoke in favor of the proposals and the benefits of the temperance cause. One member made an unsuccessful attempt to amend the resolutions, stating that while he was no friend of intemperance, he did not believe in abridging "the natural liberties of man." In the end, Condict's proposals were adopted. It turned out to be just one phase in a long struggle to end the spirit ration.[12]

After Levi Woodbury replaced Branch in the Navy Department, he issued a circular on June 15, 1831, stating that all persons who voluntarily relinquished the spirit part of their rations were to be paid for it at the rate of 6¢ per ration. By this method the friends of temperance hoped to encourage the sailor to renounce his grog voluntarily. Woodbury's action won praise from various quarters, and some in the navy began to collect money in lieu of their liquor ration.[13]

A Surgeon General and a Medical Bureau

Having made their position on the liquor ration clear, the medical officers of the navy now turned their attention to urgent matters in their own domain. Early in his tenure Secretary Branch asked Surgeon Heermann to prepare a report on the medical department of the navy. In sending his report of January 1830 to Branch, Heermann spoke of the "radical unsoundness and imperfection" of the existing system. The power to requisition medical supplies had been left too much to naval officers, the purchase to navy agents, and the examination of accounts to the Board of Navy Commissioners. At the same time the only limit on surgeons' demands, was their own discretion, and they were not accountable in the way other officers were for public property. The result was much waste and expense in the matter of medicines and storage chests.

To solve these problems, Heermann recommended the creation of a medical bureau headed by a surgeon general, with one assistant, one accounting and copying clerk, and a messenger. It would be the duty of the surgeon general, as the head of the medical bureau, to purchase on the best terms available all the drugs, medicines, instruments, hospital stores, furniture, and utensils for health care in the navy. He would make an estimate of the necessity, quality, and kind of all such items for every ship and part of the naval service. The bureau would be responsible for a strict accounting of expenditures and the keeping of receipts. It would preserve all articles deposited by surgeons of ships that returned to port or were dismantled. With the consent and by the special order of the secretary, the surgeon general would inspect and report on the hospital departments of stations, navy yards, and ships in port. The compensation of the surgeon general, his assistant, and the employees of the medical bureau would be left to the discretion of the Congress.[14]

Seeing merit in these suggestions, Branch drafted a bill for the establishment of a medical bureau and sent it to Heermann for comment. Heermann pointed out that in the draft bill the appointment of the surgeon general came from the Navy Department and the tenure was temporary, an arrangement that would not work well. If a junior officer were selected and placed over his senior in terms of the dates of the respective commissions, there would be conflicts and pretensions that would not be resolved even with a presidential appointment. As it was, officers did not comply graciously with orders and regulations issued by a commander of the same rank as themselves, whereas in an organization based on distinctive and graduated rank, they did comply. Without such an organization there would be subtle and systematic opposition to orders from the head of the medical bureau. Also, since officers of the same grade would anticipate holding a bureau appointment themselves by turns, they would be less likely to respect the authority of the head of the bureau. What was needed was a position created by an act of Congress with the same rank, compensation, and authority as that established in the army in 1818.[15]

Branch had the idea that he might appoint as surgeon general someone who had no connection with the navy and seems to have used Richard H. Bradford, the secretary of the Naval Hospital Fund, in some such advisory capacity. Bradford wrote to Surgeon William P. C. Barton to seek his advice on the most urgent problems in the area of naval medicine. Barton responded that in his opinion there was much to be done "in bringing to a state of economized system the whole of the medical concerns of the navy; especially those afloat, & those concerning the hospital and pension department." He noted specifically the method of supplying hospital stores, "including expensive liquors on ship board." Later Bradford told Barton of his plan to make a synopsis of the medical reports in the custody of the Navy Department. Barton applauded this suggestion and noted the value of such records, adding that no surgeon had published anything on his experiences since his own work in 1814. With official encouragement, perhaps more would do so. For a brief period things looked encouraging to Barton and perhaps to other surgeons. But as soon as Branch learned that a non-naval surgeon general would not be tolerated in the service, he abandoned the idea. Bradford's influence had declined by the time Branch left office.[16]

A bill to create the position of surgeon general was introduced in the Senate on February 16, 1830, by Robert Y. Hayne of South Carolina. By the time it was sent to the Navy Department for comment, Branch was gone and Woodbury was in charge. He took a more cautious approach to the subject than his predecessor. Woodbury said that while he preferred to have the office of surgeon general created, he thought it better to avoid the appearance of doing so. He suggested changing the title of the bill from the specific one to the more general "In Relation to the Medical Department of the Navy." His draft called for the detailing from time to time of a suitable person to supervise the health of navy seamen in warships, hospitals, and naval stations. For these additional duties the designated surgeon would receive double rations on shore, as well as fuel and house rent. There appears to have been little support on the part of Hayne for such a watered down version of the bill, and the proposal languished. Woodbury made reference to the pending bill for a naval medical bureau in his annual report in November 1833. If nothing was done during the current session of Congress, he intended to have one of the older surgeons, attached to either the Washington Navy Yard or the marine barracks, "detailed and employed in performing many of the duties contemplated for a surgeon general."[17]

In March 1834, Woodbury approached Surgeon Thomas Harris about the possibility of appointing him to superintend the medical affairs of the navy. Harris was apparently interested but did not want to leave Philadelphia. Woodbury wanted someone in Washington who would be available to give advice on medical matters, as well as work in the hospital in the navy yard. When Harris turned him down, Woodbury turned to Surgeon Bailey Washington, who had been in the navy since 1813. At the end of June 1834, Woodbury ordered Surgeon Washington to report to the Washington Navy Yard, where he would attend to the sick, and at the same time he would have duties at the Navy Department pertaining to all matters connected with the medical corps over which the secretary had jurisdiction. Washington was to be particularly concerned about subjects related to the health of crews of ships and of those men attached to naval hospitals and stations. He was to see to it that each surgeon and assistant surgeon prepared reports on the diseases and casualties within his area of responsibility and noted the probable causes of the problems, methods of treatment, and results. From time to time, Washington was to report to the secretary on how well the surgeons and assistant surgeons performed their duties. In addition, he was to superintend the selection and purchase of all drugs, medicines, surgical instruments, hospital stores, and furniture. He was to furnish estimates of the quality and kinds of medical and surgical supplies that were necessary for any vessel or any surgeon. When a ship returned from a cruise, Washington was to see that all articles deposited by the medical officers of the vessel were preserved. He would also be expected to perform any other duties that the secretary might assign to him which would promote the interests of the service and the attainment of professional knowledge for the advantage of the medical corps of the navy. For this extra duty at the Navy Department, Washington was to receive $1.50 a day in addition to the allowance he received as the surgeon at the navy yard.[18] Unfortunately we have only fragmentary information on how often Washington was called upon for advice and no the details of any opposition to his advisory role.

One of the first tasks assigned to Washington was to review the book by Dr. William Beaumont, *Experiments and Observations on the Gastric Juice and the Physiology of Digestion*, published in 1833. Beaumont was an army surgeon at Ft. Michilmackinac, which was located on an island between Lake Huron and Lake Michigan. He was called upon to treat a French-Canadian trapper who, in June 1822, had been accidentally wounded in the

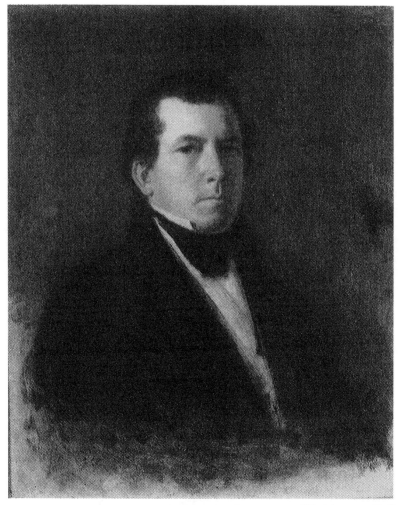

Surgeon Bailey Washington. Smithsonian Institution, Washington, D.C.

side by a shotgun fired at close range. With his chest torn open and lower lung, diaphragm, and stomach badly lacerated, as well as a portion of his flesh burned, the trapper was not expected to survive. Beaumont did the best he could to clean and dress the wound and make his patient comfortable. The trapper survived, but after a year in a military hospital, his wound was still open. The army authorities felt that they had done all they could and wanted to send him home to Canada. Beaumont believed that the journey would probably kill the patient, so he took him into his home and continued to treat him for another two years.

The wound finally healed, but the trapper had a permanent gastric fistula just below his left nipple, through which it was possible for Beaumont to look directly into the man's stomach. This unusual circumstance allowed Beaumont to undertake a series of experiments which enabled him to determine how long it took the trapper to digest various foods and what his gastric juice did to them. The patient objected to these experiments, and for a few years they were interrupted when the patient went home to Canada. Further experiments ceased in 1834 when he returned home for good. Although Beaumont wanted to carry out more experiments, the bulk of his work was finished, and he publicized his findings in book form. This book provided the basis for an understanding of the digestive process.

Surgeon Thomas Boyd acquired a copy of Beaumont's book and presented it to Captain Isaac Hull, the commandant of the Washington Navy Yard, as something of possible value to the navy. Hull sent the book to Surgeon Washington for his views and recommendations. The matter took on a new urgency when Beaumont asked the Navy Department to buy 100 copies of his book. Woodbury asked Washington for his opinion. The surgeon replied, in part,

> As an encouragement to those who may be called upon to take charge of cases apparently hopeless to perserve in their efforts to heal their patients, and to contribute towards the advancement of Medical Science whenever an opportunity may offer, it would be proper to extend the subscription of the Department; but as it is questionable whether our contingent fund could with strict propriety be applied to this purpose, I doubt the propriety of granting the Doctor's request.[19]

So it was that the Navy Department was advised not to buy any copies of the Beaumont book.

When Commodore Lewis Warrington reported from Norfolk that the *Java* had cases of cholera on board and that he sought advice on what to do about it, Secretary Dickerson turned the matter over to Surgeon Washington. The surgeon recommended a series of preventive steps:

> That the men be carefully protected from intemperance—from fruits and vegetables—and from all unnecessary exposure and hard labour,—that the Java be well cleaned and kept dry, and that the chlorides of Lime and soda be freely used, and that the officers see that the men are properly clothed and that they do not sleep on deck, and that all hands be fully impressed with the necessity of reporting without delay to the Medical officers as soon as the slightest symptoms of cholera manifest themselves.

Dickerson ordered Warrington to give this advice to the surgeon in charge of the cholera patients.[20]

On the other hand, when Lieutenant John White wanted to take the *Grampus* into a cold climate for "frosting" in order to minimize the risk of disease in the ship during its regular assignment, Surgeon Washington objected. Instead he urged that the decayed wood in the vessel be removed and that the ship be ventilated and fumigated. The secretary forwarded the recommendation to the lieutenant's commanding officers.[21]

When Secretary Woodbury described the duties that he wished Washington to assume, they included superintending the purchase of all drugs, medicines, and instruments for the use of the navy. Consequently, in January 1834, Washington asked Secretary Dickerson for permission to visit several navy yards and confer with druggists in the larger cities. Dickerson disapproved the trips because, he said, they were not a part of Washington's duties.[22] It was apparent that Dickerson had a narrower view of the role of the medical advisor than Woodbury.

In May 1835, Surgeon Washington asked to be relieved of his duties at the Navy Department and the navy yard, and his request was endorsed by Commodore Hull. Secretary Dickerson relieved him of his duties at the yard but not at the department. The secretary asked him to stay on until a successor could be selected, but he apparently gave up the effort to replace Washington, and on May 28, 1836, the surgeon was ordered to join the Mediterranean Squadron as its fleet surgeon. It was an assignment that Washington welcomed.[23]

The question of creating the post of surgeon general came up again in 1837, when Thomas Harris and 18 other surgeons and assistant surgeons petitioned the House and Senate to create that office. They argued that though the navy was employed in every sea and climate and medical officers were zealous in the pursuit of their duties, there was no one in Washington who was "charged with the reception of communications on medical topics, and to discriminate and determine concerning their merits, such papers are generally thrown aside at the Navy Department as useless." In other civilized nations such information was consigned to professional men and made useful to the world "by the diffusion of knowledge and the promotion of science." The medical officers argued that economy and efficiency would be promoted and the lives of officers and seamen preserved on foreign stations by having "an experienced and intelligent naval surgeon near the seat of government."[24]

Surgeon Barton was not in sympathy with this proposal, which he first heard about from his friend and former student, Assistant Surgeon Jonathan M. Foltz, who was then on duty at the Washington Navy Yard.

Barton immediately wrote Dickerson that he understood that a bill to create the position of surgeon general had been drafted, printed, and recommended to the president, the secretary, and the Senate Naval Affairs Committee, but no one had consulted him about the scheme. It was his feeling that the measure was premature. He then set forth five arguments in support of his position. These were: (1) The reputation, honor, and feelings of the medical corps were safe in the hands of the secretary; (2) only a senior medical officer should receive this appointment, for if a junior was put in the post, all the seniors would feel degraded and disgraced; (3) a navy surgeon general could not supervise the details of the daily duties of medical officers at sea; (4) no navy in the world had a surgeon general, and therefore it was not a necessary office; and (5) before a surgeon general could do any good, a medical bureau would first have to be created. He hoped that the secretary would not support the bill. If the position was created, Barton would "feel bound by self respect to claim the office, if any other than the senior surgeon of the Navy was to receive it."[25]

A month later, Barton sent Dickerson a 37-page printed pamphlet entitled *A Remonstrance against the Creation of the Office of Surgeon General of the Navy,* in which he refined and expanded his earlier views on the subject. He argued that since the duties of the surgeon general would tend to remove the appointee from active practice, any recommendations that he made would come out of a cloistered environment and would be impracticable. "The jewel of medical learning, unset in the strong cincture of *practice,* is a jewel of appreciable but unavailable value." If the Navy Department wished to send the best medical advice to surgeons afloat, it would be more economical to supply pertinent books to the ship as a part of its medical outfit. Doctors on active duty regularly sought the advice of older and more experienced colleagues in difficult cases, and the fleet surgeon was also available for consultation. He was closer to the scene of action and better able to give advice than any surgeon general, who would be thousands of miles away from a health problem. The situation was different in the U.S. Army: all of its forces were on land, and in an emergency information sent by express could reach it in a hurry.

On the matter of medical supplies, the navy agents were the best-informed people about fluctuating prices. The pending legislation seemed to visualize the surgeon general as functioning as a purveyor; this was unprofessional. In addition, legislation already in effect made it illegal for a surgeon to receive money in any amount. There was also a proviso in the bill that called for the surgeon general to keep a register of the duty assignments of surgeons and assistant surgeons and see that everyone had a regular turn at sea and shore duty. Barton regarded this as an erosion of the authority of the secretary of the navy. From Barton's point of view, all the goals of the proposed legislation to create the office of surgeon general could be attained by extending the jurisdiction of the existing board of naval examiners. In addition to determining the merits of candidates, it could advise the secretary on all medical matters.[26]

It is possible that Barton's arguments had some influence on Dickerson. The surgeon had at least raised some significant points about the need for a medical bureau and how it might function. Already there were those in Congress who felt that there was a need for a general reform of the whole naval administrative structure, especially those functions that were the responsibility of the Board of Navy Commissioners. Medical questions now began to be considered within the framework of a larger reform.

In February 1839 the House passed a resolution directing the secretary of the navy to submit a plan for the reorganization of his department on the basis of the duties now performed by the Board of Navy Commissioners, which would be assigned to separate bureaus. Secretary Paulding sent a proposal for the creation of three divisions: one for construction, one for supplies, and one for navy yards. Each would be headed by a line officer. The head of the second division was also to be designated as the inspector general of hospitals. The duties of the head of the third division included the supervision of the purchase of medical stores and drugs, but the actual purchases were to be made by a surgeon subordinate. Paulding's plan was not in strict accordance with the House resolution, which clearly contemplated the establishment of separate bureaus. The lack of logic and proper delegation of authority in this plan caused a knowledgeable observer to submit his comments to the Philadelphia *United States Gazette*, which published them in December 1839 under the pen name *Non Nauticus*. Noting that sea officers headed each of the proposed divisions, he said that such men were not knowledgeable about the quantity or quality of medicines. He asked if the president of the Medical Society of Philadelphia was not qualified to be the medical chief of the navy, or if such surgeons as Harris, Barton, Morgan, or Washington were not qualified to discharge these duties. Those involved in planning the reorganization were apparently unaware that in Great Britain and France, doctors headed the medical bureaus of the navy, and the same was true in the armies of Great Britain and the United States. "If there be one branch of the service which requires a responsible head more than another, it is the medical branch." By making the medical department subordinate to the division of subsistence, as the plan proposed, the naval committees of the House and Senate did an injustice to and insulted "the whole medical profession of the

United States." Instead the navy should have an independent medical bureau, headed by a doctor, and the service would be benefit.

To *Non Nauticus* it seemed clear that the medical bureau should be in charge of purchasing all medical and surgical stores and instruments, supervising medical requisitions and disbursements, and inspecting hospitals and collecting medical reports from which statistical information could be compiled. The medical bureau would also keep a roster of sea and shore service to make sure that in the future those duties would be shared equally. *Non Nauticus* or, perhaps, a sympathetic friend sent a copy of the published remarks to Senator Samuel Southard of the Naval Affairs Committee. With them was an unsigned note that said: "One who is fully aware how much the Naval Medical corps is indebted to your fostering care while at the head of the Navy Department, begs to call your attention to the subject of the enclosed extract."[27] Southard was well aware of the problems of the navy, and the medical aspects were only a part of a larger question. Talk of reform was in the air, but not much could be done until after the presidential election of 1840. Once that was out of the way and the Whigs controlled the presidency, changes took place.

Rules and Regulations

If nothing could be done about establishing the post of surgeon general, perhaps some steps could be taken to improve the institutional memory of the Navy Department on medical matters. In 1839, Surgeon Thomas Boyd told Secretary Paulding that it was a matter of regret that "the Vital Statistics of the Navy have not been under some uniform regulation that they might be serviceable to medical science." He pointed out that there were "no general form for returns" and each surgeon presented his information in accordance with his own views. Boyd thought that the method of reporting, as well as other duties of the medical department, should be governed by regulations.[28]

Boyd undoubtedly knew that many officers wanted an improved system of regulations. The ones drawn up by the Board of Navy Commissioners in 1818 had never been enacted into law despite the urgings of several secretaries. Many of them had been incorporated into the rules and regulations of specific navy ships by individual captains, however, and thus had the force of law on shipboard. Still, when the act of Congress of 1828 replaced the rank of surgeon's mate with that of assistant surgeon, and when the rank of hospital surgeon was recognized, there was some additional concern about the need to update the regulations. Matters relating to accountability for medicines, instruments, and equipment also needed to be addressed.

Woodbury brought these matters to the attention of the Board of Navy Commissioners in the fall of 1831 and asked for their recommendations.[29]

The board suggested that additional regulations were needed to cover the purchase or issuance of stores after they were returned to the hospital surgeon. It also thought that anything required in the medical department, whether it be medicines, instruments, utensils, furniture, or other items, should be the subject of a requisition on the medical purveyor or hospital surgeon and approved in writing by the commanding officer of the doctor requesting it. If the purveyor did not have the item in stock, the requisition was then to go to the navy agent, who was to acquire the item from a contractor, or if there was no contractor, purchase it. Nothing thus acquired was to be paid for until it had passed the inspection of the purveyor or hospital surgeon. Whoever did the inspecting was to certify that the article was of the approved quality and suitable for the naval service. The board also recommended that articles remaining on hand in a ship at the end of a cruise or elsewhere handed over to the hospital surgeon or purveyor, who would examine them. If he had any doubts about their fitness, he was to bring the matter to the attention of the commanding officer, who would then appoint three officers, two of whom would be surgeons, to survey the material. Depending upon the recommendations of the survey team, the items would be turned over to the purveyor for reissue, sold at auction, or destroyed. Finally, the board recommended that it should be the duty of the purveyor or hospital surgeon to keep every instrument and all medicines and hospital stores ready for issue and make quarterly reports of all articles on hand and all receipts for items issued.[30]

The need for a new set of rules and regulations was brought to the attention of Congress in 1832. Congress responded by passing a law in May of that year authorizing the president to constitute a board of navy officers, consisting of the navy commissioners and two post captains, who with the assistance of the attorney general were to revise and enlarge the regulations. When completed they were to be sent to the president for approval and then transmitted to Congress for enactment into law.

The board met in November, and a year later the results of their deliberations were sent to the secretary, who forwarded them to the president. Jackson approved them, and in February 1834 the Naval Affairs Committee of the House printed over a thousand copies of them. Evidently some changes were suggested, for in May 1834, Jackson sent Congress proposals for amending the laws in relation to the naval service. The chairman of the Naval Affairs Committee of the House reported a resolution to print the amended rules and regulations. Nothing more seems to have been done and Congress adjourned at the end of June.[31]

When the proposal to establish the office of surgeon general of the navy was being considered in January and February of 1838, the matter of regulations came up. The draft bill stated that as soon as practicable after his appointment, the surgeon general was to draw up and submit to the secretary a set of regulations for the medical department. When these had been approved by the president, they would be observed in the service; Congress would thus be bypassed. As I noted above, the bill to create the position of surgeon general soon died.

Secretary Paulding took up the subject again soon after he came to office in July 1838. He urged the board to look to the revision of the naval code. Various other concerns distracted the commissioners, so that they were not able to make a report until December 1840. Paulding approved of their efforts but did not send the results to Congress. The matter remained pending when Abel Upshur became secretary under the Whig party of William Henry Harrison in October 1841. He studied the recommendations but did not approve of them. So instead of sending them to Congress, he urged that a new, mixed commission be appointed, made up of civilians and naval officers, who would draft a new set of rules and regulations. Mindful of the agitation then going on in the land for the abolition of punishment by flogging, Upshur said that the new regulations must prevent an inequality in punishments, which caused discontent, brought courts-martial into disrepute, and undermined the discipline in the navy. It was absolutely necessary, he wrote, to have a system of rules and regulations that "absolutely define rank and authority, plainly prescribe duties and responsibilities, and ascertain crimes and their punishments." Unfortunately Upshur was not able to attain this goal.[32]

Pay

Medical officers had assumed that the changes made under the acts of 1828 and 1829 in regard to their pay were the start of some long-delayed attention to their needs. When this proved not to be the case, there was discontent. Other officers felt the same way. In response, Congress passed a law in March 1835 to regulate navy pay. Hereafter compensation would be defined on an annual rather than a monthly basis. A senior captain on active duty would receive $4,500 a year; if awaiting orders or on leave, he got $1,000 less a year. All other captains when in command of squadrons on foreign stations received $4,000, and when on other duty, $3,500; the sum dropped to $2,500 off duty. Commanders and masters commandant got $2,500 on sea duty; $2,100 when attached to navy yards; and $1,800 when awaiting orders or on leave. When exercising command, lieutenants earned $1,800 a year; when on other duty, $1,500; and while awaiting orders, $1,200.

In the case of medical men, the formula was more complicated. During the first 5 years after his commissioning, a surgeon received $1,000 per year. He got a $200 raise during the second five-year period, and an additional $200 during his third and fourth five-year periods. After 20 years or more of service, he received $1,800 a year. When attached to a navy yard, a recruiting rendezvous, a receiving ship, or a naval hospital, the surgeon got an additional one-fourth of his base pay. When on sea duty, he got an increase of one-third of his annual pay. A fleet surgeon got an additional one-half of his base salary. The formula for assistant surgeons was: awaiting orders, $650; at sea, $950; after passing his exams and being found qualified for surgeon, $850; at sea in the same status, $1,200; attached to a navy yard, hospital, rendezvous, or receiving ship, $950; and after being passed and stationed at any of these installations, $1,150.

The law also did away with the practice of giving an allowance to an officer for receiving or disbursing money, drawing bills, or transacting government business. In addition, no officer would be allowed servants, or the pay, clothing, and rations of servants. Henceforth officers would not receive allowances for quarters, to buy or rent furniture, for lights or fuel, or for the transportation of baggage. When traveling under orders, they would be allowed 10¢ a mile for expenses. Otherwise the stated yearly compensation was all that was allowed.[33]

If Congress thought that the medical men would be content with this formula, it soon found out otherwise. Twelve navy surgeons sent a petition to the House and Senate in December 1838. They noted that after acquiring an expensive education, followed by rigid examinations for admission to the navy and promotion, as well as being exposed to diseases in all kinds of climates, surgeons were still paid less than lieutenants. Lieutenants were usually promoted earlier in their careers than surgeons. As things now stood, navy surgeons received half the pay of their opposite numbers in the army. They asked that they be paid $1,200 a year for the first five years and $1,400 for the second, along with the current ratio of increases when serving at sea or on shore.[34]

A bill to increase the pay of the navy surgeons was passed by the House in 1838 but was not acted upon by the Senate. The matter was only partly resolved in 1848. In the meantime the cost of living in various cities and the deficiency in their pay caused some shore-based surgeons to go into private practice full or part time, depending on their duty assignments, the attitudes of their commanding officers, and their opportunities.[35]

Hospitals

In his annual report for 1830, Secretary Branch noted that the hospitals in most of the navy yards were "entirely deficient in the means of giving accommodation to the invalids of the Navy who may be so unfortunate as to require it." At most of these places, there was only temporary shelter or an old building. "The mariner who returns after long and faithful service in distant and uncongenial climates, finds no asylum prepared for his reception and recovery from diseases incident to such service, but is compelled to linger out his life in crowded and confined apartments even less favorable to his restoration than the hold of the vessel from which he had been discharged." With funds from the monthly deductions of the officers and men, as well as appropriations from Congress, two magnificent hospital buildings had been built at Philadelphia and Norfolk, but neither had been completed, and only the one at Norfolk was designed to accommodate the sick. Branch pointed out that it would be several years before enough capital was accumulated in the Navy Hospital Fund to continue building permanent hospitals. Money from the fund had also been used to buy land for hospitals at New York and Boston. These sites were important because a number of men were recruited there and needed buildings to accommodate invalids. At Pensacola the situation was much worse: there was not even a building to protect the sick form inclement weather.[36]

One might have expected that Branch, having reported these things, would recommend an appropriation to speed up the building of hospitals, but he did not. Like many nineteenth-century secretaries, he relied on the president and Congress to judge the need from what had been said and take appropriate action. Until they did so, plans proceeded slowly and in keeping with the emphasis on economy during the Jackson and Van Buren administrations.

Early in 1830, Commodore Chauncey had prepared a plan for a hospital at the Brooklyn Navy Yard, together with its estimated cost. Branch forwarded to the Board of Navy Commissioners for study, but without money to implement the plan, it remained pending. In 1831 the board studied a plan for Boston which visualized three distinct buildings, or one building with three sections. The center building was to be made of granite and would measure 160' × 35'. This would be linked to two smaller granite buildings measuring 70' × 62' which were to be placed at the ends of the center building. The estimated cost for all was $102,750. Eighteen months later the board recommended that only the right wing be built at the present time.[37]

Meanwhile the situation at Pensacola had demanded action. Commo-

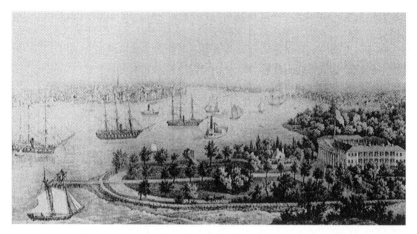

Norfolk Naval Hospital as It Appeared in 1850. Hampton Roads Naval Museum, Hampton, Va.

dore Jesse D. Elliott had called the department's attention to the fact that the old building at Barrancas which was used as a hospital was not large enough or in a proper condition for even the limited number of patients who were now there. Yet Pensacola was also supposed to be available for the sick of the West India Squadron. He urged that the building materials already on the base be used to construct a new hospital.[38] Before any action could be taken on this request, the army evacuated a base known as Cantonment Clinch, about six miles from the navy yard and two and a half from town, and turned it over to the navy. It had a hospital that was a big improvement over the one the navy had been using, so about 30 patients were moved to it. It was later determined that this building needed repairs, and approval was sought for the expenditure. The board approved the funds, but some confusion arose over orders to repair it. The board and Captain Dallas, in charge of the navy yard, understood that the money was to be spent on improving the old army hospital, but Branch apparently intended it for the building near Barrancas. The problem was resolved when Commodore Rodgers told Branch that the Barracas building was not worth repairing. Yet Branch apparently still did not have a clear idea of the situation, for in his annual report he said that there was no building at Pensacola to protect the sick from inclement weather. This was true only in relation to the grounds of the yard itself.[39]

Funds appropriated by Congress in 1832 made it possible to start building new hospitals at Pensacola, Brooklyn, and New York, and in the Charlestown district of Boston. These were designed so that they could be enlarged if the future needs of the service required it. Also, a special appropriation in 1831 provided $1,000 for public works at Norfolk, and another $31,000 voted in 1833 made it possible to finish that hospital. Woodbury reported that it was "one of the most beautiful and useful public buildings belonging to the government." The completed hospital structure was now larger than what was currently needed, so that some of the interior spaces were not finished. Additional sums that were needed to provide for the comfort of patients were taken from the general hospital fund.[40]

Woodbury was also able to report that by the end of 1833 the Naval Asylum at Philadelphia had been completed and partly furnished. But there were problems with the city and the state. The state had the power to enforce criminal and civil processes within the asylum, and the city wanted to tax the property and run a city street through it. These were eventually resolved. Nevertheless, in 1836 the Board of Navy Commissioners reported that some of the land originally set aside for the asylum had been diminished by the building of Sutherland Avenue, on the west side. Otherwise things were progressing. To complete work on appendages to the main building, build a brick wall around the property, drain the ground, plant trees, and establish a cemetery would require an additional $30,000.[41]

At Secretary Dickerson's request, the board prepared a progress report on the naval hospitals in 1836. Earlier it had been decided that the hospital in the Boston area would be built at Chelsea. A structure measuring 70' × 62', consisting of a cellar, two stories, and an attic, was nearing completion. It was estimated that a house for the surgeon would cost $19,380, of which $10,000 was needed that year.

Progress had also been made at Brooklyn, where a hospital structure measuring 100' × 48', with a basement, two stories, and an attic, had been constructed. To finish the work on the building, graduate and enclose the grounds, construct a wharf for landing patients, and repair a house for the surgeon would require $34,500, of which $16,000 was on hand.

The situation in Norfolk was good, but funds were needed to finish work on one of the wings of the hospital building and its dependent structures. A wall also needed to be built around the hospital grounds.

At Pensacola the hospital was finished, and the surgeon's residence was being completed. It was recommended that a brick wall be built around the hospital grounds. Also, since sickness was common in ships operating in the Gulf of Mexico and the West Indies, and if the navy squadron there was increased, it would be desirable to enlarge the existing hospital.

In recapitulating the costs of work at various locations, the board said

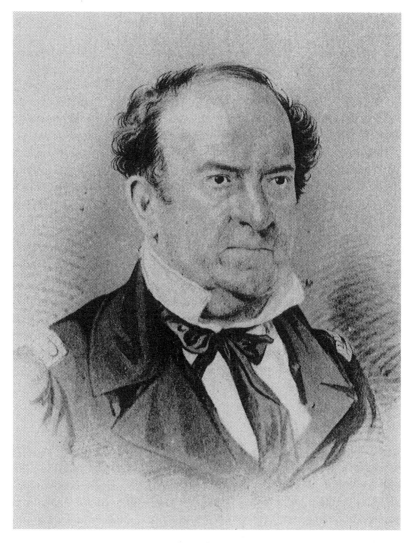

Surgeon Thomas Williamson, First Superintendent of the Naval Hospital at Norfolk, Virginia. U.S. Navy Bureau of Medicine and Surgery, Washington, D.C.

that to complete all the pending work at Chelsea, Brooklyn, Philadelphia, Norfolk, and Pensacola, a total of $156,880 was needed. It recommended that the appropriation be made collectively, so that any funds left over from one hospital could be applied to another.[42]

Congress did not accept all these recommendations, but it did supply funds so that work continued at some places. At Norfolk money was provided in 1837 to erect a sea wall to protect the shore, enclose the grounds, compete the basement, and repair damage. Small sums were appropriated in 1839, 1840, and 1841, followed by $13,750 in 1842. In Brooklyn two wings were added to the main building in 1840. Each was 79' × 49' and the same height as the main structure. A "pest house" was constructed of the same height and style for patients with pestilential diseases. The hospital was designed to accommodate 125 patients.[43]

The sums allocated for hospitals were a part of a general increase in naval appropriations which was due in part to a concern about a possible war with Great Britain over boundary disputes. But whatever the motivation, the fact remains that by the end of the Van Buren administration, the navy had five permanent hospitals in operation. In addition, the Naval Asylum in Philadelphia was providing a dignified atmosphere in which retired seamen could finish out their days. All this represented a big improvement in health care and a long overdue act of justice to the men of the navy, who had paid hospital money to the government for many years. There were still makeshift arrangements in the navy yards at Washington, Philadelphia, and Portsmouth, New Hampshire, but the number of patients requiring hospitalization was usually low. Doctors in the permanent navy hospitals were setting the standards by which medical care on shore was judged. The good reputations of the doctors and the hospitals helped to improve the morale of the enlisted men.[44]

The Size of the Navy Medical Corps

Medical officers in the navy came to the conclusion that in terms of numbers they were at a disadvantage in comparison with other line officers, so in February 1837 they sent a letter to President Jackson calling his attention to their plight. One of the interesting features of this letter is that the signers referred to themselves collectively as "the Medical Corps of the U.S. Navy." It was signed by 7 surgeons, 11 passed assistant surgeons (men who had passed the examination for assistant surgeon and were waiting for vacancies), and 1 assistant surgeon. Heading the list were the names of Surgeons William P. C. Barton and Thomas Harris.

The medical officers pointed out that between 1815 and 1836, the number of captains had increased from 32 to 40; commanders from 18 to 40; and lieutenants from 150 to 257. In contrast, the number of surgeons had decreased from 48 to 43 and assistant surgeons from 71 to 50. They noted that there was an insufficient number of medical officers to supply the warships that the last session of Congress had ordered into commission.

The pending appropriation bill called for 35 surgeons for sea service and 18 for hospitals, navy yards, recruiting duty, and in receiving ships, or a total of 53. In addition, 54 assistant surgeons were needed for sea service, and 14 for shore duty, for a total of 68 assistant and passed assistant surgeons. These figures, the medical officers continued, made no allowances for those who were incapacitated by poor health or old age or who were on leave after a long cruise. As things now stood, medical officers were more constantly employed than other ranks. There was also a greater fatality among medical officers than line officers. Therefore the number of surgeons should be increased to 70, and the same increase should be applied to the assistant and passed assistant surgeons. With these additions, "all the wants of the service could be conveniently attended to." President Jackson forwarded the letter to Secretary Dickerson for appropriate action. With the passage of time it became clear to the medical officers that no change was forthcoming.[45]

There was indeed a shortage of medical officers able to take on any duties assigned by the secretary. At the same time some who sought active service were kept waiting. Dickerson resorted to the practice of asking officers if they would welcome a particular assignment. When a medical officer asked why he had received a query about any interest he might have in a cruise to the Pacific, the secretary replied, "The difficulty, frequently, of getting officers free from objections to those distant stations, was the cause of the letter being addressed to you, as well as to others, that the Department might be apprised of your and their wishes on the subject, & as the contemplated cruise was not so generally known as to give an opportunity for *applications* for such service, if desired."[46]

The Seminole War

Some additional problems in finding suitable officers for all assignments came about as a result of the Second Seminole War, which began in Florida in December 1835. For the next seven years, the army, assisted by a small naval force, attempted to subdue a Indian population of fewer than 1,200 warriors. When the commandant of the marines took his troops from Washington to Florida in June 1836, Surgeon John A. Kearney volunteered to accompany them. The marines served alongside Brigadier General Thomas Jesup's troops in Alabama and Florida. Marines and sailors from the West India Squadron also served in the war, forming a "Mosquito fleet" of shallow-draft vessels which patrolled the rivers and coastal waterways that ran into the Everglades. Marines from the barracks lost 6 men in battle and had 22 deaths from disease before they returned to Washington in 1838. Marines from the West India Squadron lost 1 man who died of wounds and 16 who succumbed to disease. Casualties among navy men were small. By the spring of 1842, the Seminoles had been reduced to about 250 souls, and the United States announced that the war had been won.[47]

Chapter 15

Health Problems, 1829–1842

The work of the West India Squadron in suppressing pirates had brought to the attention of the Navy Department the health problems relating to that environment. After the pirates had been eliminated, routine cruises in the Caribbean sometimes brought to light serious health problems.

In 1830, Captain Jesse D. Elliott wrote from Pensacola to report the arrival of the sloop of war *Erie*. With the ship came Commander Robert M. Rose, who was suffering from debility and a deranged mind. Five days after he landed, Rose died of "an enlargement of the brain." Elliott said that Rose had been ill some time before his last assignment and that he had arrived in the West Indies from the north with an enfeebled constitution, which left him with insufficient strength for duty in the tropics. The other sick men in the *Erie* were both of the medical officers, a midshipman, and two seamen. The midshipman had since died of an unreported cause. Elliott could not estimate how long the two medical officers would be in the hospital, so he asked to have them replaced with two surgeons and two assistants. He pointed out the necessity of assigning men who had some experience with fevers in the West Indies, "for it not infrequently happens that two Surgeons do not minister alike to the disease."[1]

Elliott got his replacements, but lack of institutional memory on how to treat tropical diseases continued until Surgeon William P. C. Barton addressed the question late in 1830. His involvement with the West Indies came about as a result of Secretary Branch ordering him to sea as the surgeon of the frigate *Brandywine* under the command of Captain Henry E. Ballard. The voyage originated in New York, where many of the crew were transferred from a receiving ship with colds. Captain Isaac Chauncey, the commandant of the Brooklyn Navy Yard, and Captain Ballard worked in severe winter weather to get the ship ready for sea. Using men with colds for work in this climate resulted in the sick list growing from 15 on the day after the transfer to 58 within 10 or 11 days. "With two or three exceptions," wrote Barton, "all of these were afflicted with the diseases arising from intense and continued cold; such as frosted hands, fingers, toes and feet, chilblains, pleurisies, pneumonic affections, etc." One midshipman and five men with scarlet fever were transferred to the naval hospital "for the indispensable benefit of fire and other comforts."[2] In addition, one of Barton's assistant surgeons became ill, and he was still convalescing when the ship sailed. His other assistant was still suffering from chilblains brought on by his duty between decks. Another midshipman became "dangerously ill of a pneumonic fever," which "assumed the typhoid type" during the continuing bad weather. He was still recovering very slowly when the ship left New York.[3] In Barton's opinion, this officer and another midshipman with scarlet fever owed their lives to their transfer to the larger and more comfortable quarters of the captain's cabin. The sick assistant surgeon was also moved there. Sixteen other sick seamen were sent back to the receiving ship and placed under the care of the surgeon of the navy yard. Nevertheless, the sick list continued at 35–57 up to the time of sailing. There were also "numbrous applicants with slighter catarrh affections" who were treated but not placed on the sick list.[4] Several of the older midshipmen were doing duty although they still had colds and chilblains, and seven were on the sick list.

This state of affairs at the commencement of a scheduled cruise in the West Indies disturbed Surgeon Barton. He wrote to Captain Ballard and reviewed the health situation between January and March 10, when the ship was on the eve of dropping its pilot off Sandy Hook. He considered the crew "especially predisposed" to suffer during the shift from winter to the very warm weather of the West Indies during the unhealthy season. Their condition would make them vulnerable to tropical diseases, and therefore he recommended that the frigate remain at sea until the end of June or the beginning of July and avoid such unhealthy ports as Havana. Otherwise, he feared, there would be "a disastrous result of the cruise." Captain Ballard forwarded Barton's letter to the Navy Department, where it would seem that no one paid any particular attention to it.[5]

The *Brandywine* sailed to the West Indies, cruised around Cuba, and anchored in Havana early in April 1830. During the voyage from New York, four men had died and several others were in a dangerous state, but the general health of the crew had improved. Ballard's reason for stopping in Havana was to wait for the arrival of Commodore Jesse D. Elliott, the squadron commander, from Key West and to overhaul his ship in a more congenial climate. After leaving Havana, the ship touched at Santo Domingo, Vera Cruz, Tampico, and Pensacola. Further duty had to be curtailed because of the sick on board. When the *Brandywine* reached Hampton Roads on July 7, 1830, the total number of men on the sick list who had been treated was 488. The ship had sailed with 483 officers and men and 4 passengers.

According to Barton, most of these cases were of

> typhoid, pneumonia, scarlet fever, low fever of tertian and quartan types, diarrhoea and rheumatism, diseases generated by dampness. When this dampness became a heated moisture, as it soon did in the West Indies, the causes of fever were of extremely dangerous aspect, and the pneumonia and anginose affection general, and excessively distressing and difficult to manage. Sore throats running to ulceration, with dejected spirits and low state of the system, accompanied more or less, all the cases.

He attributed the sickness mainly to a severe winter, a foul hold and lower apartments, and "a bilged well," as well as the fact that the *Brandywine* was "a damp, ill-ventilated and wet ship," which should not have been sent to the tropics. Yet there were only 10 deaths, and only 2 of these were due to fever, but not yellow fever.[6]

On Barton's recommendation all hands were removed from the ship. Those who had completed their terms of service were paid off, and those who had not were transferred to another ship. All the officers were allowed to live elsewhere for weeks while the ship was ventilated. The stores were removed and fires lit below decks to dry the timbers. Those assigned to work in the ship were relieved every hour. The hold broke open and it was found to be extremely foul. A carpenter's yeoman, who had lived continually below the berth deck, was sent to the hospital, where he died three days later. Accompanying him to the hospital was Assistant Surgeon Gustavus R. B. Horner, who was still suffering from a fever; he recovered sufficiently to be sent home. Henry S. Coulter, the senior assistant surgeon, also went on leave. Barton himself had a slight attack of the same fever that afflicted Horner, but he was not hospitalized. Two other officers who were among the last to leave the ship were ill when they headed for their homes. From his residence on the James River in Virginia, one of them wrote to Barton asking for his advice in treating the "low fever" from which he suffered. The ship's boatswain left for New York in a weakened state. These cases convinced Barton that he had done the right thing in recommending that the men leave the ship as quickly as possible. Despite his advance warning about the health of the crew, his letter from Norfolk accompanied by his list of the sick in the *Brandywine* caused much concern in the Navy Department, for the ship had been gone for barely six months. Barton was asked to send a report with as much detail as he thought necessary on what means could be used to protect the health of seamen in the interval between enlistment and the beginning of a cruise. The department noted with pleasure that during the voyage the officers in the steerage abstained from the spirit ration and hoped that their example would be followed by others. As for Barton himself, the department assured him that his professional services during the cruise would be "properly estimated."[7]

Encouraged by this sign of confidence in his work, Barton sent the requested report. In it he referred to his long experience in Philadelphia examining recruits. During that time he also had taken advantage of every opportunity to talk to foreign medical and line officers, merchants, and others in order to learn from their experiences. He pointed out that in the Spanish navy, duty in the West Indies was rewarded with double pay. In the British navy, duty off the coast of Africa or in the East Indies meant increased pay and rapid promotion. Both the British and the Spanish navies counted a cruise of any duration in the West Indies as equivalent to double service elsewhere. As for the specific reasons for the *Brandywine's* high rate of sickness, Barton believed that the practice of salting a ship to preserve its timbers tended to create dampness and an unhealthy environment. The humid condition was worsened by too much wetting of the gun and spar decks, some of it due to weather, but most of it to scrubbing. For Barton the only way to arrest sickness in such an environment was to free everyone from it as soon as possible.

Barton said that he stood ready to make suggestions for improving the health of officers and men which the department could enforce through regulations. These regulations would involve the necessity of commanders consulting frequently with their medical officers and in all practical things, pursuing their advice, without argument, murmur, or contention. "It will be in vain to place a medical man of character (as none other can now get into the navy or be promoted) in a situation where his advice is neither asked for or followed; and his suggestions for health or life, either condemned or derided, or half executed, or complained of in execution."[8] Was the captain of a ship competent to decide on the safety of communication with shore in an unhealthy foreign port without any consultation with his medical officer? Or suppose that he denied his medical officer the right to go ashore to gather scientific and other information but allowed himself or others to go, risking their bringing back disease to the ship. How could such problems be overcome? In the Spanish and British navies, said Barton, the opinion of the medical officer on matters of health admitted of no appeal or opposition. It should be the same in the U.S. Navy.

Barton had raised some fundamental questions about who was ultimately responsible for the health of the ship's crew, questions that challenged the authority and pretensions of the line officers and could not easily be resolved, even by a secretary resolute enough to see the issue through to a conclusion. Branch had shown a willingness to take controversial stands, but he was not ready to make a decision on the points raised by Barton. When he had completed the transfer of his sick to the hospital, Barton requested and received a leave of absence.

En route to Philadelphia he stopped in Washington, where he saw Secretary Branch and met Richard H. Bradford, the secretary of the Naval Hospital Fund. The latter and Barton found they had common interests, and after Barton returned to Philadelphia, the two corresponded. Bradford told Barton of his plan to make a synopsis of the medical reports in the custody of the Navy Department, and Barton endorsed the proposal, emphasizing the value of such records. "There is no surgeon of observation or talent who makes a cruise, but might derive from it, some useful experience for others who are to sail in the same seas and under the same sun; and he ought not to be content with the mere performance of ship duty; but ought to give the result of such experience, to the Department, or to the public under the auspices of the Department." Many things had struck him during his recent cruise which he thought might be published in a small volume "touching the prophylactic and medical discipline of officers and crews, in that clime, which, if the Department has confidence sufficient in my ability to perform, I would wish to issue under its auspices." He asked Bradford to try to ascertain if Branch would encourage such a project.[9]

It is known that Bradford told Barton that the proposed book might be of use to the merchant service as well as the navy, but just how much hope he held out for official encouragement is not clear. Barton believed that the book might be profitable for himself, and he began to write it with his accustomed gusto. In September 1830 he published *Hints for Medical Officers Cruising in the West Indies.* For his fellow medical officers, he drew upon and expanded the information previously sent to the secretary, and in an appendix he printed the text of his prophetic letter to Branch written before the *Brandywine* put to sea. Among other things, he declared that yellow fever was not contagious, an argument advanced by Benjamin Rush and other medical writers some years earlier.[10] Barton also declared himself an advocate of temperance, and he felt that doctors ought to set a good example in this regard. When he saw a medical officer drink brandy, "I fear and mistrust his professional efficiency and skill." On an examining board for medical officers, he continued, he would never vote for the promotion of any surgeon addicted to alcohol.[11]

While Barton was on leave, events were unfolding in Norfolk and with the *Brandywine* which would soon affect his plans. The new naval hospital was now far enough along to allow for the transfer of patients from the older facility in Gosport. When this subject was first broached, Surgeon Thomas Williamson, who was in charge at Gosport, wrote to Bradford, the secretary of the Naval Hospital Fund, that the proposed transfer would cost about $100, which would be spent on the repair of camp cots and the purchase of chairs, tables, washstands, basins, and some extra sheets and pillowcases. He pointed out that the furniture then being used at Gosport was not adaptable to the new hospital; for example, the cots were not very durable. At that time the patient load consisted of 2 officers and 16 men. Most of them had chronic diseases, but there were two insane men, whose situation was made worse by the lack of proper cells. The attendants consisted of a steward, a cook, two washerwomen, two nurses, and one ordinary seaman from a ship out of commission, who acted as a gardener and also helped out in the hospital when the patient load was heavy. There was also a boy from a ship in ordinary, who tended the gate to the hospital and carried medicines to nurses and requisitions for provisions. Williamson did not see how he could function with a smaller staff, especially if the sick list increased. Also, he requested a small boat and two men to carry provisions and other items to the hospital. When not on boat duty, the men would remove rubbish from the hospital and keep up the property. Before the patients could be transferred, a few laborers would be needed to clean up an accumulation of rubbish in the north wing of the new hospital. After consulting with Nash Legrand, the navy agent, the surgeon believed that an additional $200 would allow the north wing to be fixed up sufficiently to accommodate 30 or 40 sick men.[12]

Surgeon Williamson was able to see most of these plans to completion before he was ordered to the *Brandywine* for a cruise. To replace him at Norfolk, Secretary Branch chose Surgeon Barton, who did not welcome the assignment. Earlier he had avoided another tour of sea duty, and he did all he could to get his Norfolk orders changed, citing family responsibilities and his work in Philadelphia. But Barton had also built a reputation for his ideas on hospitals and his recent suggestions on health care growing out of his service in the *Brandywine*. Therefore it is not surprising that Branch wanted the best man he could find to supervise the newly completed hospital at Norfolk. So, in the end, Branch prevailed and Barton took up his duties in Norfolk in late October 1830.[13]

As soon as Barton had explored his new surroundings, he began to write letters drawing attention to problems and suggesting changes. He renewed Williamson's request for a boat and crew for the use of the hospital. Looking over the list of expenditures, and knowing that sick men did not each much, he began to suspect abuses and fraud; upon investigating, he found that this was indeed the case, and he sent a detailed report of his findings to the secretary. From September 1 to October 31, 1830, the total cost of food for the hospital was $437.07. An allowance of 25¢ a day was provided for rations, so for the 36 patients fed over a 61-day period, the allotted amount was $549; thus a saving had been made. But when Barton examined the wages of the staff and the costs of medicine and fuel, he came up with a total expenditure of $238.64 more than the income from the Naval Hospital Fund, and he projected this into an annual deficit of $1,431.66.

To cut this deficit, he discharged the washerwomen, laborers, and a messenger. In his view, the 25¢ a day allowed for rations must also be applied to administrative costs. This made it necessary to feed the patients on half the value of the ration. Barton showed that by buying provisions in quantity, savings could be made. He would also put out the washing on a piecework basis and thus save wages, rations, soap, and fuel. In his quarterly report submitted in December 1830, Barton showed that his economies would save $744 a year in the feeding of 36 patients. An analysis of his figures shows that the patients received 2,500–3,000 calories per day at a cost of 4⅙¢ a meal. Barton's report was sent to both Branch and Secretary of the Treasury Samuel D. Ingham in their capacities as commissioners of navy hospitals. Both expressed appreciation for Barton's work in cutting expenditures and improving the general arrangement of duties.[14]

Nevertheless, it seems clear that Barton's rigid approach to economy would eventually get to sensitive areas such as perquisites, the care of dependents, and the cost of completing the naval hospital. So he was ordered to Philadelphia to sit on boards of examination for medical officers. At first this was listed as a leave of absence, with Surgeon Jonathan Cowdery acting in his stead, but later Secretary Woodbury found it convenient to bring Surgeon Thomas Williamson back and place him in charge of the hospital again.[15]

As for Barton, he was happy to be back in his beloved Philadelphia, where he continued to pursue his teaching and medical practice. The Navy Department was apparently willing to leave him alone. But he did not forget the needs of the naval medical service, as witnessed by his letter to the secretary in 1833 calling attention to the arrival of a Dr. Burroughs from Manila. Barton said that Burroughs had a limited quantity of oil of camphor and oil of cajuput. This was the first importation of these items to the United States, and Barton thought that the navy should buy and test them. The oil of camphor was said to be a remedy for cholera, and it could be purchased from Burroughs for $15.00 a bottle. A bottle of cajuput sold for $22.00. Acting on Barton's suggestion, Woodbury approved the purchase of two bottles of each, their contents to be divided into smaller bottles for distribution. The largest number of bottles would go to the navy hospitals at New York and Norfolk and the rest to ships on active service. How the testing was carried out and what the results were are unknown to this writer.[16]

Later in that year, Barton again wrote to Woodbury informing him that he had just published a book on botany and asking if the Navy Department would purchase enough copies to supply every surgeon and assistant surgeon in the service. Woodbury referred the matter to the Board of Navy Commissioners, and they recommended that the book not be purchased because heretofore the department had not furnished libraries to the medical service. Woodbury endorsed this response in his reply to Barton.[17]

During Secretary Dickerson's tenure, Barton was offered the post of fleet surgeon with the Pacific Squadron under Captain Henry E. Ballard. He declined on the grounds that he was the sole support of his 77-year-old mother and other members of the family. Also, he had served with Ballard in the *Brandywine,* and their relationship in regard to matters of health care was not always pleasant. In light of the record of the *Brandywine,* it is of interest that while on duty in the Pacific during two and a half years, Ballard's flagship, the ship of the line *North Carolina,* lost 26 men out of a total complement of more than 800; 4 were killed in accidents, and the rest died of unspecified diseases. It should be noted, however, that the *North Carolina* and the rest of the ships in the squadron were anchored off Callao, Peru, for nine months while observing the enforcement of the blockade of that port in the war between Peru and Chile.[18]

Through the years, Barton continued to serve on the navy examining board and thus had an important influence on the type of men admitted to and promoted in the medical establishment. He had also become increasingly interested in the problem of the quality and cost of medicines furnished to the service. One solution would be to centralize supplies. So in 1831 he suggested to the secretary of the navy the establishment of the office of medical purveyor in Philadelphia. This would be the point from which all medical instruments and supplies would be sent to the navy, as well as the center for the return of surpluses in those categories. Barton viewed himself as the likely holder of the proposed office. Secretary Woodbury referred Barton's proposal to the Board of Navy Commissioners for comment. That body disapproved of the suggestion on the grounds of the increased costs and risks in transporting medical supplies and equipment to ships, as well as the expense of hiring additional clerks. After receiving the board's report, Woodbury told them that he thought there was merit in Barton's proposal. But in light of the board's opinions and the recent rejection by the Congress of a bill to create the position of surgeon general, Woodbury did not feel justified in pursuing the subject.[19]

Secretary Paulding showed an appreciation for Barton's medical experience when he asked him in 1839 for his recommendations on recruiting and the physical standards for recruits. Barton had had an interest in this subject from as far back as the War of 1812. He pointed out that the responsibility for examining recruits was first and foremost with the recruiting surgeon. Some surgeons had been lax in performing this duty, knowing that a second examination would take place before the men went to sea. But some of the medical officers who made the second examination were also lax, so that unfit men were admitted to the service. Barton recommended ending this system of divided responsibility and making the surgeon who did the initial examination responsible. This and similar recommendations by other surgeons represented a growing effort on the part of naval surgeons to improve their profession.[20]

An earlier manifestation of this spirit can be seen in the West India Squadron after Barton left it. A concern about ships being the source of disease led the Navy Department to order experiments in the use of chloride of lime as a disinfectant and prophylactic in the squadron. It was to be sprinkled on the timbers and in the bilges to sweeten and purify the ship. Quarterly reports on the experiment were to be forwarded to the Navy Department. George S. Sproston, who had served as an assistant surgeon in the *Brandywine* under Barton, was now the fleet surgeon of the West India Squadron and in charge of the experiment. He reported that there were 40 cases of fever in the flagship *Erie* but that there was no epidemic of malignant fever. He believed that the use of chloride of lime had reduced the risk of fever throughout the squadron.

Sproston's enthusiasm for the chemical was not shared by Surgeon Robert J. Dodd of the schooner *Shark*. He found that it had an offensive odor and caused some men to vomit and a number to complain about a pain in the head and a sick feeling that lasted from 10 to 15 minutes. Dodd wondered if the use of lime were not better adapted to larger ships than a schooner such as the *Shark*, and he sent his observations to Sproston. The senior surgeon tended to dismiss Dodd's comments as a single exception to the rule in the squadron. But he told Dodd to continue to use the lime and send "more experimental detail, and circumstantial statement of the facts" that led him to his conclusions. He was also reminded that the orders required quarterly reports and that one was now due from him. Meanwhile he forwarded copies of Dodd's letter and his own response to the secretary. Sproston said that while there was not a single case of malignant fever in the navy where chloride of lime had been used steadily, it alone could not be considered sufficient for the preservation of a sound atmosphere.[21] Presumably the experiments continued, at least until the end of Secretary Branch's tenure, but the final results are not known to this writer. They must have been generally positive, for chloride of lime was used until the Civil War.

Health Reports

The discussions in Congress and in the navy on the proposed duties of a surgeon general and the need to keep statistical records on health care evidently resulted in some attempts to preserve the quarterly reports sent by surgeons to the Navy Department. Although it is unusual to find reports on a ship or station for a whole year or more, there are some fragmentary returns that provide some insights into the health problems of the navy during the Jacksonian years.

The *Hudson* started the quarter ending December 31, 1829, with 23 patients left over from the previous quarter, but their ailments are not listed. There were 118 new admissions. Out of the total of 141 cases, 123 were cured, 6 were sent to the United States, and 13 remained sick. There was only one death, and that was from chronic diarrhea. Surgeon Andrew Cook reported that most of his cases were of only a few days' duration. The most dangerous cases were of dysentery, biliary colic (resulting from the accumulation of bile in the intestines or the passages of the bile duct), erysipelas (a skin rash with associated heat and pain), and cholera morbus (severe diarrhea). Of the 13 patients then in a convalescent state, none was in a dangerous condition. Cook's breakdown of the main ailments treated during the quarter shows catarrh, 21 cases; wounds, 12; vertigo, 10; diarrhea, 9; hemorrhoids and dysentery, 7 each; abcesses and contusions, 6 each; cholera morbus and fever, 5 each; dislocations, 4; and burns and tumors, 3 each.[22]

Barton's report on the navy hospital at Norfolk in December 1830 showed only 22 patients. Five of these were listed as convalescent and 3 others as incurable or nearly so. Those in the latter category included one ordinary seaman described as "Insane (probably for life)," one seaman suffering from "phthisis pulmonaris," or consumption, and another man with partial blindness. Nine others were in the hospital but not undergoing treatment:

three did duty at the hospital; one operated the boat; another, who was partly paralyzed, acted as a clerk; and a third functioned as the doorkeeper. Also included in the total were five marines who were awaiting their discharges from the Marine Corps.[23]

Surgeon Jonathan Cowdery sent a report of the sick from the Mediterranean Squadron who had arrived in the *Lexington* in November 1831. This showed 39 patients from six warships. Most had been recommended for discharge as unfit for service and capable of providing for themselves. Only 9 needed hospitalization, their ailments including a single case each of rupture, stricture of the urethra, rheumatism, ophthalmia, syphilis, an ulcerated leg, the loss of the use of an arm, a compound fracture of a thigh bone resulting from a wound, and one disease that cannot be deciphered.[24]

The report of Surgeon Waters Smith from the *St. Louis* for April–June 1830 shows 66 cases, of which 15 were of catarrh; 6 of rheumatism; 5 of fever; 4 of ophthalmia; 4 of stomach disorders; 1 of a wound; 1 of syphilis; and the rest of assorted ailments. Of the 5 fever cases, Smith said that 4 were of the intermittent type. All but one of the fevers occurred when the men enlisted on the western coast of South America.

A return from the hospital at Portsmouth, Virginia, for an unidentified quarter of 1831 showed 30 patients remaining from the last report. There were 41 new admissions, 35 patients were discharged, 36 remained at the end of the quarter, and 4 died. Of the deaths, one each was due to consumption, chronic diarrhea, dropsy, and smallpox.[25]

The most complete and comprehensive account of the medical record of a single navy ship in the decade of the 1830s was that prepared by Surgeon Jonathan Foltz. During the course of a circumnavigation of the world in 1831–32, the frigate *Potomac* and its crew of 502 were exposed to many different climates ranging from 40° north to 57° south latitude. As accurately as could be ascertained, the average age of the crew was 31. When the ship sailed from New York on August 24, 1831, everyone appeared to be in good health except one officer, who was suffering from tracheal phthisis, or inflammation of the trachea. Foltz recorded the temperatures every day at noon, when the ship's day began, and the number and nature of the ailments on the sick list. Early in the voyage the men landed on the west coast of the island of Sumatra and assaulted the town of Quallah Battoo in retaliation for an earlier attack on a U.S. merchant ship. Two Americans died and 11 others were wounded. The wounded were placed on the gun deck while they were undergoing treatment, and they recovered rapidly. The rest of the voyage was a routine cruise. When it was completed, Surgeon Foltz calculated that the *Potomac* had traveled over 61,000 miles, had been to sea 514 days, and had crossed the equator six times. During that time not a spar had been carried away and no lives had been lost as the result of accidents. The daily average number on sick report was 28. There had been 25 deaths, including the 2 in the attack on Quallah Battoo. Of the remainder, 16 were due to dysentery; 3 to phthisis (tuberculosis); and 1 each to hepatitis, concealed hernia, hydrocephalus, and fractured vertebrae. With the average complement of 490 officers and men, the annual death rate was 2.08 percent. This, said Foltz, was much lower than in the same number of adults on shore.[26]

Examples from other fragmentary records might be cited, but they would confirm that there were few deaths and that navy doctors treated a variety of ailments more or less successfully and in accordance with the medical thinking of the time. There were few instances of a large number of cases of a single disease, especially of infectious types. The health situation in the navy was generally good, and this impression seems to be reinforced by the lack of adverse comment in the annual reports and letters from the various ships.

The largest loss of life during these years was due to accidents, notably the loss of the sloop of war *Hornet* off Tampico, Mexico, in September 1829, in which 141 men died. One of those who perished was Surgeon William Birchmore, who was one of the early group of doctors who had to pass through the examination process before being promoted to surgeon. He seems to have been a man of learning and sensitivity who might have made a name for himself if he had been spared. Other losses included the one-gun *Sylph*, which was engaged in the protection of the timber trade when it disappeared in 1831, taking about eight men to their graves. The pilot boat *Sea Gull* sank in April 1839 with a loss of 15 men.[27]

The Wilkes Exploring Expedition

Perhaps nothing better illustrates the general health of the navy during the Jacksonian years than the experience of the Wilkes Exploring Expedition during 1838–42. This expedition consisted of the sloops of war *Vincennes* and *Peacock*, the brig of war *Porpoise*, the pilot schooners *Flying Fish* and *Sea Gull*, and the store ship *Relief*. The ships were manned by 83 officers and 342 men under the command of Lieutenant Charles Wilkes. During the time it was at sea, the expedition explored and surveyed islands in the Pacific Ocean, a part of Antarctica, and the northwest coast of North America from Puget Sound to parts of California. The officers and men were thus exposed to every climate.[28]

The medical duties of the whole squadron were assigned to the surgeons and assistant surgeons of each ship in rotation, so that everyone would have the opportunity to go ashore at the various locations and make his own observations. A medical journal kept by Assistant Surgeon Silas Holmes of the *Peacock* offers invaluable information on the health of the members of the expedition. Also, Dr. Holmes was one of the few officers who did not run afoul of Wilkes. His easygoing, optimistic outlook saved him from some difficulties, but he also had problems in trying to make his superiors aware of threats to the health of the crews.

After sailing from Norfolk in August 1838, Holmes noted early in the voyage that he had only one man on the sick list, who had a protracted disease and should not have been enlisted. When the expedition made its first stop on the island of Maderia, off Morocco, he was discharged, along with a few other seamen. They were replaced by men who enlisted in Maderia. When the ship departed from Maderia, Holmes noted that the sick list was higher than usual, but he attributed this to excessive indulgence by the men while on shore. They were restored to duty after a few days.

In mid-October 1838, Holmes and Surgeon J. Frederick Sickles examined the *Peacock*'s men in the crew's quarters and vaccinated 14 who had not received that treatment previously. Presumably this was an instance of compulsory vaccination. Additional measures to prevent scurvy were taken in late January 1839 after the ships left Rio de Janeiro. Two bottles of lemon juice were assigned to each mess, and pickles were also dispensed. As the ship headed southward toward the Antarctic and the weather became colder and wetter, extra clothing was issued and stoves were kept lit below decks where men could warm and dry themselves.

A man fell asleep while on one of the main topsail yards and fell into the water. He was rescued, brought back to the ship nearly lifeless, and resuscitated. The next day he was worse and had trouble breathing. Holmes noted that he had a rash over the whole of his thorax. When he died, Holmes wanted to do an autopsy to determine the precise nature of the injury, but Surgeon Sickles did not consider it necessary.

Continuing to sail southward, they entered the Antarctic Circle, and hot coffee was served to the deck watches. Men were sent ashore from the *Porpoise* at Good Success Bay to hunt for game and pick wild celery and "scurvey [*sic*] grapes," and were later unable to get off from land. Two boats were sent to rescue them, and one capsized, but its two crewmen were rescued. Wilkes decided to send the *Peacock* and the *Flying Fish* deeper into the Antarctic. The *Peacock* was slowed by fog and icebergs, but the *Flying Fish* made it as far as 70° south before turning back. When it reached the spot where the *Peacock* was waiting, it reported that it had one sick man on board. Assistant Surgeon Holmes entered a boat and went to the ship, where he found a man who about two weeks earlier had been knocked down by a tiller and broken one or more ribs. Since his injury he had been judiciously treated by a lieutenant. The injured man was transferred to the *Peacock*. Many of the crew of the *Flying Fish* "were suffering from rheumatic pains so common to seamen, especially when much exposed to cold and moisture."

The squadron sailed for Valparaiso, Chile. Off that coast the *Sea Gull* was lost in a gale. In the *Peacock,* Assistant Surgeon Holmes was looking forward to a trip to the interior of Chile, but he had to cancel his plans when Surgeon Sickles and a number of other men in the squadron became sick. Sickles was transferred to the *Relief* along with other sick men and was replaced in the *Peacock* by Assistant Surgeon James C. Palmer, who had previously been attached to the *Relief* and whose commission was earlier than that of Holmes. One of the sick men sent back from the *Relief* to the *Peacock* was a seaman who subsequently died; upon examining the body, Holmes concluded that the cause was peritonitis. Holmes also had to treat one of the ship's boys, who contracted smallpox while ashore in Lima. When his condition was discovered, he was transferred to a hospital ashore, the U.S. consul was advised of his case, and the doctors acquired smallpox vaccine in Lima to vaccinate all the crew of the *Peacock*.

After leaving Callao, Peru, another case of smallpox appeared. The surgeon and assistant surgeon again vaccinated everyone on board except those who had had smallpox and who could show the resulting marks on their bodies. The man with smallpox recovered quickly. In the *Vincennes* a marine died of "inflammation of the brain," and in the *Porpoise* an ordinary seamen died of pneumonia. For most of this part of the voyage, a few men in the squadron suffered from dysentery, diarrhea, and venereal disease. The average number on the sick list of the *Peacock* was six. In early August 1840, when the surface temperature of the sea reached 77°, the officers and crew were issued life preservers and "allowed to bathe."

From Peru the expedition charted the coral atolls in the Paumoto group and surveyed the Samoan Islands before sailing to Sydney, Australia. By this time there was a considerable amount of disaffection in the squadron. Wilkes decided to send the slow-sailing *Relief* home with the sick and the discontented. En route to Sydney two men died in the *Relief,* presumably from illness; while the ship was there, another died of consumption.

When Dr. Sickles was sent to the *Relief,* Passed Assistant Surgeon Edward Gilchrist, then attached to the *Vincennes* and next in seniority, sought the position of fleet surgeon. Wilkes would not grant this request because he considered Gilchrist overrated as a medical man and believed him to be the ringleader of a cabal of anti-Wilkes officers. In addition, Wilkes found the doctor lacking in feeling for the objects of the expedition. Gilchrist persisted in his claim and asked permission to live ashore in Sydney. When this was refused, the doctor wrote a letter to Wilkes which the latter regarded as disrespectful. Gilchrist would not apologize for the letter or withdraw it, so Wilkes suspended him from duty and confined him to the ship. Later, health reasons made Wilkes decide to let Gilchrist go ashore. If Wilkes could have replaced him easily with another assistant surgeon, he would have sent the doctor home.

Another doctor who sought a promotion was Assistant Surgeon Charles F. B. Guillou of the *Porpoise,* but he did not go through channels but instead wrote directly to the secretary of the navy. Wilkes ignored his request. Guillou next got into trouble with Lieutenant Cadwalader Ringgold, commander of the *Porpoise,* over a requisition for medical supplies made in a slovenly manner and the loss of a mortar and pestle. The result of all of this was a transfer of some of the medical officers. Guillou was sent to the *Peacock* to serve under Dr. Palmer, and Assistant Surgeon Holmes took Guillou's place in the *Porpoise.* Guillou and his supporters considered this a demotion. With the departure of Dr. Gilchrist, Assistant Surgeon John L. Fox moved up to become the acting surgeon of the *Vincennes,* the flagship, with John S. Whittle as assistant surgeon.

Leaving Sydney on December 26, 1839, the expedition headed for the Antarctic to make further explorations. The crew continued to be healthy. In late January, Holmes had four on his sick list, three of them cases of venereal disease picked up in Sydney but not reported by the men until the disease reached an advanced stage. Their cases gave Holmes a great deal of trouble before the men recovered. In the opinion of Dr. Holmes, the general good health that prevailed in the *Porpoise* was due almost entirely to the regulations of Captain Ringgold. "All hands are never called [on deck], so that the watch below are never disturbed: every man on deck is forced to be clad in warm and dry clothing; hot Coffee is served out nearly every night; advantage is taken of every fair day to air the bedding and ventilate the berth deck, and every measure is adopted which can tend to increase the comfort of the crew. I serve out each week, lime juice to the ship's company."[29]

Operating independently, the ships of the squadron made their own explorations of the Antarctic waters. They had to cope with gales, ice, and cold weather. The *Peacock* damaged its rudder in the ice and departed for Sydney to make repairs. The *Porpoise* searched for a way through an ice barrier and got as far south as 64° 66¹ before turning and heading for New Zealand. As the *Vincennes* made its own probe of the ice barrier, a gunner slipped on an icy deck and fell, breaking some ribs. Aloft a man on a

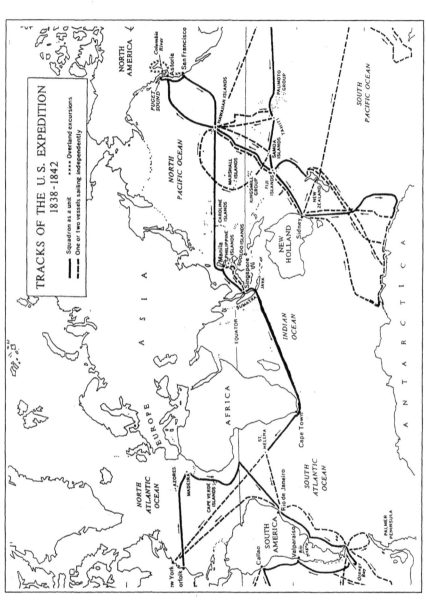

Map Showing Tracks of the U.S. Exploring Expedition, 1838–42. American Philosophical Society, Philadelphia.

yardarm had a sail blown over him and he could not move. When his plight was ascertained, a line was thrown around his body and he was hauled in to the mast top and then lowered. Several men who were exhausted by cold, fatigue, and excitement had to be carried below. Drs. Fox and Whittle advised Wilkes that the ship was in danger because of the poor health of the crew. By this time, Dr. Gilchrist had been restored to duty and recommended that the ship return at once to a milder climate. But Wilkes continued to probe the barrier for another three weeks. He discovered land on January 19, 1840, and on this he based his claim that he had discovered a continent. Then on February 21 he turned back and reached Sydney on March 11.

In Antarctic waters the sick list of the *Vincennes* rose to 23. Men suffered from rheumatism and coughs, and a few had frostbitten hands and toes. Wilkes himself and three of his servants became ill in part from breathing carbolic acid gas from the charcoal stoves. All the sick recovered.

The squadron reassembled in New Zealand and proceed to Fiji. During the survey of those islands, one man in the *Porpoise* was accidentally shot in the side by a musket at close range. He recovered. Two officers were murdered by the natives, and a seaman was wounded. The Americans attacked Fiji warriors and a village and forced the natives to seek peace. During the attack two seamen were wounded and an officer suffered a minor eye injury when a pistol was fired too close to his face.

After Fiji the vessels separated to perform individual tasks before reassembling in the Hawaiian Islands. During this work shortages of food and water made it necessary to reduce the daily rations, but the health of the men continued to be good. One of those who did not feel well was Dr. Whittle, whose liver and stomach troubles were aggravated by the dry ship's biscuits, which contained worms, and salty food. When the squadron reached Honolulu, it was to be a time for resting the men and refitting the ships.

For those who would reenlist to finish the work of exploration, Wilkes offered a 25 percent increase in pay, three months' advance wages, and two weeks of liberty. All reenlisted except 23 men, whose places were taken by Hawaiians. For most, the time in Hawaii was a busy one as preparations were made to continue the survey work, which was now behind schedule. While in Honolulu, Wilkes asked his officers to turn in to him the journals they had kept thus far in the expedition. Dr. Guillou refused on the grounds that it contained private information. Wilkes regarded this as impertinence and suspended him. Wilkes wanted to dismiss him and send him home, but the doctor insisted that if he departed it would be under orders and at government expense. Guillou later turned in his journal after cutting out some pages.

On November 15, 1840, the *Porpoise* left Hawaii to resume survey work as far south as Tahiti. The *Peacock* and the *Flying Fish* had to survey a number of islands in the central Pacific, and Wilkes, in the *Vincennes,* was to study a volcano on the island of Hawaii. In late December one of the Hawaiian crew members in the *Porpoise* died of chronic dysentery; food had to be reduced by one-quarter so that there would be enough to last until Tahiti. On the return to Hawaii, food again was short. Yet for most of this time, the sick list remained at three or four more or less permanent invalids.

While the *Porpoise* was being overhauled, Assistant Surgeon Holmes sent a "respectful paper" to Captain Ringgold pointing out that the crew needed time for rest after their incessant labors. The doctor feared for their health as they entered unhealthy areas while suffering from exposure and fatigue. Ringgold paid no attention; he was driven by Wilkes's schedule, and on April 5, 1841, the *Porpoise* and the *Vincennes* sailed for the Pacific northwest.

Three days later the fears of Dr. Holmes came true. His sick list went from six to eight, seven of whom were petty officers. Four were suffering from a form of typhoid fever that Holmes believed was brought on by fatigue and exposure. Holmes considered eight cases out a crew of 52 men a large list. As their situation became worse, he requested a consultation with Dr. Fox of the *Vincennes,* who came over by boat on three occasions to consult with Holmes before the men eventually recovered.

By late April the ships were off the Columbia River. Preparations for the survey work in the Pacific northwest began. Holmes went ashore to attend the daughter of a farmer who had fractured her thigh, and he gave the girl's family a plan of treatment they could follow. The *Peacock* and the *Flying Fish* reached the mouth of the river, and the *Peacock* was wrecked trying to enter the channel in late June. The *Porpoise* went to Ft. Vancouver, Washington, and then began survey work on the Columbia River. During this interval the sick list of the *Porpoise* varied from 10 to 27 men. Most of the patients were Hawaiians transferred from the *Peacock,* who did not have sufficient clothing for the climate. They suffered from ague and fever but all recovered.

A party under Lieutenant George F. Emmons left for survey work in California even though Emmons was suffering from intermittent fever and some of the men still showed traces of malaria. When they returned, several were still struggling to overcome intermittent fever.

Meanwhile other members of the squadron had also been busy. To replace the *Peacock,* a brig was purchased from the Hudson's Bay Company and renamed the *Oregon.* Dr. Holmes was named the ship's medical officer, Acting Surgeon Fox took his place in the *Porpoise*, and Dr. Palmer transferred to the *Vincennes*. Dr. Guillou, who had been under arrest in the *Porpoise*, went on board the *Oregon* and later transferred to the *Flying Fish*.

After some final work in the Pacific, the expedition headed for home, reaching New York in late June and early July 1842. It had accomplished some important scientific work, and in so doing it had established an excellent health record. Although exposed to many climates and diseases, the expedition lost only 27 men. Of that number, 15 were lost with the *Sea Gull*. The total also includes one marine in the *Vincennes* who died of an internal injury and a sailor from the *Peacock* who was presumably murdered by natives in the Drummond Islands. Disease appears to have killed only 7.

The expedition also pointed up some longstanding problems between line and staff officers. Medical officers who had tried to make their health concerns known were generally disregarded. There was conflict in other areas as well. When he got home, Dr. Guillou faced a court-martial on six charges. The court found him guilty on four—disrespect, disobedience, neglect of duty, and disobedience of orders—and sentenced him to be dismissed. Secretary Ushur believed the sentence was too harsh. Guillou was told to collect letters attesting to his high moral character, professional skill, and attention to duty, which were sent to President John Tyler, who decided to commute Guillou's sentence to suspension of pay and emoluments for 12 months from the date of the sentence.

Wilkes was court-martialed also and found guilty only of illegal punishment of enlisted men; for this he was publicly reprimanded by the secretary.[30] On all other charges the court found him not guilty or the charges not proven.

Chapter 16

The Growth of Professionalism

Since the time of the Quasi-War, there had been individuals who were concerned about creating a professional environment within which the medical men of the navy would operate. From the Navy Department's viewpoint, the official conduct prescribed was set forth in navy regulations. The earliest of these were promulgated by individual captains, and they touched on matters of health without making any specific reference to the surgeon or surgeon's mate. Thus the series of articles promulgated by Captain James Sever for the frigate *Congress* in 1800 state that the upper and gun decks must be washed every morning at 5:00 A.M. in the summer; that the hammocks should be brought up and aired at 7:00 A.M. unless the weather was bad; and that grog and meals should be served at designated times. A lieutenant and the sailing master were to make frequent inspections of the berth and orlop decks, the cockpit, and the passages to the storerooms, and they were to direct that these be cleaned as often as required. There was also a reference to the need for economy and the avoidance of waste in the expenditure of public stores, and while these matters had medical aspects, the surgeons are never mentioned.[1]

The duties of the surgeon are set forth for the first time in the navy regulations issued in 1802. These state that the surgeon was to inspect and take care of the items necessary for the use of the sick men. If they were not good, he must tell the captain; otherwise he must see that they were dispensed. He was to visit the sick at least twice a day and more often if necessary, and he was to make sure that the surgeon's mates did their duty, so that none of the sick "want due attendance and relief." In difficult cases the surgeon was to consult with the other surgeons in the squadron. He was to inform the captain daily about the condition of his patients. When the sick were to be transferred to a hospital, he was to go with them to the surgeon in charge of that facility and give to him an account of the time and manner of their illnesses and the methods of treatment that had been followed. No sick men were to be sent to the hospital unless their illnesses or the number of sick on board were such that they could not be cared for on the ship. The situation requiring the transfer was to be certified by the surgeon before the patients were moved. If the surgeon of the hospital ascertained that the patients could have been cured on the ship with a little extra time, the surgeon of the ship was to be fined $10 for each improper transfer.

Before a battle, the surgeon was to see that his mates and assistants were ready with everything that might be needed to stop bleeding and dress wounds. Stores needed by the medical department were to be issued on a requisition from the surgeon, and he would be responsible for their proper use. He must keep a regular account of the receipts and expenditures and send a report on them to the accountant of the navy at the end of every cruise.

The surgeon was to keep a daybook of his practice consisting of the names of his patients, their ailments, the dates when they became ill and when they recovered, the date and place of transfer or death, and the method of treatment followed. From this record he was to make two journals, one of his surgical practice and one of his physical, to be sent to the Navy Department at the conclusion of a voyage.[2]

No separate or specific duties were set forth for the surgeons' mates except as noted above. The presumption is that they would perform the duties assigned to them by the surgeons. In these regulations as in those of individual ships, certain health-related duties, such as those relating to the cleansing of the ship or the men, as well as those relating to food, were assigned to the captain or to other officers.

These regulations remained the guidelines for many years, though individual captains could supplement them through rules for a specific ship or station or in accordance with the views of the secretary of the navy in a given situation. As has been noted earlier, the attempt to expand the regulations and have Congress enact them into law went on for many years. That effort was renewed after the Whig party won the election of 1840. In the meantime the Navy Department did what it could to bring order to the situation. When the rank of assistant surgeon replaced that of surgeon's mate in 1828 and when the ranks of hospital surgeon and fleet surgeon were established, presumably additional clarifications were needed. But in the absence of regulations, anything that the secretary of the navy needed to have done could be covered in orders to individual officers or in circulars.

One example of this was Secretary Southard's decision in 1829 to do away with the practice of giving surgeons an allowance for preserving, compounding, and delivering medicines to a squadron. The change in the allowance was not known to Surgeon Benjamin F. Bache, who submitted a bill for these services in the West India Squadron in 1831. The news of the rejection was given to Bache by his commanding officer, Captain Alexander J. Dallas, who was then in charge of the navy yard at Pensacola. Dallas did as he was ordered but wrote to Secretary Woodbury that he regretted this decision because both the government and the naval service would suffer a loss "from the want of someone to take charge of the medicines &c." Woodbury took exception to this and told the captain that the Navy Department expected "that every duty connected with the preservation of the medical instruments, and the preparation of medicines, at the different yards, as well as attention to the sick, will be promptly and faithfully performed, by the Medical Officers stationed at them." These things were "considered part of their general duty." Despite this ruling, Bache persisted and asked Dallas to rescind his order since it did not come within the scope of the duties of the surgeon of the navy yard. Dallas presumably stood firm and followed the Navy Department's guidelines, but it was yet another indication of the need for a body of regulations to cover all such contingencies. In the short term the situation was a source of discontent to Bache and perhaps others who performed similar duties.[3]

Three years later, Woodbury issued an order to the commanding officers of all squadrons and stations to have the senior surgeon under them start keeping records on the weather. He was to keep a journal in which he recorded readings of the thermometer and barometer at sunrise, noon, and sunset each day "and oftener if found convenient; or in case of any sudden and great change." The journal was to include information on "gales, storms and hurricanes, with their directions, time of commencement and termination and a brief statement of the effects, immediate or remote, supposed to be produced by any of the important changes, on the health of officers and men." In addition to the journal, separate reports on the subject were to be submitted monthly to the Navy Department along with any remarks that the commanding officer deemed important. By this order the secretary hoped to begin collecting weather information in the same way as the army did.[4]

Medical care for non-naval persons was a problem that arose from time to time. Dr. Waterhouse's problems with the commanding officer of the Boston navy yard were noted earlier. Most surgeons and mates seem to have gone along with the need to treat without charge such civilians as the wives and children of officers, as well as those of enlisted men attached to a navy yard or station. The earlier custom of allowing enlisted men to bring women with them on voyages was done away with early in the nineteenth century, except for Captain Decatur's brief experiment in using two women as nurses. But when navy ships carried diplomatic and consular officers and their families to their foreign posts, the surgeons often had to supply medical aid to them. When their commanding officers would allow it, some surgeons also had a civilian practice in their off-duty hours. An interesting twist in the story of the care of dependents took place in 1831 when the children of Captain Dallas needed to be vaccinated. His mother-in-law acquired "genuine vaccine matter taken from the arm of a healthy child related to you." This was delivered to the Navy Department in a "cork secured in sealing wax," which was sent to Dallas in Pensacola. John Boyle, the chief clerk of the department, who was then acting Secretary of the Navy, expressed the hope to Dallas that the vaccine would protect his children from smallpox. If any of the vaccine was left after the needs of the captain's family had been supplied, wrote Boyle, "have the goodness to cause it to be employed in protecting from the ravages of a loathsome disease those engaged in the naval service under your command." It is not known whether the navy men ever got any benefit from this vaccine.[5]

Attempts to get formal orders requiring vaccination of recruits and other persons at risk in the navy were successful in 1826. As has been noted in other connections, medical officers who had earlier asked for guidance in specific instances were left to their own devices. We know from Surgeon Usher Parsons that Commodore Oliver Hazard Perry ordered his men to be vaccinated in 1815. Probably some other captains did the same, but the details have not been preserved.[6]

A similar situation prevailed in regard to the use of lemon juice to prevent scurvy. As early as the Quasi-War, some officers were aware of its utility and its use in the Royal Navy, yet as late as the War of 1812, Surgeon Barton was trying to get Secretary Hamilton to make its use mandatory. Barton failed, but it is believed that at least some ships acquired lemon juice through Surgeon John Bullus when he went on to become the navy agent at New York in 1808.[7]

When it came to determining how medical duties were to be divided, the surgeon and his mates most likely worked out their own arrangements, the details of which, with one exception, have been lost. That exception is a letter of instruction that Surgeon William Barnwell Jr. gave to John Fitzhugh Jr. and David S. Edwards, his surgeon's mates in the frigate *Congress* in May 1819. Barnwell designated his remarks not as orders but as "observations relative to your duties." These might make it necessary for both mates to be on duty at the same time, but they were free to work out the arrangements that were most agreeable to themselves. The first observation was that they should be in the sick bay by 9:00 A.M. and be ready to attend to any cases. These included "giving the directions for the application of poultices or fomentations, changing and dressing blisters," and taking care of trivial cases that did not belong on the sick list. They were to see that their attendants had "clean rollers, warm water, adhesive plaster," and other items in readiness to dress ulcers and wounds. Medicines in general use or likely to be needed during the day should be prepared ahead of time.

For the care of patients during the day, the mates were "to have such medicines, food, or drinks, given to the patients" for whom they were prescribed and report to the surgeon directly or through an attendant "any remarkable change which may have occurred in any of the patients, for which you may not wish to prescribe." The mates must also be attentive in checking the cleanliness of copper pots used for cooking food and must report to the lieutenant any negligence on the part of the cook. A list of the sick was to be posted on the binnacle by 11:00 A.M., as well as a list of patients who were taking cathartics, wines, brandy, or porter to whom the daily grog ration should not be issued. In addition, the grog should be stopped in "any cases where an antiphlogistic regimen is necessary."

The mates were also to see that the bedding and furniture of the patients were kept in good order. The sick bay was to be whitewashed at least once every two weeks. Mates were to keep accounts of the expenditure of hospital stores and guard against any waste or abuse. Finally, they were to keep a journal in which they recorded the name, rank, disease, and dates of admission and discharge of every person on the sick list.[8] Through these "observations," Barnwell was able to suggest to his subordinates the range and detail of their obligations.

Contributions to Knowledge

In the meantime navy surgeons were drawing upon their experiences to make contributions to medical or scientific knowledge. Beginning in December 1800, Surgeon Edward Cutbush began keeping a record of the temperatures of the air and sea, including those in the Gulf Stream. When John Vaughn of the American Philosophical Society expressed interest in this, Cutbush promised to send him a copy of his journal. The surgeon did so in July 1801, with the last entry on May 20 of that year. This was added to the society's collections.[9]

A more ambitious work appeared under Cutbush's name in 1808 as *Observations on the Means of Preserving the Health of Soldiers and Sailors; and on the Duties of the Medical Department of the Army and the Navy: With Remarks on Hospitals and Their Internal Arrangement*. This small book was full of practical information that could be applied by army or navy surgeons in dealing with the sick. The Navy Department would have done well to purchase a number of copies for distribution to ships, navy yards, and hospitals, but secretaries did not think of that; even if they had, there was always a question of how to pay for such books.

Two years after Cutbush's book appeared, Surgeon Jonathan Cowdery contributed an article to the *Medical Repository*, "On the Efficacy of Alkalies to preserve Cleanliness and Health on ship-board, and on the Usefulness of Acid Fumigations for those purposes." He drew upon his experience as the surgeon of the brig *Angus*, 18 guns, with a crew of 130, beginning with and assignment to Norfolk followed by cruises along the coast from Florida to New York in the summer of 1808 and off the coast of New England in the fall and winter. In the course of 15 months, the crew was exposed to the summer heat of the South and the extreme cold of a northern winter, but not a man was lost. Cowdery attributed this to having the men sleep in hammocks with clean, dry, comfortable blankets and mattresses and never in the open or on deck. Whenever water was foul, it was purified by unslacked lime or with pulverized charcoal. The provisions were examined frequently and anything tainted thrown overboard. Attention was paid to the cleanliness of the men, who were clothed according to the climate.

Additional safeguards included the frequent whitewashing of the interior of the ship with new lime. The decks were cleaned with sand and lime. The berth deck was never washed except in fine weather, and then it was completely dried before men were allowed to sleep there. Wind sails were placed at the hatchways to channel fresh air to the decks below. Although there were a few cases of typhoid fever in the South, with "modern remedies" and the alkalizing plan, the patients soon recovered. In the North, when men came down with catarrhs, pneumonia, and rheumatism, the usual remedies had little effect until stoves were placed between decks and fires started to warm the area. Proper nourishment and good nursing helped to bring about a complete recovery.

In his discussion of the best means of fumigating a ship, Cowdery indicated an awareness of the works of Drs. James Lind, J. Carmichael Smyth, and Guyton de Morveu, a Swedish chemist.[10]

If the experiments in foreign navies stimulated Cowdery, it was the situation in New Orleans that inspired Surgeon Lewis Heermann to write his book. The defense in Louisiana involved the use of gunboats, and these usually operated without any medical man on board. To help them to cope with their health problems, Heermann published a work for nonmedical navy men assigned to gunboat duty. The first section described the contents of the medical chest, beginning with castor oil and ending with bandages. Each entry was numbered, from 1 to 50. In the second section he discussed health problems, from apoplexy to wounds, indicating how much and in what fashion the numbered contents of the medical chest should be applied. Thus in a discussion of scurvy, he describes the symptoms and then says that for treatment a "nutritive diet supersedes all other medicines, but No. 3 [bark] and No. 15 [elixer of vitrol] may be given with advantage. Porter or small beer, made from a decoction of rice, hops, or barley, with molasses and porter, and fermented for three to five days is grateful and of advantage." Anyone following Heermann's guidance would first look under *bark* to see how it should be prepared, and then under *elixer of vitrol* to determine how the taste and efficacy of the bark would be improved with drops of no. 15. On the other hand, if a reader encountered a disease where bleeding was recommended, he would be wise to turn first to the entry for *lancet* in order to learn how it should be done. Slightly more than two pages were devoted to the use of the lancet in bleeding procedures. Here one learned that a properly managed lancet need not go more than an eighth of an inch below the skin.[11] It would be interesting to know if any officers attached to gunboats actually used Heermann's book and if so, how carefully its directions were followed.

The need for line officers to seek the advice of surgeons on matters of health was one of the deeply held convictions of Surgeon William P. C. Barton of Philadelphia. He got his first chance to expound his views when Secretary of the Navy Hamilton asked him to draw up a system of rules for the proposed marine hospital in Washington. Taking advantage of a cruise to Europe in 1811, Barton studied the hospitals for seamen in Great Britain at Greenwich, Haslar, near Portsmouth, Plymouth, Chelsea, Deal, Yarmouth, the Isle of Wight, and Paignton. From there he moved on to an examination of the regulations, procedures, and victualing of French hospitals. With a basic knowledge of European practices as background, Barton went on to discuss guidelines for the location, construction, heating, ventilating, washing, and administration of the proposed hospital. The duties of everyone were described, from the governor, surgeon, dispenser, steward, matron, nurses, various assistants, and chaplain down to the guards. Barton left nothing to chance. He made recommendations on the construction of fireplaces, stoves, victualing, bedding, and the paper forms that were to be used in administration.

This information more than fulfilled the secretary's request for a code of regulations for the hospital. But Barton did more. In the second part of the volume he discussed what needed to be done to systematize the medical department of the navy, drawing upon his observations of the Royal Navy as well his own experiences. He recommended the elimination of the venereal fee and the grog ration, limitation of the wet scrubbing of decks, improvements in the ventilation and warming of ships, and the introduction of lemons and limes into the diet of seamen. Barton also advocated a pay raise for surgeons and mates to put them on a par with their colleagues in the army, a board of examiners for the appointment and promotion of surgeons and mates, and a more rigid examination of recruits. Indeed, his recommendations correctly forecast the path of reform for more than 20 years. All these ideas and recommendations were set forth in his book, *A Treatise Containing a Plan for the Internal Organization and Government of Marine Hospitals in the United States, Together With a Scheme for Amending and Systematizing the Medical Department of the Navy*, which was first published in 1814.

A second and revised edition was published in 1817 in which Barton lamented that even though his suggestions had been endorsed by prominent officers such as Decatur, Porter, and Rodgers and tested in the Royal Navy, the secretary had refused to issue an order or a circular to regularize the use of lime juice. From what we know of the later views of Secretaries Hamilton and Jones about Barton, it would seem that they would go to great lengths to avoid acknowledging any contribution from him. Whether or not his book was widely read by his fellow surgeons, Barton deserves credit for anticipating all their concerns and their efforts to change things.

The 1817 edition was partly responsible for court-martial proceedings against Barton. Surgeon Thomas Harris was replaced by Barton as the head of the naval hospital in the Philadelphia Navy Yard in November 1817 following a visit by Barton to President James Monroe in Washington. Feeling aggrieved, Harris charged Barton with "conduct unbecoming to an officer and gentleman" and supported the charge with two specifications: that the book on marine hospitals had falsely degraded the character and reputation of Surgeon Edward Cutbush, who had previously been in charge of the naval hospital in Philadelphia; and that Barton had "insidiously solicited and procured" the hospital appointment for himself. The court ruled that Barton did not need to answer or refute the first specification; the second was sustained only to a certain extent. The court stated that it was impressed by the number and weight of the testimonials to Barton's talents, usefulness, and deportment. President Monroe also provided answers to questions that the court had sent to him. In the end the court sentenced Barton to be reprimanded by the secretary of the navy.[12] The result seems to have been a longstanding emnity by Harris and some others against Barton.

As was noted earlier, Barton's brief cruise in the *Brandywine* provided the basis for his 1830 publication, *Hints for Medical Officers Cruising in the West Indies*. Again drawing on British practices as well as his own experiences, he provided a useful text for all officers whose duties took them to the West Indies. But again it is difficult to know how widely read the book was in naval circles. Barton hoped that his books would encourage other navy surgeons to write about their experiences, but apparently it did not. Many of them could not afford to buy books, and probably there were some who would not even if they could spare the money. Still others who might have had the desire to write possibly could not find the time or energy. Between 1814 and 1833, Barton published four books on botany, and in 1836 he reedited a work on the subject by his late uncle, Benjamin Smith Barton, to which he added a biography of the author. Barton tried unsuccessfully to have the Navy Department buy and distribute his uncle's work to its medical officers. His *Polemic* against the creation of the office of surgeon general has been noted elsewhere. Barton was also active on the Philadelphia medical scene. He was the professor of botany at the University of Pennsylvania and held a fellowship in the College of Physicians in Philadelphia until 1822. Barton also worked to obtain a charter for the Jefferson Medical College, which was established in 1825, and he subsequently joined the faculty as professor of botany.[13]

Meanwhile Harris too was active in medical circles. In 1826 he was invited to become the professor of surgery at the Medical Institute, a non–degree-granting medical school in Philadelphia, a connection that benefited the naval medical officers whom he prepared for examinations. Harris's reputation led to his appointment as surgeon at the Pennsylvania Hospital in 1829. In his naval capacity he served as president of the board of examiners of surgeons and surgeon's mates. In 1831 he delivered an address before the Philadelphia Medical Society on the importance of exercise which was subsequently published, and a case report by him on the resectioning of an elbow joint appeared in the New York *Medical Examiner* in 1842.[14]

From time to time other naval medical officers contributed case reports to medical journals, and some of these have been noted elsewhere. Others were beginning to receive recognition for their work in the field of medicine. Surgeon Elnathan Judson received an honorary M.A. degree from Brown University in 1818, followed by an M.D. from Dartmouth in 1823 and an M.A. from Hamilton College that same year. By a unanimous vote of the trustees in 1825, Surgeon Edward Cutbush was elected professor of chemistry in the Medical Department of Columbian College, later the George Washington University. He served in that capacity for two years in addition to his duties at the Washington Navy Yard. Secretary Southard was invited to attend his first lecture, but whether he did so is not known. When Cutbush resigned his professorship in 1827, the board of trustees adopted a resolution by unanimous vote thanking him for "the ability and assiduity" with which he discharged his duties.[15]

Cutbush's willingness to share his knowledge had been exceeded by that of Surgeon Usher Parsons. A desire to spread practical information on the means of preserving the health of sailors in both the naval and merchant services led Parsons to publish a small volume in 1820 called *The Sailor's Physician*. In it he classified diseases as general and local. The first included fevers, scurvy, jaundice, dropsy, dyspepsia, epilepsy, apoplexy, lockjaw, smallpox, and measles. Local diseases were those that affected a particular part of the body, for example, the head, neck, or chest. The intention was that the officer, who did not know diseases but was well aware of what part of a sailor's body was affected, could turn to that portion of the book which applied to his ailment and then read the symptoms for the various diseases that pertained. Only the diseases common to seafaring people were included, and only the most constant and invariable of symptoms. The remedies were limited to those items commonly found in a ship's medical chest. Technical terms were avoided and common terms were used when speaking of medicines.

On the subject of medicines, Parsons admitted that many valuable remedies were omitted either because of expense or because they were unsafe in the hands of inexperienced persons. These included arsenic for fever and ague, "corrosive sublimate for gonorrhoea, syphilis, and some other complaints, and the concentrated acids in a variety of of diseases." Similarly, when discussing symptoms, Parsons writes that the pulse, "which is the grand index to constitutional affections with an experienced physician, is little understood by others," so that it is not referred to in his book except in connection with diseases "where the morbid change it undergoes is great, and obvious to a common observer." In such cases the person doing the prescribing should compare the patient's pulse with his own or that of another healthy individual.

When discussing yellow fever, Parsons indicates how the medical thinking had changed since Benjamin Rush's day in regard to bleeding. Now the great majority of practitioners who treated the diseases in ships and in the West Indies agreed that the most that could be said for it was that "where the patient is young and corpulent, and there is a hard throbbing pulse with violent pain in the head and back, it may be advisable to draw a small quantity of blood in the first twelve hours, but that it is not safe to take any after this period."

In cases of scurvy "the most celebrated and infallible remedies, are succulent fruits, of which oranges, lemons, limes and apples, are the best." Unfortunately these were hard to preserve on long voyages and difficult to find when most needed. As a result, Parsons relied on potatoes, which were cheap and easy to get in almost any port. "I rarely use any other remedy in a man of war, and always lay in a stock of them with the hospital stores purposely for the cure of Scurvy. Whenever a scorbutic patient reports himself unfit for duty, I direct him to abstain from all salted food, and to commence eating raw potatoes scraped and mixed with vinegar, to the quantity of one to three pounds of the potatoes a day, according as they may agree with his stomach and bowels. The dish is very agreeable, resembling salad or sliced cabbage." It was probable that cabbages and turnips were as valuable as potatoes and that a cabbage preparation, "krout," was a "highly reputed anti-scorbutic" that could be kept for years. If no vegetables or lemon juice could be had, the patient should take 10 grains of nitre dissolved in vinegar and sweetened.

This practical approach to health problems was popular, and the book was reprinted in 1824. For a third edition, which appeared in 1842, Parsons rewrote the work, adding new diseases, and retitled it *Physician for Ships*. A fourth edition followed in 1852, by which time Parsons no longer had any connection with the navy, having resigned his commission in April 1823.[16]

If Parsons had demonstrated that there was a market for nontechnical books, another naval surgeon observed that narratives of travels were popular, and he decided to put his own experience to use. William S. W. Ruschenberger was commissioned as an assistant surgeon in 1826, and he served in the *Brandywine* with the Pacific Squadron in 1826–29. When he returned, he received his M.D. degree from the University of Pennsylvania in 1830 and was promoted to surgeon the following year. Next came another assignment to the Pacific Squadron in the sloop *Falmouth* in 1832–34. As a result of the latter voyage he published a book in 1834, under the pseudonym "An Officer of the United States Navy," entitled *Three Years in the Pacific*. Fifty years after its appearance, Ruschenberger wrote that he used a pseudonym in case it was a failure. This resolution may have been reinforced when the doctor received a reprimand from Secretary Southard for an article attributed to him which appeared in a Chilean newspaper. The article was concerned with the death and funeral of a marine officer which, in Southard's eyes, depreciated the character and standing of the

U.S. minister to Chile. In any case, except for a brief description of hospitals in Lima, there is nothing in the book to suggest an interest in health. And, as he says in his preface, "the author has avoided obtruding himself upon the attention of the reader, and has indulged in but few reflections; being content to present naked facts, and allow each one to dress them for himself, and draw his own conclusions."[17]

Despite this approach, or perhaps because of it, the book apparently did well. Ruschenberger was designated fleet surgeon of the East India Squadron in 1836, which was charged with a diplomatic mission. The sloop *Peacock* carried Edmund Roberts, a special agent of the United States, who was to try to negotiate a trade treaty with the rulers of Siam, Cochin-China, and Japan. Roberts was successful in signing a treaty with Siam and Muscat, but he died in Macao in 1836 before he could finish his mission. From Ruschenberger's point of view, it was an interesting cruise, and he published his account of it in 1838 in *A Voyage Around the World*. The title page carried his name and rank as well as the information that he was the author of *Three Years in the Pacific*. In this book, Ruschenberger tells of the deaths of Roberts and Lieutenant Archibald S. Campbell, the commanding officer of the schooner *Enterprise*, of a disease contracted at Bangkok which he does not name. He tells us that the sick of the *Peacock* and the *Enterprise* were sent ashore at Macao, where a large house served as a temporary hospital until the ships were ready to sail, but he gives no indication of their ailments. In another chapter he describes the funeral of the acting purser of the *Enterprise*, who also became ill in Bangkok. After this the crew "long saddened by scenes of sickness and death, now resumed its wonted cheerfulness," after having been silent since the ship left Bombay.[18] Thus there are few medical details in the narrative. The lack of such information frustrates a historian, but Ruschenberger's books were popular with the reading public of his day, and they helped to make him well known.

Enlarging the Horizons of Medical Men

Since the time of the Barbary Wars, the Navy Department had generally been receptive to requests by medical officers for leave to take courses. Thus in 1805, Surgeon's Mate Joseph New was given five months' leave to attend medical lectures in Philadelphia. A year later, Surgeon Larkin Griffin received a furlough to attend a course of chemical lectures in that same city. Other officers similarly were given time off to study in Philadelphia or elsewhere. Surgeon Usher Parsons, for example, got permission to attend medical lectures in Boston in 1818. At first there were only a few requests, but in the years following the War of 1812, when many medical officers were not on active duty, the number slowly grew.[19]

After Surgeon Harris began teaching his refresher course, and when he got his students free access to seven lectures at the University of Pennsylvania medical school, many junior officers sought assignments in Philadelphia. Spending time under the guidance of Harris became one of the best ways of preparing for the examination for promotion to surgeon. Harris was justifiably proud of the program he had arranged. "It is now the most complete course of medical & surgical instruction in this country, and perhaps in the world. The course continues ten months in the year—six months in lectures, and the remaining four in examinations and familiar illustrations." Medical officers who took the courses were full of praise for them. From this program a uniformity of training was emerging that owed much to the University of Pennsylvania, Harris, and his connection with the Medical Institute in Philadelphia. And as Harris pointed out to Secretary Woodbury, he did all of this on the pay of an ordinary navy surgeon.[20]

The improved quality of navy surgeons and assistant surgeons was also due to the system of examinations that began in 1824. In the case of the army, regular examinations for entry and promotion did not begin until 1834. By the 1830s virtually all of those accepted for commissions in the navy as assistant surgeons had college or medical school educations as well as practical experience. While there continued to be turnover due to deaths and resignations, a number of competent men were electing to remain in the service.

Study in Europe

As the knowledge of their profession grew, more navy doctors became interested in studying the medical practices and teaching in Europe. In 1806, Surgeon Lewis Heermann requested an 18-month leave of absence to study hospitals in Europe and "in order to obtain that improvement which those seminaries offer to a professional man, and which is so necessary to the officers who devote their services to their country." Secretary Smith granted this request. While Heermann was in England, the *Chesapeake* incident took place. Fearing that there would be a war, he asked for orders to return if his services were needed. The war scare passed, but by the time Heermann was ready to return, a shortage of U.S. ships due to the embargo delayed his departure. He did not report his arrival in Norfolk until August 1808. Just what Heermann learned in Europe and how or if it affected his practice cannot be ascertained from existing records. Presumably observations and consultations improved his knowledge of his profession. Whatever the reality was, his medical skills were soon needed. The departure of Dr. Cowdery in the *Argus* resulted in a shortage of medical men at Norfolk, and Heermann immediately applied for and got the duty at that station.[21]

When Surgeon Usher Parsons was on duty in the Mediterranean in 1819, he asked to be detached from his ship to travel and to return to the United States because of a chronic disease of the liver. His request was granted, and he visited the hospitals, museums, and universities at Palermo and hospitals at Naples before he left the ship at Leghorn. From there he visited the hospital and medical school at Florence and several hospitals in Rome and enjoyed sightseeing in Rome, Leghorn, Genoa, Switzerland, Nice, and Marseilles. He continued up the Rhone valley to Lyons and Paris, where he toured hospitals and met with French physicians. He did not find the French doctors to be either neat, scientific, or successful in their treatment of ulcers and wounds. Some surgeons were caring individuals, while other showed great inhumanity.

While in Paris he took advantage of the opportunity to buy medical books and instruments including a stethoscope that had been designed, examined, and used by René Théophile Hyacinthe Laennec, the inventor. His stay in Paris also provided an opportunity to meet Humphrey Davy, the English physicist and chemist, who was passing through town. He also met another Englishman, William Clift, the conservator of the Royal College of Surgeons, who had been a pupil of the famous British surgeon John Hunter. The friendship with Clift was to last a lifetime.

From Paris, Parsons traveled to London, where he met a number of eminent surgeons, including Sir Ashley Cooper, studied a museum maintained at the College of Surgeons, attended lectures and meetings, and visited hospitals. He sailed for the United States in December 1819. After his return, Parsons was assigned to duty with the marine guard at the Boston Navy Yard until he went on leave in April 1822. He got married and involved in the medical scene in Providence, Rhode Island, so that when he was ordered to sea a year later, he decided to resign. As a result, there were few opportunities to apply the knowledge he acquired in Europe for the direct benefit of the sick of the navy.[22]

Other surgeons who were attached to the Mediterranean Squadron took advantage of their time in Europe to visit hospitals and medical schools in Italy and France. How much they absorbed depended on where they went, what they saw, and how long they could be spared from their duties. But the generally healthy condition of the squadron made such leaves more likely as time went on. When the newly appointed fleet surgeon Lewis Heermann wished to visit Europe again in 1830, the secretary of the navy was most cooperative, ordering him to the *Concord* for duty in the Mediterranean. His orders went on, "Should you think proper to visit Europe for the purpose of inspecting military hospitals and acquiring other professional information, you are at liberty to leave the Concord at any port you may prefer; and after having accomplished the object in view, you will avail yourself of the first favorable opportunity of joining the flag ship of the squadron and reporting to Commodore James Biddle."[23]

Heermann availed himself of this opportunity to leave the ship in Great Britain. He visited hospitals in London and the Royal Hospital at Haslar, near Portsmouth, where sailors of the British navy were treated. From there he traveled to France, stopping in Rouen, Paris, Mayenne, Chalons, Verdun, and Metz, and to Prussia, where he visited Saarbrücken. In the German states he visited a number of places, including Frankfurt, Berlin, Leipzig, and Dresden, before moving on to Vienna, Prague, Milan, Innsbruck, Verona, Genoa, and Marseilles. After this 187-day journey, he boarded the sloop of war *Fairfield* at Marseilles and sailed to Port Mahon.

It was Heermann's intention to write a report of his observations, but shortly after he reached Port Mahon, he became ill. He sailed in the *Brandywine* but was still sick, and he was transferred to the British civil hospital at Gibraltar. Here he was placed under the care of Dr. Frederick Dix, surgeon of the British Ninety-fourth Infantry Regiment. When he recovered sufficiently, he sailed for the United States and landed in New Haven in September 1831. Delayed by illnesses and bad weather, he did not reach New Orleans until a year later. He died there in August 1833, the promised report on European hospitals never finished.[24]

A younger generation of navy doctors now felt that there was more utility in a concentrated period of study in one place, such as Paris, than a grand tour in the fashion of Parsons and Heermann. The first to do this seems to have been Assistant Surgeon Lewis A. Wolfley. As a young man of 18 years, he had obtained a license to practice in Ohio after a brief apprenticeship. He then spent a year at the Ohio Medical College, where he completed courses in anatomy, chemistry and pharmacy, obstetrics, physiology, surgery, materia medica, and the theory and practice of medicine. This background enabled him to pass the entrance examination for the navy and be commissioned as an assistant surgeon in June 1832. Before reporting for duty, he resigned his position as secretary of the 13th district of the Medical Society of Ohio, a post to which he had been elected less than two months before. Service in the West Indies in the sloop *St. Louis* followed. After about four months on duty, a combination of seasickness, physical exhaustion, and homesickness resulted in his being transferred to the naval hospital at Cantonment Clinch in Pensacola.

Shore duty and presumably a lighter patient load helped Wolfley to adjust to the navy, and in May 1833 he was ordered to the ship of the line *Delaware* for duty in the Mediterranean. En route to that station, Wolfley dealt with the normal run of shipboard medical problems, but on such a large ship, the burdens were shared with other junior medical officers, as well as the surgeon. Nevertheless, Wolfley was none too happy at sea and applied for leave to continue his medical education in France. This was granted by Secretary Dickerson and Wolfley arrived in Paris in December 1835.

For the next 11 months, Wolfley paid French surgeons and physicians for the privilege of attending certain lectures and operations at hospitals where they taught, thereby improving his knowledge of clinical procedures and surgical techniques. He also paid Armand Velpeau, the surgeon at the charity hospital (La Charité) for a private course in dissection. From another he learned how to use a stethoscope, and he attended lectures on skin diseases and rheumatism, strangulated inguinal hernia, gastritis, gonorrheal ophthalmia, heart problems, and the pseudo science of phrenology. While Wolfley learned a great deal, he was not uncritical of what he saw and heard. In his journal he wrote, "From what I have observed in the Hospitals of Paris I am more and more convinced, daily, that small diseases bro[ugh]t into the Hospitals should be treated without cutting more than can possibly be helped, as there is a manifest tendency in almost all cases where there is a solution of continuity to become erysipelatous & gangrenous—patients frequently dying after an amputation of a finger or toe."[25]

The costs of advanced study and of acquiring improved techniques were borne entirely by Wolfley from his own limited resources. When his leave was up, he rejoined his ship in the Mediterranean, and he later returned home on furlough. Subsequently he was assigned to the naval asylum in Philadelphia. He was promoted to surgeon in July 1841 and went to sea again in 1843. In all his assignments after his return from France, Wolfley presumably applied the knowledge he had acquired in Paris.[26]

Available data suggest that the general good health of the Mediterranean Squadron made it possible for other young doctors who were so disposed to improve their medical education in Europe. This, in turn, slowly helped to improve the medical expertise, outlook, and professionalism of the whole medical service.

Chapter 17

Establishment of
the Bureau of Medicine
and Surgery

By 1840 the Navy Department had on its rolls 61 surgeons, 17 passed assistant surgeons, and 53 assistant surgeons. Of the surgeons, 23 were assigned to duties on shore in the United States; 1 was in charge of the naval hospital at Port Mahon, on the island of Minorca; 19 were at sea; 16 were at home awaiting orders; and 3 were on leave. Of the passed assistant surgeons, 8 were at sea; 6 were assigned in the United States; 2 were awaiting orders; and 1 was on leave. Of the assistant surgeons, 37 were on sea duty; 8 had shore stations; 6 were standing by for orders; and 2 were on leave.

A surgeon and an assistant surgeon were attached to the receiving ships at Boston, New York, and Norfolk, and a surgeon to each of the recruiting stations at Boston, New York, Philadelphia, Baltimore, and Norfolk. The navy yard at Portsmouth, New Hampshire, had a surgeon assigned to it, whereas the yards at Boston, New York, Philadelphia, and Washington each had an assistant surgeon; Norfolk had a surgeon and two assistants, who also helped out at the hospital if needed. The naval asylum at Philadelphia required a surgeon and an assistant surgeon, a steward, two nurses, two washers, and one cook, all of whom were also expected to help out in the hospital at busy times. A similar situation prevailed in the case of the medical staff at the Washington Navy Yard. At Pensacola a surgeon and an assistant surgeon were assigned to the navy yard, and they were expected to attend to the marines and the men in the receiving ship, if one was stationed there. Naval stations at Baltimore and Charleston had only one surgeon assigned to them. Thus less than one-third of the surgeons were at sea, while slightly more than one-third had shore assignments. The passed assistant surgeons were almost evenly divided between sea and shore duty. Yet more than one-half of the assistant surgeons were practicing at sea.[1]

As this increasingly complex system evolved, the senior medical officers felt a growing need for improved arrangements in regard to the requisition and quality of medicines, the authority to implement recommendations on matters of health, and greater fairness in the assignment of sea and shore duties. On land or sea the medical men were under the control of line officers, and they began to feel that until one of their members was on duty at the Navy Department, the interests of the medical community would never be adequately represented. Informal arrangements such as calling upon the surgeon of the Washington Navy Yard for advice in specific instances were not enough. There had to be a continuous presence and the opportunity to meet with the secretary. The need to deal with such problems had led to proposals for a surgeon general, but such a position had not been established. New opportunities to address these questions arose as the result of a series of magazine articles by a line officer.

Discontent over the way in which the Board of Navy Commissioners functioned had long been apparent among line officers. Criticisms of the board had been expressed in print before, but it remained for Lieutenant Matthew Fontaine Maury to deliver the most devastating assault. Writing in the *Southern Literary Messenger* under the pen name of Harry Bluff, Maury dissected the administrative failures of the board in a series of articles published between April 1840 and June 1841. As a line officer might be expected to do, Maury discussed such topics as promotion, the lack of a sufficient naval force afloat, the waste of money involved in repairing ships, discipline, and other matters, but he also had some thoughts about medicine.

"To its corps of Surgeons the Navy points with pride—for it can boast of some of the most eminent physicians in the country." He noted some of the published works of Barton, Harris, Ruschenberger, and Horner and declared that the authors were held in high repute both at home and abroad.

> Yet such are the anomalies of the present system, that the Navy-Board are required to make rules according to which these men shall treat the sick. And what is still more extraordinary, when one of these Surgeons is ordered to sea, it rests with a Captain to say what medicines shall be laid in for the cruise. The Surgeon's schedule of medicines, like the model and drawings of the [naval ship] Constructor, must be submitted to the inspection of, and is subject to be altered by, officers who know nothing of the art; and the former too frequently finds the pen of authority drawn across this or that item, in his list of articles for the hospital.

Given this situation, wrote Maury, surgeons were forced to resort to artifices to get what they needed. One solution was to give the Latin name of the desired item.[2]

Maury went on to say that some months earlier, navy surgeons complained that the regulations regarding the physical requirements of recruits were so vague that they did not state what constituted a disability. Baldness, dandruff, and ringworm could be interpreted as barring men from the service. "The holding of officers of one profession responsible for the duties of another, which they have never studied, and do not understand, (which is frequently done under the present system,) is not only unwise, but mischievous." It exposed the meddling officer to ridicule and diminished respect for laws and regulations.

To bring about the needed changes, Maury advocated the establishment of a navy medical bureau. Under its jurisdiction a national dispensary would be established where medicines for naval use would be prepared under the direction of a surgeon in chief. Maury thought that small quantities of medicines should be put in glass bottles and sealed with glass stoppers; at the end of a voyage, any unopened bottles would be returned to the dispensary. Under the existing system, "the medicines that are now condemned and sold as unfit for use, are bought up by the apothecaries, repacked, and frequently again sold to the Navy as fresh and good." If a national dispensary did nothing else but correct this system, it would be reason enough to establish one.[3]

Maury's articles were a devastating attack on the waste and mismanagement in the navy. While the Board of Navy Commissioners was the target of most his criticisms, his pieces underscored the lack of adequate supervision by the secretaries of the navy and the naval committees of Congress. Also, the articles appeared before, during, and after the presidential election of 1840, in which the Democrats under President Martin Van Buren were discredited and William Henry Harrison, the Whig party's candidate, became president. For his secretary of the navy, Harrison chose Judge Abel Parker Upshur of Virginia. Upshur was undoubtedly familiar with the charges that Maury had leveled against the navy commissioners, but he was also a man who looked into matters on his own and drew his own conclusions. In his first annual report to the president, Upshur said: "I have had but a short experience in this Department; but a short experience is enough to display its defects, even to the most superficial observation. It is, in truth, not organized at all." He recommended a series of changes, most of them relating to ships, gunnery, promotion, rules and regulations, and similar topics, but some referring in passing to health and hospitals.[4]

Upshur noted with pleasure that the officers and crews of ships on duty in the East Indies were in good health but expressed concern that those cruising off the African coast suffered severely from the climate. Many additional precautions were necessary to protect the men engaged in suppressing the slave trade, he said, but he did not indicate what they were. In addition, the Naval Hospital Fund was gradually increasing and currently totaled $217,907.53. Upshur recommended that he be given the authority to invest the surplus over current obligations in an interest-bearing fund. The interest could be used advantageously to promote the comfort of seamen.

Upshur's current recommendations were "the mere outlines of the many important subjects to which I desire to invite your attention." If Congress chose to act to reform the naval establishment, the secretary was prepared to provide it with all the information it needed.[5] Congress was moved to take action. Upshur's report, coming on the heels of Maury's articles, left little room for complacency. There were a number of naval matters that required attention, and the reform of the Navy Department itself was one of them. During the second session of the Twenty-seventh Congress, several bills were introduced to deal with such things as dry docks, midshipmen, the pay of pursers and engineers, and the redefinition of the daily navy ration, in which the grog portion was reduced to one gill. Only persons at least 21 years of age could receive it. Those who chose to relinquish the daily ration of spirits would be paid for it according to an established rate. Thus the long agitation against the issuing of liquor on the same basis as food had resulted in some modifications. Young men would presumably be less likely to acquire a taste for alcohol, and those older individuals who might consider giving up the spirit ration now had a monetary incentive. Tea, coffee, and cocoa were to be included in the ration as options for those who gave up their grog.[6]

Congress also addressed the care of the insane. The sum of $10,000 was appropriated to alter an old jail so that it could accommodate the mentally ill in the District of Columbia.[7] While this subject was not one to which Upshur called the attention of the president and the Congress, it was of concern, for the insane in the navy were becoming a problem in the various navy hospitals. At an earlier time, two officers had been turned over to the care of the Philadelphia Hospital. By the 1840s there were both officers and enlisted men with mental disorders. While considering what to do about the problem, Upshur wrote to a Dr. Dunbar in Baltimore to inquire about arrangements and rates in that city.[8] Eventually the navy would rely on the establishment in the District of Columbia to care for its mentally ill, but that story belongs to a later period. The question of their

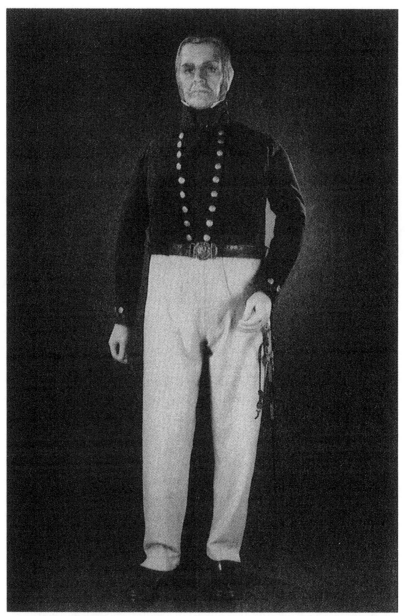

Dress Uniform of Surgeon Bailey Washington, 1841. Smithsonian Institution, Washington, D.C.

care is noted here as yet another aspect of Upshur's wide-ranging concern about problems in his department.

On matters more specific to the immediate needs of the navy, the Congress had much to consider. To ensure a smoother and more logical distribution of duties, Upshur suggested that the Board of Navy Commissioners be replaced by six specialized bureaus. In 1839, Secretary Paulding, at the request of the Congress, had submitted a similar plan, but Upshur had some ideas that he wished to incorporate in the proposed legislation, which he said was "indispensable to the due administration of the Department, and . . . cannot be longer delayed without serious injury to the service."[9]

The reorganization bill was introduced in the House of Representatives by Henry A. Wise, a Virginia Democrat, on February 9, 1842, and it was referred to the Committee of the Whole House. To call attention to the need for a medical bureau, Surgeon Thomas Harris wrote to Wise in March in the Congressman's capacity as chairman of the House Committee on Naval Affairs. Nevertheless, the reorganization bill remained pending. The Senate passed its own version on August 8 and sent it to the House, which did not consider it until the end of the month. Amendments were added and the bill was passed by a vote of 117 to 35. The Senate objected to the amendments and so notified the House, which stood by its version and referred the matter back to the Senate. It was now the last day of the second session of the Twenty-seventh Congress, and in the rush to adjourn, the Senate was persuaded to accept the bill as amended by the House. That same day the measure went to the White House, where President Tyler signed it into law.[10]

The new law called for the abolition of the Board of Navy Commissioners and the reorganization of the Navy Department into five bureaus. These were to have jurisdiction over yards and docks; construction equipment and repair; provisions and clothing; ordnance and hydrography; and medicine and surgery. Navy captains were to head the bureaus of yards and docks and ordnance and hydrography, and they were to be paid $3,500 a year in lieu of all other compensation. A skillful naval constructor was to be chosen to head the Bureau of Construction, Equipment, and Repair, and a suitable person would head the Bureau of Provisions and Clothing, each at an annual salary of $3,000. A surgeon was to be placed in charge of the Bureau of Medicine and Surgery and his annual compensation was to be $2,500.[11] So, while the bureaus were theoretically equal, there was a great disparity in compensation. By paying the head of the medical bureau less than his colleagues, the Congress had placed him and his area of expertise on the lowest level of importance. Yet it was important that the bureau was finally established.

When it came to the selection of a head for the medical bureau, the secretary had few options. Jonathan Cowdery was the ranking surgeon, but he was 75 years old and had been largely inactive for many years. Next in seniority was Surgeon William P. C. Barton of Philadelphia, who was offered the post. Earlier he had argued against the concept of a surgeon general, but now he was ready to head the new bureau. Shortly afterward he moved to Washington to take up his new duties. A new phase in the history of navy medicine was about to begin.[12]

Health problems of those who went to sea were among the earliest concerns of the government of the United States. Congress was slow to address them, but an important step was taken when it established a marine hospital and a system of prepaid health insurance. The seizure of seamen from U.S. ships by the pirates of North Africa resulted in efforts to ransom the unfortunate men and the building of naval vessels. Diplomacy and the payment of ransom eventually resolved the problems of those in captivity. A new assault on American commerce came from the French and resulted in the creation of the U.S. Navy.

During the war the prepaid health insurance program for those in the merchant service was extended to cover the men of the navy. The navy emerged from the brief and successful Quasi-War with a smaller peacetime organization and the beginnings of a medical corps. The war with France was followed by an attempt to eliminate the menace to commerce posed by attacks by the Barbary pirates. Before the naval campaigns in the Mediterranean had been completed, it had become necessary to establish a temporary hospital at Syracuse under the direction of Surgeon Edward Cutbush. It was invaluable experience for a young doctor which was soon to be applied in the United States.

With the settlement of the problems with the Barbary pirates, the United States found itself increasingly involved in arguments with Great Britain over the issue of neutral rights. During these same years the attention of the Congress was directed toward the inadequate health care in marine hospitals and navy yards, and it passed a law in 1811 authorizing the establishment of a separate navy hospital in Washington. Suggestions were solicited from ranking surgeons about the organization and management of this hospital, and Benjamin Latrobe, a prominent architect, designed the structure. But before the hospital could be built, the War of 1812 began.

Doctors on shipboard and in navy yards and shore installations treated the battle wounded and the sick in much the same environment as they had in peacetime. But in places such as Sacket's Harbor and New York, there were more sick sailors than was usually the case. On the whole, surgeons and surgeon's mates of the navy performed satisfactorily despite the lack of adequate hospital facilities. The experience of the war also underscored the need for changes in the way medical men were perceived and paid. After the war a group of senior navy surgeons sought to convince the Navy Department of the need for an increase in pay, better methods of selection and promotion of medical men, and permanent hospitals. Before these needs could be met, Congress and the various presidents had to determine what the peacetime role of the navy should be and what size and type of force was needed to carry out that mission. The medical needs of the service were postponed until the larger questions could be resolved. In the meantime dissatisfaction with the existing situation led to turnover in the medical ranks. It was not until 1828 that legislation was enacted to improve the pay and status of doctors. The first permanent naval hospital was built in 1830, and in succeeding years others came into operation, thereby improving the working conditions and morale of the doctors and the chances of recovery of the patients. Other efforts to define by law the duties of medical officers were frustrated by the refusal of Congress to pass the necessary legislation.

Preliminary investigations into the state of origin of medical officers warranted or commissioned through the War of 1812 show that the largest number of applicants came from Maryland, followed by Massachusetts, New York, and Virginia.[13] During the years immediately following the War of 1812, there were few opportunities for young medical officers to join the navy until death, resignations and improved conditions of service created vacancies and a new environment in which to pursue a career. Beginning in 1824, entrance and promotion depended on passing examinations administered by navy doctors. In this way the professional standards of the service were gradually raised. Prior to the War of 1812, the number of officers with medical degrees was comparatively small; by the 1830s those without medical degrees were becoming the exception to the rule. Adding to this growth of professionalism was the establishment of a school in Philadelphia which helped medical officers to prepare for their examinations. They not only learned navy administrative procedures but through a cooperative arrangement with the University of Pennsylvania and the Medical Institute, were exposed to the best medical education available in the United States. This exposure helped to keep them abreast of developments in the civilian medical world and to widen their professional horizons and contacts.

Building on this foundation, navy medical men began to take advantage of their assignments in European waters to visit medical schools on the

Continent to observe the teaching, the care of patients, and the hospital arrangements. Some were able to audit classes for varying periods of time. These visits enabled navy doctors to compare what they had learned in the United States with what was being taught in Europe and to judge what methods and approaches could be applied to their own service. One of the first places to apply such knowledge was at the naval hospital at Port Mahon, on the island of Minorca. From the earliest days of the service, some navy doctors shared their experiences with their civilian colleagues. Through case reports in professional journals, they passed on their descriptions of unusual cases and their methods of treatment.

A few navy doctors preserved a record of their experiences in book form. The publication of these works not only enhanced the public and professional reputations of individual doctors but also added luster to naval medicine in general.

Improvements in the rank, status, pay, environment, and working conditions of doctors in the navy encouraged some men to make it a career, thereby strengthening the organizational identification of their corps. Others, who left the service for civilian careers, were often proud of their identification with the navy as a phase in their professional education. For those who were in the navy in 1842 when the Board of Navy Commissioners was abolished and replaced by a bureau system, the establishment of the Bureau of Medicine and Surgery was a high point in the drive for better recognition of the health concerns of the service. Now, at long last, there would be a doctor on duty in Washington, close to the secretary, who could represent the interests of the medical community in relations with the Congress and the rest of the navy. There was hope that such an arrangement would improve the quality of medicines used in the navy, lead to further advances in the care of patients and a better recognition by line officers of the professional judgments of their medical shipmates, and result in a fairer method of rotation between sea and shore assignments. How these worked out in practice is the subject of another study.

In their efforts to deal with illnesses in shore environments, navy medical officers implemented decisions that established precedents reflecting the service's attitude toward public health concerns. When Congress established the system of deductions from the pay of merchant and navy seamen to pay for their hospital care ashore, it apparently expected that it would be on a pay-as-you-go basis. But Congress did not build the hospitals as soon as they were needed by both the merchant service and the navy, and the navy's funds were misappropriated. By the time Congress corrected the situation and separate navy hospitals were being built, precedents and procedures had been established in the makeshift hospitals in the various navy yards. In theory the medical men attached to a navy yard dealt only with navy men and illnesses and injuries incurred in the line of duty. In practice they treated officers and enlisted personnel and their families, civilian employees of the yard, and any slaves whose labor was used in the yard. And if the commandant was agreeable, medical officers moonlighted in private practice in adjacent civilian communities. Hence the expertise of government doctors was made available to a wide range of people. Navy doctors would probably not have seen many of these types of case if they had not made themselves available in the working-class neighborhoods adjacent to the yards.

Also, the doctor was not dependent on income from such patients for his livelihood. What the impact of such proximity and expertise was on the public health of those living near a yard, or employed in it, cannot be determined, but it seems likely that it was beneficial. In addition it led to a conclusion on the part of some naval officers and secretaries that since the government's medical men were available and their services were needed, humanitarian considerations seemed to dictate that they be used for the public good. Persons in the yard, both civilian and naval, were treated without payment. Those civilians outside of the yard who were treated apparently paid moderate fees. Thus many of the yards were important for the medical influence on the community as well as their economic impact.

It had taken the government 48 years to move from the first authorization for floating surgeons and surgeon's mates, envisioned in the act of 1794, to the organizational plateau represented by the establishment of the Bureau of Medicine and Surgery. Now that these painful preliminaries were past, the navy would soon take on new responsibilities with the Mexican War and the increased involvement of the United States in the world. All of these matters had their impacts on the health and well being of the men of the navy. By this time the naval doctors had acquired considerable expertise in what worked and what did not in matters of preserving and restoring health. Armed with this knowledge and confident of their professional abilities, the medical men of the navy felt fully prepared for the challenges that lay ahead.

Abbreviations

AF	Area File of the Naval Records Collections, 1775–1910, Microcopy M-625, National Archives, Washington, D. C.
ASP:NA	U.S. Congress, *American State Papers: Naval Affairs,* ser. 6, 4 vols., a subsection of *American State Papers: Documents, Legislative and Executive,* 38 vols. (Washington, D.C., 1832–61).
CL	Letters Received by the Secretaries of the Navy: Captains' Letters 1805–61, Microcopy M-125, National Archives, Washington, D.C.
GLB	General Letterbook or Miscellaneous Letters Sent by the Secretary of the Navy, Microcopy M-209, National Archives, Washington, D.C.
HSP	Historical Society of Pennsylvania, Philadelphia.
LBNC	Letterbook of the Board of Navy Commissioners, Record Group 45, National Archives, Washington, D.C.
LC	Library of Congress, Washington, D.C.
LO	Letters Sent by the Secretary of the Navy to Officers, 1798–1868, Microcopy M-149, National Archives, Washington, D.C.
ML	Miscellaneous Letters Received by the Secretary of the Navy, 1801–84, Microcopy M-124, National Archives, Washington, D.C.
NA	National Archives, Washington, D.C.
NYHS	New York Historical Society, New York.
NYPL	New York Public Library, New York.
OL	Letters Received by the Secretary of the Navy from Officers below the the Rank of Commander, 1802–84, Microcopy M-148, National Archives, Washington, D.C.
RG	Record Group.
RGCM	Records of General Courts-Martial and Courts of Inquiry of the Navy Department, 1799–1867, Microcopy M-273, National Archives, Washington, D.C.
USND	United States Navy Department, Washington, D.C.
USNIP	*United States Naval Institute Proceedings,* Annapolis, Md.
ZB File	Biographical Information on American Navy Officers, Navy Operational Archives, Naval Historical Center, Washington Navy Yard, Washington, D.C.

Notes

Chapter 1
The Health, Welfare, and Safety of Seamen

1. Worthington C. Ford et al., eds., *Journals of the Continental Congress, 1774–1789*, 24:813, 821–28; 26:176–77, 180–85, 355–56; 27:357–62, 368–72; *Papers of Thomas Jefferson*, ed. Julian P. Boyd et al., 7:497; 8:208–9, 235, 238; 9:88 (hereafter cited as Boyd, *Jefferson Papers*). The sum recommended by Franklin, Adams, and Jay as compensation to Pecquet is equivalent to approximately $9,500 in 1993 dollars. I am grateful to Professor John McCusker of Trinity University for this computation. The amount Pecquet actually received has not been determined.

2. Samuel Flagg Bemis, *Diplomatic History of the United States*, 65–70; Merrill Jensen, *New Nation*, 168–69, 174–76. For details of the relationship of foreign trade to the movement for the Constitution, see Frederick W. Marks III, *Independence on Trial*. For the texts of the treaties negotiated during the Confederation period, see Hunter Miller, ed., *Treaties and Other International Acts of the United States of America, 1776–1863*, 2:3, 45, 59, 123, 165, 185.

3. Boyd, *Jefferson Papers*, 17:244–49; William Barnes and John Heath Morgan, *Foreign Service of the United States*, 31–36, 57–60.

4. Boyd, *Jefferson Papers*, 17:423–24.

5. Ibid., 177–78.

6. *U.S. Statutes at Large*, 1:254–57.

7. USND, *Naval Documents Related to the United States Wars with the Barbary Powers*, 1:1–6, 14–15, 29 (hereafter cited as USND, *Barbary Wars*). Buboes are a sign of bubonic plague.

8. Ibid., 18–22 (for ransoms demanded for individual captives in 1785, see p. 1).

9. Ibid., 34–35, 47–49, 56–58.

10. Ibid., 69–70; Charles W. Goldsborough, *United States Naval Chronicle*, 56n. For a discussion of the political, economic, and diplomatic aspects of the act of 1794, see Marshall Smelser, *Congress Founds the Navy, 1787–1798*, chap. 4; Craig L. Symonds, *Navalists and Antinavalists*, chap. 2.

11. John Davis, Comptroller, Treasury Department, to Jedediah Huntington, Philadelphia, September 1795. The text of this letter is printed in item 99 in *Doris Harris Autograph Catalog No. 24*, Los Angeles, December 1978.

12. USND, *Barbary Wars*, 1:98, 107–17, 202, 208–10; *Gazette of the United States*, February 9, 1798. The sickness seems to have been smallpox, not bubonic plague.

13. USND, *Naval Documents Related to the Quasi-War between the United States and France*, 1:25 (hereafter cited as USND, *Quasi-War*).

14. Ibid., 21, 46, 48.

15. Robert Straus, *Medical Care for Seamen*, 17–21; J. J. Keevil, Christopher Lloyd, and Jack L. S. Coulter, *Medicine in the Navy, 1200–1900*, 3:189–208; William

Palmer, ed. and comp., *Calendar of Virginia State Papers and Other Manuscripts
. . . Preserved . . . at Richmond,* 4:362; 5:130, 139, 444–46; 7:392–93; 9:116, 132–33,
136, 184; William Waller Hening, comp., *Statutes at Large, Being a Collection of
the Laws of Virginia,* 10:379–86; 11:161–62; 12:438–42, 494–95; 13:133–35, 158–59,
223–24.

16. Augustus W. Greeley, *Public Documents of Early Congresses,* 92; *Annals of
Congress,* 1st Cong., 1:685 (July 20, 1789); *House Journal,* 1st Cong., 1st sess., 1:364;
William A. Baker, *History of the Boston Marine Society, 1742–1967,* 63–65.

17. *Papers of Alexander Hamilton,* ed. Harold C. Syrett et al., 11:294–96; Straus,
Medical Care for Seamen, 25.

18. Straus, *Medical Care for Seamen,* 25–26; U.S. Congress, *American State
Papers, Foreign Relations,* 1:761–66; *Finance,* 1:497; *Senate Journal,* 5th Cong., 1st
sess., 16–17.

19. *Annals of Congress,* 5th Cong., 2d sess., 2:1383–93. The debate was also
published in two Philadelphia newspapers, *Gazette of the United States,* April 13,
14, 1798, and *Carey's United States Recorder,* April 14, 1798.

20. *Annals of Congress,* 5th Cong., 2d sess., 2:1383–93.

21. *U.S. Statutes at Large,* 1:605–6.

22. Ibid., 1:729; Straus, *Medical Care for Seamen,* 29–31; Henry W. Farnam,
Chapters in the History of Social Legislation in the United States to 1860, 232–34.

23. *U.S. Statutes at Large,* 1:729.

Chapter 2
The Quasi-War with France

1. For background on the Quasi-War see Alexander De Conde, *Quasi-War,*
chap. 1; Michael A. Palmer, *Stoddert's War,* introduction. Naval documents relating
to the conflict are published in USND, *Quasi-War.*

2. *U.S. Statutes at Large,* 1:350–51.

3. Smelser, *Congress Founds the Navy,* 35–86; Symonds, *Navalists and Antinavalists,* 17–65; *U.S. Statutes at Large,* 1:523. The act of 1797 is reprinted in
USND, *Quasi-War,* 1:7–9.

4. Francis B. Heitman, *Historical Register and Dictionary of the United States
Army,* 1:456.

5. Gillasspy's notebook is in the Rare Book Room, Van Pelt Library, University
of Pennsylvania, Philadelphia. Bound with it is a copy of Benjamin Rush, *Syllabus
of a Course of Lectures on the Institutes of Medicine.* The inscription quoted is
inside the cover of the syllabus, but the printed pages of the book are interspersed
with Gillasspy's handwritten notes. Rush's lectures began on February 1, 1798.
Barton's lecture is no. 5 in the notebook; Rush's are nos. 3 and 4.

6. McHenry to Barry, August 30, 1797, USND, *Quasi-War,* 1:16.

7. For an account of the illness in the ship, see William Bell Clark, *Gallant John
Barry, 1745–1803,* 388–92. McHenry to Tench Francis, September 11, 1797, Correspondence on Naval Affairs When the Navy Was under the War Department,
1794–1798, M-739, roll 1. NA. The hospital in question was probably the local

marine hospital, but it could also have referred to rented houses near the river where patients could be kept in isolation.

8. Barry to McHenry, September 13, 1797, John Barry Correspondence, John S. Barnes Collection, NYHS, McHenry to Lieutenant John McRea, May 11, 1798, LO.

9. Gillasspy to Barry, September 15, 1797; Francis to Barry, September 13, 1797; Meade to Barry, October 8, 1797, Barry Correspondence. The law of July 1, 1797, providing for naval armament also stipulated the ration of food. Every day the men were to receive one pound of bread, supplemented in accordance with the following schedule: Sunday, one and one-half pounds of beef and a half-pint of rice; Monday, one pound of pork, a half-pint of peas or beans, and four ounces of cheese; Tuesday, one and one-half pounds of beef, one pound of potatoes or turnips, and pudding; Wednesday, two ounces of butter or six ounces of molasses, four ounces of cheese, and a half-pint of rice; Thursday, one pound of pork and a half-pint of peas or beans; Friday, one pound of salt fish, two ounces of butter or one gill of oil, and one pound of potatoes; Saturday, one pound of pork, a half-pint of peas or beans, and four ounces of cheese. In addition, the men received a half-pint of distilled spirits or one quart of beer per day. In serving something not on this list or out of sequence, Gillasspy was technically violating the law.

10. War Department to Gillasspy, September 22, 1797, Correspondence on Naval Affairs when the Navy was under the War Department, 1794–1798, M-739, roll 1, NA. For biographical data see "John Bullus," ZB File. Information on his days in Reading may be found in Bullus to Benjamin Rush, July 23 and September 12, [1797?], Benjamin Rush Manuscript Correspondence, Library Company of Philadelphia Collection, vol. 1A, and "Yellow Fever," pt. 3. HSP.

11. Gillasspy to Barry, October 3, 11, 16, 1797, Barry Correspondence.

12. Gillasspy to Barry, November 21, 26, 1797, Barry Correspondence.

13. Truxtun to Gross, August 30, 1797, USND, *Quasi-War*, 1:13; Rush to Truxtun, October 4, 1797, Correspondence of Benjamin Rush, M.D., 1793–1813, Dreer Collection, HSP.

14. Heitman, *Historical Register*, 1:187; "George Balfour," ZB File; USND, *Quasi-War*, 7:316; USND, *Barbary Wars, vol. 7, Personnel and Ships' Data*, Richard C. Holcomb, *Century with Norfolk Naval Hospital, 1830–1930*, 67.

15. USND, *Quasi-War*, 8:333; Stoddert to Orr, October 24, 1799, LO. The muster roll of the *Constellation* in *Quasi-War*, 1:304 shows him as an ex-regimental warrant officer, but he is not listed in Heitman *Historical Register* as an army officer.

16. McHenry to Truxtun, March 16, 1798, USND, *Quasi-War*, 1:42–43.

17. Higginson to McHenry, June 6, 1798, USND, *Quasi-War*, 1:107.

18. *U.S. Statutes at Large*, 2:553, reprinted in USND, *Quasi-War*, 1:59–60.

19. USND, *Quasi-War*, 1:46.

20. Ibid., 58

21. Ibid., 59–60. For the most recent assessment of Stoddert, see Palmer, *Stoddert's War*. An earlier evaluation is John J. Carrigg is in Paolo E. Coletta, ed., *American Secretaries of the Navy*, 1:59–75; and Carrigg, "Benjamin Stoddert and the Foundation of the American Navy" (Ph.D. diss., Georgetown University, 1952).

22. USND, *Quasi-War*, 1:51–63, 67–68, 72, 74.

23. Ibid., 77.

24. Ibid., 87–88, 91.

25. Ibid., 92–93, 104–95, 118.

26. *U.S. Statutes at Large*, 2:569, reprinted in USND, *Quasi-War*, 1:127. The Revenue Cutter Service and the Life-Saving Service were combined in 1915 to form the U.S. Coast Guard.

27. *U.S. Statutes at Large*, 1:627, 699, reprinted in USND, *Quasi-War*, 1:516–17.

28. *U.S. Statutes at Large*, 2:594, reprinted in USND, *Quasi-War*, 1:188–89.

29. USND, *Quasi-War*, 1:175–76, 183, 231, 258; Palmer, *Stoddert's War*, 30–31.

30. USND, *Quasi-War*, 1:189–94, 442, 336, 377, 430; Palmer, *Stoddert's War*, 36–43.

31. Palmer, *Stoddert's War*, 72–106.

32. USND, *Quasi-War*, 3:110–11, 169–70; Palmer, *Stoddert's War*, 105–6.

33. USND, *Quasi-War*, 3:177, 187–88, 276, 336.

34. Palmer, *Stoddert's War*, 225, 233–39.

35. Whitfield J. Bell Jr., "Medical Practice in Colonial America," *Bulletin of the History of Medicine* 31 (1957):442–53; Genevieve Miller, "Physician in 1776," *Journal of the American Medical Association* 236 (1976):26–30; Richard H. Shryock, "Significance of Medicine in American History," *American Historical Review* 62 (1956):81–87. On the influence of the care and teaching at the Royal Infirmary of Edinburgh, see Guenter B. Risse, *Hospital Life in Enlightenment Scotland.* By 1795 seamen of the Royal Navy were being regularly admitted to this hospital. For a discussion of quacks and alleged quacks, see Peter Benes, "Itinerant Physicians, Healers, and Surgeon-Dentists in New England and New York, 1720–1825, "in Benes, ed, *Medicine and Healing*, 95–112.

36. Henry E. Sigerest, "Boerhaave's Influence upon American Medicine," in Felix Marti-Ibanez, ed., *Henry E. Siqerest*, 203–9. Sigerest says that at the time of the American Revolution it is estimated that there were at most 3,500 physicians in the colonies, of whom only 400 had medical degree. William G. Rothstein, *American Medical Schools*, 28–29.

37. J. Worth Estes, "Therapeutic Practice in Colonial New England," in Philip Cash et al., eds., *Medicine in Colonial Massachusetts, 1620–1820* 289–93; Estes, "Medical Skills in Colonial New England," *New England Historical and Genealogical Register* 134 (1980):259–75; Estes, "Practice of Medicine in Eighteenth-Century Massachusetts," *New England Journal of Medicine* 305 (1981):1040–47; Estes, "Patterns of Drug Usage in Colonial America," *New York State Journal of Medicine* 87 (1987):37–45; J. Worth Estes, "Quantitative Observations of Fever and its Treatment before the Advent of Short Clinical Thermometers," *Medical History* 35 (1991):189–216; Miller, "Physician in 1776," 26–30.

38. Rothstein, *American Medical Schools*, 31–32.

39. Those appointed surgeon were Joseph Anthony, June 20; George Wright, June 27; Larkin Thorndyke, July 3; Thomas Rowland, July 25; Thomas Reynolds, September 10; Jeffrey D. Shanley, September 10; John K. Read, Jr., September 12; Nathaniel Bradstreet, September 23; and Joseph Lee, October 10. Asa Sargent was appointed surgeon by Captain Edward Preble and began duty on July 18, 1798. His commission was not delivered until June 15, 1799. He served in the revenue cutter

Pickering, which was lost at sea in January 1800. Appointments as surgeon's mates went to William Turner, June 7; Samuel Anderson, July 2; Henry Wells, July 25; Hanson Catlett, August 3; John Hart, September 10; and Thomas Oliver Hunt Carpenter, October 13.

40. Secretary of the Navy Stoddert to Samuel Anderson, July 2, 1798, USND, *Quasi-War,* 1:160; 7:315. Anderson's commission was forwarded on July 13, 1799.

41. USND, *Quasi-War,* 7:332, 346.

42. The alphabetical listing of all officers in USND, *Quasi-War,* 7:315–58 includes the ships in which they served. The three mates who were promoted in less than a year were Richard C. Shannon, who served in the revenue cutter *Scammel;* Benjamin Shurtleff of the revenue cutter *Merrimack;* and Daniel Hughes of the *Ganges.* See USND, *Quasi-War,* 6:283, 290; Edward W. Callahan, ed., *List of Officers of the Navy of the United States and of the Marine Corps,* 174.

43. Information from the Harvard University Archives.

44. St. Medard to Secretary of the Navy Smith Thompson, May 29, 1820, OL; USND, *Quasi-War,* 7:348.

45. Clifford K. Shipton, "Amos Windship," in *Biographical Sketches of Those Who Attended Harvard College in the Classes of 1768–1771,* 17, 673–79; RGCM, roll 3, case 7.

46. F. L. Pleadwell, "Edward Cutbush, M.D.," *Annals of Medical History* 5 (1923):337–86.

47. USND, *Quasi-War,* 7:334, 337, 339, 348–49, 355.

48. Silas Talbot Papers, G. W. Blunt White Library, Mystic Seaport, Mystic, Conn.

49. The promotions went to Samuel Anderson, James Dodge, and Charles Webb. Those appointed surgeon were John Goddard, John Howell, and Walter Buchanan. The 22 mates were Benjamin G. Harris, Jonathan Cowdery, William Turk, Francis Le Barron, William Frost, Charles Webb, Thomas D. Prince, Starling Archer, Robert B. Stark, Hugh Aitken, Daniel McCormick Jr., James H. Bradford, Thomas H. M. Fendall, Zephaniah Jennings, John P. Fisher, Samuel E. Willett, Henry Gardner, and John H. Perkins. Charles F. Thornton declined the appointment. In addition, Thomas Starke was appointed temporarily as surgeon's mate by Captain Alexander Murray of the *Insurgente.* Abraham Solis served as the surgeon's mate in the *Herald* during 1800, and Alexander McWilliams as a surgeon's mate in the *United States* in late 1800 and early 1801, but his commission was not dated until February 1802. Most of these men had brief careers, but Charles Webb probably had the most rapid series of changes between his appointment as a surgeon's mate in March 1800, promotion to surgeon the following November, and court-martial and dismissal eight months after that. See USND, *Quasi-War,* 7:315–57.

50. F. L. Pleadwell and W. M. Kerr, "Jonathan Cowdery," *United States Naval Medical Bulletin* 17 (1922):83–84; "Jonathan Cowdery," ZB File.

51. USND, *Quasi-War,* 7:320.

52. Lewis Heermann was appointed surgeon's mate in September 1801. Larkin Griffin served as an acting surgeon's mate in the *Maryland* in 1801 but was not commissioned until September 1802. William C. Smith was an acting surgeon's

mate in the *President* but was not commissioned until June 1802. Daniel Osgood served as a surgeon's mate in the *Warren* but was not commissioned. USND, *Quasi-War,* 7:331–32, 343, 350.

53. F. L. Pleadwell and F. Lester "Lewis Heermann," *Annals of Medical History* 5 (1923):121–27, 138.

54. Stoddert to Captain Richard Dale, May 11, 1798; McHenry to the lieutenant of the marines in the *Constellation,* March 10, 1798, USND, *Quasi-War,* 1:41, 72.

55. For information on civilian medical practices of the time, I am grateful to Dr. Worth Estes of the Boston University School of Medicine.

56. USND, *Quasi-War,* 7:364–71. For details of the *Constitution,* I am indebted to Commander Tyrone G. Martin, USN (Ret.), a former captain and the author of a history of the ship.

57. Truxtun to Stoddert, June 24, August 11, 1798, USND, *Quasi-War,* 1:155.

58. Truxtun to Lieutenant John Rodgers and others, July 1, 1798, USND, *Quasi-War,* 1:155.

59. Isaac Henry to Hugh Henry, June 18, 1799, Isaac Henry Papers, William R. Perkins Library, Duke University, Durham, N.C.

60. RGCM, case 7.

61. Ibid., case 10.

62. Ibid., case 16. The charges against Marshall and his statement of defense are printed in USND, *Quasi-War,* 7:178–79, 259–61.

63. RGCM, case 5.

64. Ibid., case 12; USND, *Quasi-War,* 7:203–4.

65. USND, *Quasi-War,* 7:33, 148–49.

66. *U.S. Statutes at Large,* 2:110–11. This law is reprinted in USND, *Quasi-War,* 7:134–35. The list of surgeons and surgeon's mates to be retained is on p. 136 of this volume.

67. USND, *Quasi-War,* 7:315–58; USND, *Barbary Wars.*

Chapter 3
Medicine and Health in the Quasi-War

1. James Lind, *An Essay on the Most Effective Means of Preserving the Health of Seamen,* was published in 1752 and reprinted in 1762 and 1779. The last edition also carried a reprint of his *Two Papers on Fever and Infections,* which first appeared in 1763 and went through three editions during his lifetime as well as being printed abroad in translation. But his specific recommendations on the prevention of scurvy were not adopted by the British Admiralty until 1795. Lind's *Essay on Diseases Incidental to Europeans in Hot Climates, With the Method for Preventing their Fatal Consequences* was published in 1768 and went through six editions by 1806. The first U.S. edition did not appear until 1811. It was the standard treatise on the subject for 50 years.

Gilbert Blane published *A Short Account of the Most Effective Means of Preserving the Health of Seamen* in 1780 and distributed it to the captains of the fleet to which he was attached. His *Observations on the Diseases Incident to Seamen,* first published in 1789, went through a second edition that same year and a third in 1799. See Christopher Lloyd, ed., *Health of Seamen*, 2–5, 132–34; Blane's observations on the diseases common to seamen are on p. 151. Blane sent a copy of his book, presumably the third edition, to President John Adams on September 13, 1799, which Adams acknowledged on May 18, 1800. It is not known what happened to this book. Adams may have sent it to the Library of Congress, where it was subsequently lost in a fire, or it may have been sent to the Navy Department. Robert Adams, editor in chief, Adams Papers, to the author, September 23, 1981.

2. Loblolly boys were sick bay attendants, so named for the porridge they served to the sick. In the Royal Navy the loblolly boy banged a mortar and pestle to announce sick call. See Keevil, Lloyd, and Coulter, *Medicine and the Navy*, 1:219; 3:27–28, 64.

3. Balfour to Richard Rush, August 15, 1798, Rush Correspondence, "Yellow Fever," pt. 3.

4. Barry to Stoddert, July 26, 1798, two letters: Letters Received by the Fourth Auditor and Accountant of the Navy, 1795–1798, 1:65–66, RG 217, NA; Eugene S. Ferguson, *Truxtun of the "Constellation*," 141; USND, *Quasi-War*, 1:135.

5. USND, *Quasi-War*, 1:240, 264, 251.

6. Keevil Lloyd, and Coulter, *Medicine in the Navy*, 3:71.

7. USND, *Quasi-War*, 1:304–15.

8. Ibid., 304, 309; 312; 2:335, 337–39. During the battle, Seaman Neil Harvey became terrified and ran from his gun. Lieutenant Andrew Sterret, believing the man to be a coward, ran him through with his sword. Harvey was subsequently carried on the muster list as killed in action. USND, *Quasi-War*, 1:306; Ferguson, *Truxtun of the "Constellation*," 164.

9. USND, *Quasi-War*, 2:330, 345, 351, 355, 357–58, 411, 427.

10. USND, *Quasi-War*, 5:161–63; Isaac Henry to Hugh Henry, February 3, 1800, AF. M-625, NA.

11. John Hoxse, *Yankee Tar*, 70–71.

12. USND, *Quasi-War*, 5:208.

13. Hoxse, *Yankee Tar*, 79–80.

14. USND, *Quasi-War*, 5:118–19; Callahan, *List of Officers*, 452.

15. USND, *Quasi-War*, 5:3–4. 226–27. Edward Stevens, the U.S. consul general at Santo Domingo, reported that a French passenger was wounded by a spent ball and Lieutenant David Porter received a slight contusion in the arm from a musket ball. Lieutenant William Maley, the commander of the *Experiment*, reported Porter's wound.

16. USND, *Quasi-War*, 2:4, 11, 268, 281, 301, 316, 318, 351, 375, 413, 419; 3:152, 290, 297, 300, 311, 409. Commander Martin, a former captain of the USS *Constitution* and the historian of the ship, has entered the data from the ship's logs into a computer database and has provided me with a printout of the casualty figures cited. See Martin, "The Captain's Clerk" (database). Tryon, N.C.: Timonier Publications, 1989.

17. Ibid., 4:260.

18. Ibid., 6:335, 368.

19. Ibid., 167, 263–64.

20. Ibid., 264.

21. Ibid., 5:322, 414, 455–56.

22. Ibid., 421. For information on the mutiny and the court of inquiry, see pp. 65–66, 414–15, 419, 421, 436, 451–56, 492–93.

23. For a fuller account of Dr. Field's case, see Harold D. Langley, "Edward Field," *Connecticut Medicine* 46 (1982):667–72.

24. Charles Morris to Thomas Turner, May 30, 1800, General Accounting Office Records, Letters Received by the Accountant of the Navy, 3, RG 217, NA.

25. Charles Morris to Field, July 12, 1801, James Sever Papers, LC. For the sentence of the court-martial and Truxton's views, see USND, *Quasi-War,* 5:520–21.

26. USND, *Quasi-War,* 5:580–81; 6:107–8, 137–38, 303–4, 343–44; Langley, "Edward Field," 669–70.

27. USND, *Quasi-War,* 5:300.

28. "Journal of the USS *Essex,* August 5, 1800," Edward Preble Papers, LC; Christopher McKee, *Edward Preble,* 72.

29. McKee, *Edward Preble,* 74–79; USND, *Quasi-War,* 6:2, 2, 76. On June 1, 1800, Preble reported the death of unknown causes of Midshipman William H. Williams. That same day, 10 men were reported sick. "Journal of the USS *Essex,*" Preble Papers, LC.

30. Orr to Preble, June 25, 1800, Letterbook, vol. 23, Preble Papers. Lind wrote, "When ships are necessarily obliged to put into such unhealthy ports, the first precaution to be taken is, to anchor at as great a distance from the shore as can be done, and to prefer the open sea, where the anchorage is safe, to running up into rivers or bays unclosed with the land, and especially where there are high mountains, that may interrupt the salutary current of sea breezes." See Lloyd, *Health of Seamen,* 55.

31. USND, *Quasi-War,* 7:339.

32. "Journal of the USS Essex," vol. 35, July 1, September 11, 14, 1800, Preble Papers, LC.

33. Preble to Smith, September 15, 1800, Letterbook, vol. 23, Preble Papers, LC.

34. Of the seven deaths reported, two were identified as men belonging to the main topmasts, and death may have resulted from falls. The same may be true of a man who was identified as belonging to the forecastle starboard watch. For each of these days there is no entry in regard to sickness aboard. When Seaman Charles Swed died on October 12, 1800, Preble noted that he had been sick every since he came on board in Batavia. This is the only death clearly associated with illness. Two others seem likely because the ship was then off Java. On Preble's digestive disorders, see McKee, *Edward Preble,* 88.

35. Balfour to Rush, August 15, 1798, Rush Correspondence, 37:10–12. If Balfour's measurements were correct, it meant that Seaman Foss lost about 60–65 percent of his blood, and this seems unlikely. Similar doubts exist in the case of gunner Morgan. See David C. Sabiston Jr., ed., *Davis-Christopher Textbook of Surgery,* 120–22.

36. John Rush to Dr. Coxe, August 17, 1804, *Medical and Agricultural Register* 1 (1806–7):34–37.

37. Anderson to Rush, April 21, 1800, Rush Correspondence, vol. 24, pt. 4.

38. USND, *Quasi-War,* 6:172, 201, 217; Secretary of the Navy B. W. Crownin-shield to B. Smith, May 6, 1816, GLB. The symptoms noted could also have been the result of meningitis or a stroke. Baker's "derangement" increased, and he was confined to a hospital in 1801. The captain's inability to support his family was a source of much distress to his wife, who was left with seven children to raise. The settlement of the captain's accounts in October 1801 brought her the sum of $197.40, and in August of that year she began receiving his pension of $37.50 a month until his death in 1820. For this information on Baker's subsequent history I am grateful to Christopher McKee.

39. "Some Observations Taken on Board the U.S. Frigate Philadelphia During her Cruise in the Year 1800—and After Leaving her. By Benjamin G. Harris, Surgeon's Mate," Navy Department Records, Subject File MV, box 1, RG 45, NA. Harris left the ship on December 10, 1800, when he accepted a position on shore at Monserrat, a British possession in the Leeward Islands. See also Kenneth Carpenter, *History of Scurvy and Vitamin C,* 75–97.

40. Stoddert to Surgeon William Graham, December 6, 1800, roll 4, LO. In the British navy the fee was originally 15 shillings for a marine and 30 shillings for a seaman but was later set at 15 shillings for all. The result of the fines was that seamen refused to report the disease in its early stages and tried to avoid payment. The practice of collecting fees was ended in 1795 thanks to the efforts of Dr. Thomas Trotter. See Lloyd and Coulter, *Medicine in the Navy, 1200–1900,* 3:357–58.

41. Catlett to Rush, October 25, 1807, Rush Correspondence, 3:30.

42. Hawthorne to Stoddert, December 15, 1800, General Accounting Office Records, Letters Received by the Accountant of the Navy, 5:339, RG 217, M-117, roll 124, NA.

43. Jacobs to Thomas Turner, July 15, 1800, General Accounting Office Records, Letters Received by the Accountant of the Navy, 4:148, RG 217, M-1187, roll 124, NA.

44. General Accounting Office Records, Journal no. 1, Accountant of the Navy Office, RG 217, NA: Rush to William Winder, Accountant of the Navy, December 3, 1798, General Accounting Office Records, Letters Received by the Accountant of the Navy, 1:223, RG 217, NA.

45. Talbot to Commodore John Barry, November 24, 1800, Huntington Library Collection. Most likely Barry referred this letter to the secretary of the navy who, in turn, forwarded it to the accountant in the Treasury Department who dealt with navy matters.

46. Higginson to Thomas Turner, August 20, 1800; Jesse V. Lewis to Turner, August 20, 1800, General Accounting Office Records, Letters Received by the Accountant of the Navy, 4:209, 217, RG 217, NA.

47. USND, *Quasi-War,* 1:362–63.

48. Ibid., 406.

49. General Accounting Office Records, Journal no. 1, Fourth Auditor's Records, RG 217, NA.

50. Turner to Albertus, September 7, 1802, General Accounting Office Records, Letter Book of the Accountant of the Navy, 75, RG 217, NA.

51. Stoddart to Geddes, April 12, 1800, roll 3, LO.

52. James and Eben Watson to Thomas Turner, September 3, 1800, Letters Received by the Accountant of the Navy, 5:79, RG 217, NA.

53. Turner to James and Eben Watson, September 20, 1800; Turner to John Hoxse, September 20, 1800; John Hoxse to Turner, September 22, 1800; Turner to James and Eben Watson, October 1, 1800; James and Eben Watson to Turner, October 7, 1800; Turner to Gibbs and Channing, October 23, 1800; Gibbs and Channing to Turner, November 10, 1800, General Accounting Office Records, Letters Received by the Accountant of the Navy, vol. 5; Letter Book of the Accountant of the Navy, RG 217, NA.

54. USND, *Quasi-War,* 1:558, 579; 2:47.

55. Ibid., 3:288.

56. Ibid., 1:312.

57. Harold D. Langley, "Respect for Civilian Authority," *American Neptune* 40 (1980):23–37.

58. Louis H. Roddis, "Naval and Marine Corps Casualties," *Military Surgeon* 99 (1946):305–10; U.S. Department of Commerce, *Historical Statistics of the United States, Colonial Times to 1970,* 2:1135–36, 1143. The strength of the U.S. Navy during the Quasi-War is a matter of dispute. Volume 7 of the Navy Department's volumes on the *Quasi-War* contains an admittedly incomplete listing of officers, acting officers, and petty officers which totals 1,149. If we deduct the petty and warrant officers and count the master's mates as officers, the total is 976. If we deduct the master's mates, the total is 911 officers. The same volume also lists 63 marine officers and 7 Revenue Cutter Service officers after deducting 2 petty officers and 7 mates from the latter service. Thus 911 naval officers, 63 marines, and 7 Revenue Cutter officers bring the total to 981 for the whole period of the war. A similar problem exists in relation to the total force employed. Secretary Stoddert's report of December 24, 1798 shows 4,170 men, of whom 660 (220 each) are listed as the complements of ships that were under construction, the *General Greene,* the *Connecticut* and the *Adams.* But volume 7 of the *Quasi-War* documents shows the complement of the *Connecticut* as 180, not 220, which is the case with the other two ships. No figures are given in Stoddert's report for other ships being built by the public or for the Revenue Cutters *Diligence, Scammel,* and *South Carolina.* If we list all the ships operated by the navy during the Quasi-War, omit the galleys operated by the War Department, and record the official complements of the vessels selected, we get a grand total of 7,621. Of course this assumes that the authorized strength was the actual strength, does not allow for deaths and transfers, and assumes that all the ships were in active service at the same time. If many of the ships operated well below their authorized strength, that is not reflected in the surviving documentation known to the writer.

Chapter 4
The Barbary Wars

1. Cutbush to James Rees, June 23, October 2, 1801; Samuel Smith to Cutbush, June 13, 1801, and Cutbush's note on same written about 1830, Edward Cutbush Manuscripts, Josiah Trent Collection, Medical Center Library, Duke University.

2. For the political and diplomatic background of the Barbary Wars see Ray W. Irwin, *Diplomatic Relations of the United States with the Barbary Powers 1776–1816;* James A. Field Jr., *America and the Mediterranean World, 1776–1882,* chap. 2; Symonds, *Navalists and Antinavalists,* 90–96; Dumas Malone, *Jefferson the President: First Term, 1801–1805,* chap. 6, and pp. 262–63.

3. The naval side of the question may be found in Gardner W. Allen, *Our Navy and the Barbary Corsairs;* Harold and Margaret Sprout, *Rise of American Naval Power, 1776–1918,* 55–61; Roger C. Anderson, *Naval Wars in the Levant, 559–1853;* Dudley W. Knox, *History of the United States Navy,* chap. 6; Charles Oscar Paullin, *Commodore John Rodgers,* chaps. 6, 7; McKee, *Edward Preble,* chaps. 6–16; David F. Long, *Ready to Hazard,* chaps. 3–5; Long, *Nothing Too Daring,* 15–35; Linda M. Maloney, *Captain from Connecticut,* chaps. 4, 5. Documents on naval operations may be found in USND, *Barbary Wars.*

4. USND, *Barbary Wars,* 1:497–99, 534–35, 548–49, 552–56, 560–61, 568–69, 570, 580, 584–85, 590, 593–94, 608.

5. Ibid., 569, 573, 587, 596.

6. Ibid., 606–907.

7. Ibid., 607.

8. Ibid., 613, 621, 623–24, 627–28, 633–37.

9. Ibid., 628–32, 634–36, 638, 584, 607, 435, 595–96.

10. Ibid., 2:20, 51–52, 76, 83, 92, 99–100, 118–19, 130, 136, 261, 389–90.

11. USND, *Naval Regulations Issued by Command of the President of the United States of America, January 25, 1802,* 16–17.

12. USND, *Barbary Wars,* 2:102, 170, 173, 209, 217–19, 236, 242.

13. Ibid., 161–62, 173, 236–37, 257–58, 296–97, 306–7.

14. Ibid., 293–94, 300, 302, 311, 324.

15. Ibid., 325, 328–29, 333. The *Constellation* 's log for November 29, 1802, shows, "Crew very sickly—upwards of 100 on the list with violent colds." Fears of spreading disease made some authorities reluctant to allow burials ashore. In view of the limited funds available to the consul, it may not have been possible to procure a grave site ashore.

16. Ibid., 324–25, 328, 331–32, 334. Murray was delayed at Gibraltar by bad weather, and while he was directing the veering out of cable in a storm, his left thumb and a finger were nearly torn off by a badly fastened ring rope. Murray does not mention receiving medical treatment. Twelve days later, he told Morris that his thumb and finger had nearly healed, but the sinews had contracted and he had lost the use of the injured digits. See USND, *Barbary Wars,* 2:342, 344.

17. Ibid., 350.

18. Ibid., 350–55.

19. Ibid., 355; USND, *Barbary Wars: Personnel and Ships' Data,* 14; Paullin, *Commodore John Rodgers,* 103–4. Davis returned to the navy during the War of 1812.

20. USND, *Barbary Wars,* 2:301, 385, 387–88, 398–99.

21. Ibid., 408–9, 425–26, 430, 432, 435–37, 439–40, 457–58, 465–66, 474–77, 503–4, 512–14, 523–32; 3:45–46; McKee, *Edward Preble,* 146–47, 158. Morris actually turned his command over to John Rodgers, who subsequently released it to Preble.

22. J. Worth Estes, "Naval Medicine in the Age of Sail," *Bulletin of the History of Medicine* 56 (1982):238–53. See also the USS *Constitution* Museum pamphlet *Naval Medicine in the Early Nineteenth Century*, 5–6.

23. For background details not in Estes, "Naval Medicine in the Age of Sail," see USND, *Barbary Wars*, 2:403.

24. Estes, "Naval Medicine in the Age of Sail," 249.

25. USND, *Barbary Wars*, 2:203, 215, 236, 270, 329.

26. Ibid., 5:61–71.

27. McKee, *Edward Preble*, 196–99; USND, *Barbary Wars*, 5:230–37. The quotation from Heermann is from Pleadwell and Kerr, "Lewis Heermann," 119.

28. USND, *Barbary Wars*, 4:295–309. These actions are discussed in detail in McKee, *Edward Preble*, chaps. 14, 15.

29. USND, *Barbary Wars*, 5:163, 194, 205–7.

30. Ibid., 547–58, 553–55; Maloney, *Captain from Connecticut* 107–10. The story of the expedition against Derne is well told in Louis B. Wright and Julia H. Macleod, *First Americans in North Africa*, chap. 7.

31. McKee, *Edward Preble*, 312–16; Maloney, *Captain from Connecticut*, 111–14; Paullin, *Commodore John Rodgers*, 134–36.

32. Wright and Macleod, 176–93; McKee, *Edward Preble*, 331–35. For a brief review of the views of scholars on the treaty, see Long, *Ready to Hazard*, 98, as well as his own assessment in Long, *Gold Braid and Foreign Relations*, 31–32, 36.

33. Bainbridge's captivity is treated in Long, *Ready to Hazard*, chap. 5. Jonathan Cowdery's account is in his *American Captives in Tripoli*. His diary entries are reproduced in USND, *Barbary Wars* beginning with 4:61–65. On his value to the pasha and his treatment of a Tripolitan officer, see Long, *Ready to Hazard*, 81–82.

34. William Ray, *Horrors of Slavery*, 86–87, 97, 160. Ray was also critical of Bainbridge and said that he trusted his subordinate officers too much. While preparing his book, Ray wrote to Bainbridge for information, and the commodore did not reply. When Ray's book was published, Bainbridge produced letters from members of the crew while in captivity seeking his help for better treatment for them. See USND, *Barbary Wars*, 4:240–44; Cowdery's notes on the mistreatment of prisoners are in 5:3, 100, 174, 176–77, 334; 6:43, 74, 77. Cowdery reports that when he took his final farewell of the pasha, the ruler was deeply affected. See USND, *Barbary Wars*, 6:96.

35. USND, *Barbary Wars*, 2:106.

36. Ibid., 123.

37. Ibid., 1:476.

38. Ibid., 3:160–62, 166. One of the reasons why Gibraltar and Malta were less desirable than formerly was the resumption of war between Great Britain and France in May 1803, due in part to Britain's refusal to turn Malta over to the Order of the Knights of Malta as promised in the Treaty of Amiens in 1802. Spain allied itself with France, and Britain was joined by Austria, Russia, and Sweden. On the matter of the health of Preble's men, the shortage of crew members may have resulted in more space for those who remained and thus lessened the risks of infection.

39. Ibid., 3:209, 215.

40. Ibid., 214–15, 243–45, 351, 355, 375.

41. Ibid., 4:121, 142, 171, 498, 507–10, 512–13. The brig *Scourge* may have been used temporarily as a hospital ship. John H. Beall was commissioned as a surgeon's mate on April 28, 1804, and served in the *Congress* and the *Constellation* during the Barbary Wars. On December 2, 1805, he was furloughed, and in 1807 he was assigned to the Norfolk station. He resigned from the navy on October 15, 1807. See USND, *Barbary Wars: Personnel and Ships' Data,* 4

42. USND, *Barbary Wars,* 4:135; 5:49–50. John W. Dorsey was commissioned as a surgeon's mate on July 16, 1803. He served in the Mediterranean in 1803–5 in the *Argus* and the *Vixen*. Assigned to the naval rendezvous (recruiting duty) at Fell's Point, Maryland, in 1807, he resigned on July 9 of that year. See USND, *Barbary Wars: Personnel and Ships' Data,* 16. Dorsey had been ill since he went to sea, and he looked forward to shore duty. See USND, *Barbary Wars,* 4:498.

43. USND, *Barbary Wars,* 5:133–34.

44. Ibid., 137, 164. Portugal's longstanding economic ties with Great Britain made it logical to assume that English-made surgical instruments might be available in Lisbon.

45. Cutbush to Secretary of the Navy John Branch, June 15, 1829, "Edward Cutbush," ZB File; Captains Samuel Barron and John Rodgers to Cutbush, November 10, 1804, USND, *Barbary Wars,* 5:133–34. These orders specify that the house being used as a hospital was to accommodate 100 men but that immediately arrangements were necessary for 75 men. On Schoolfield see USND, *Barbary Wars: Personnel and Ships' Data,* 48.

46. Records of the Legislative Branch, House Committee on Naval Affairs, various subjects, H.R. 19A, D 15.7, NA. For the work of the hospital, see USND, *Barbary Wars,* 6:47, 51, 110, 175–77, 180; on closing down the hospital, 242, 405, 414, 430.

47. Cutbush to John Branch, June 15, 1829, "Edward Cutbush," ZB File. The hospital was turned over to British troops on the promise that they would restore it to the condition in which the Americans received it. Perishable items in the hospital were sold before the house was turned over to the British. The whole process of breaking up the establishment was complicated by the resignation of George Dyson as navy agent at Syracuse due to postwar cutbacks. The work of liquidating assets was not completed until mid-August 1807. See USND, *Barbary Wars,* 6:505, 552.

48. USND, *Barbary Wars,* 6:152.

49. Ibid., 224.

50. Ibid., 255.

51. Ibid., 292–95. In the Royal Navy it was the policy to have the surgeon advise all the men who had not had smallpox, or who were doubtful about whether they had had it, to be inoculated. See Lloyd and Coulter, *Medicine in the Navy,* 4:210. In 1804, Captain Isaac Chauncey ordered his crew to be inoculated, and Commodore Preble probably did the same.

52. See Log of the *John Adams,* December 30, 1804, NA; Preble Papers, January 14, 1805, vol. 32.

53. USND, *Barbary Wars,* 6:501–2.

54. Secretary of the Navy Robert Smith to Jacques, October 7, 1801; Smith to

Captain Alexander Murray, February 6, 1802, LO; USND, *Barbary Wars: Personnel and Ships' Data,* 28.

55. USND, *Barbary Wars: Personnel and Ships' Data,* 2, 5, 12, 22, 25.

56. Tisdale to Lieutenant Stephen Decatur, August 5, 1803; Decatur to Robert Smith, August 21, 1803, OL; Smith to Tisdale, April 16, 1804; Smith to Dorsey, July 16, August 8, 27, 1803, LO.

57. Balfour to Smith, April 12, 1804, OL.

58. USND, *Barbary Wars: Personnel and Ships' Data,* 45, 57, 14, 16, 13, 53, 59, 7, 36.

59. *Barbary Wars: Personnel and Ships' Data,* 1–59. Those appointed as surgeons were: Thomas Babbitt of Massachusetts in 1804; James Dodge of New York, who had served as a surgeon's mate in the Quasi-War and had been discharged at the end of it; Thomas Ewell of the District of Columbia in 1805; John Ridgely of Maryland in 1803; William Rogers of Maryland in 1804 after having previously served as a surgeon's mate in 1802–3 and resigned; James M. Taylor of Maryland in 1805; and Thomas Triplett of Virginia, who had served as a surgeon during the Quasi-War, resigned in July 1804, and been reinstated as a surgeon on May 6, 1806. Surgeon's mates who were promoted to surgeon were: Nathaniel T. Weems of Maryland in 1803 after 10 months' service; Patrick Sim of Maryland in 1805 after 20 months' service; and Samuel D. Heap of Pennsylvania in 1807 after 7 months.

The third diplomatic appointment was for Surgeon John Ridgely, commissioned in 1803, who became the U.S. chargé d'affaires at Tripoli.

In addition, commissions as surgeon's mates were offered to three other men, but they were declined. Walter W. Buchanan declined a surgeon's commission. William C. Smith, who acted as a surgeon's mate in the *President* in the Mediterranean from June 1801 to May 1802, was commissioned as such on June 1, 1802, and resigned on July 13 of that year. See *Barbary Wars: Personnel and Ships' Data.* For assistance in identifying and confirming the states from which various individuals came, I am grateful to Christopher McKee.

60. Roddis, "Naval and Marine Corps Casualties," 307; Estes, "Naval Medicine in the Age of Sail"; USS *Constitution* Museum, *Naval Medicine in the Early Nineteenth Century;* USND, *Barbary Wars.* For information on the mortality of the officer corps, see Christopher McKee, *A Gentlemanly and Honorable Profession,* chap. 32; McKee, "The Pathology of a Profession," *War and Society* 3 (1985): 1–25. See also Estes, "Naval Medicine in the Age of Sail"; USS *Constitution* Museum, *Naval Medicine in the Early Nineteenth Century;* USND, *Barbary Wars;* Louis H. Roddis, "Naval and Marine Corps Casualties in the Wars of the United States," *Military Surgeon* 99 (1946):307.

Chapter 5
New Orleans

1. The diplomatic background of the Louisiana Purchase may be found in standard works in diplomatic history, such as Robert H. Ferrell, *American Diplomacy,* as well as in more recent surveys such as that by Howard Jones, *Course of Ameri-*

can Diplomacy, vol. 1, chap. 3. More detailed monographs are Alexander De-Conde, *This Affair of Louisiana;* John G. Clark, *New Orleans, 1718–1812,* chaps. 11, 12; Irving Brant, *James Madison: Secretary of State, 1800–1809,* 65, 69, 71, 73, 75, 77–78, 82, 96–97, 100, 107, 117, 125, 156–69; Malone, *Jefferson: First Term,* chaps. 14–16.

2. Watkins to Rush, June 24, 1800, Rush Correspondence, 19:40–42.

3. U.S. Congress, *American State Papers,* Commerce and Navigation, 1:493.

4. *Annals of Congress,* 7th Cong., 1st sess., 721.

5. Dunbar Roland, ed., *Mississippi Territorial Archives, 1798–1803,* 421–22.

6. *Annals of Congress,* 7th Cong., 1st sess., 261, 302–3, 721, 1372–74; *House Journal,* 7th Cong., 1st sess., 180, 192–94.

7. *Annals of Congress,* 7th Cong., 1st sess., 261, 302–3, 721, 1372–74; *House Journal,* 7th Cong., 1st sess., 237–40.

8. *U.S. Statutes at Large,* 2:192–93.

9. Jefferson to Gallatin, August 14, 1802; Gallatin to Jefferson, August 19, 1802; Clark to Gallatin, August 15, 1802, Jefferson Papers, LC; William E. Rooney, "New Orleans Marine Hospital, 1802–1861" (M.A. thesis, Tulane University, 1950), 10–15.

10. Bache to Jefferson, March 29, 1803, Jefferson Papers, LC; Rooney, "New Orleans Marine Hospital," 16.

11. William E. Rooney, "Thomas Jefferson and the New Orleans Marine Hospital," *Journal of Southern History* 22 (1956), 174–75.

12. Brant, *Madison: Secretary of State, 1800–1809,* chaps. 8, 9, 10; Malone, *Jefferson: First Term,* chaps. 15, 16.

13. Rooney, "Jefferson and the New Orleans Marine Hospital," 175–77; Dunbar Roland, ed., *Official Letterbooks of William C. C. Claiborne, 1801–1816,* 2:23–24. See also John Salvaggio, *New Orleans Charity Hospital.*

14. Rooney, "Jefferson and the New Orleans Marine Hospital," 178–80; Rooney, "New Orleans Marine Hospital," 20–26.

15. Jefferson appointed two representatives of the U.S. government to take possession of New Orleans: William C. C. Claiborne, the youthful Governor of Mississippi Territory, and Brigadier General James Wilkinson, the general in chief of the U.S. Army. Wilkinson detached three companies of artillery from the garrison at Fort Adams, located seven miles below Natchez, and with mounted militia under Claiborne set out for New Orleans for the transfer ceremonies. Several months passed before Congress passed the legislation giving territorial status to Louisiana. See James Ripley Jacobs, *Beginning of the U.S. Army, 1783–1812;* 309–11; Allan R. Millett, *Semper Fidelis,* 40–41.

16. Rogers to Jefferson, October 1807, ML; Robert Smith to Rogers, March 13, 1804, LO.

17. Rogers to Jefferson, October 1807, ML.

18. Rogers to Smith, May 10, 1804, Letters Received by the Secretary of War, Unregistered Series, M-222, roll 1, NA.

19. Ibid. For more on the problem of food supplies in New Orleans during this period, see Clark, *New Orleans, 1718–1812,* 233–38, 246, 250–51, 257–61, 268–69.

20. Kilty to Smith, January 1, 1805, ML.

21. Smith to Rogers, January 2, 1805, LO.

22. Ibid.; Rogers to Smith, March 28, 1805, OL.

23. Rogers to Smith, September 2, 1805, with enclosure from Captain Carmick, OL.

24. Rogers to Jefferson, October 1807, ML.

25. Rogers to Smith, September 2, 1805, OL.

26. Turner to Smith, September 2, 1805, ML.

27. Rogers to Jefferson, October 1807, ML.

28. Rogers to Smith, November 1, 1805, OL.

29. Rogers to Smith, June 11, 1806, OL; Smith to Rogers, July 16, 1806, LO.

30. Rogers to Smith, November 5, December 11, 1806, OL.

31. Rogers to Smith, December 11, 1806, OL; Spence to "My Dear Polly," January 1, 30, February 13, 27, 1807, Keith Spence Papers, Spence-Lowell Collection, Huntington Library, San Marino, Calif.

32. Thomas Perkins Abernathy, *Burr Conspiracy;* for the Louisiana and Mississippi aspects, see chaps. 11, 13. The quotation is from *Louisiana Gazette,* December 6, 1806.

33. Shaw to Rogers, December 1, 1806; Rogers to Shaw, December 4, 1806, RGCM, no. 35, roll 4; Rogers to Smith, December 11, 1806, OL.

34. Shaw to Rogers, December 16, 1806, RGCM, no. 35, roll 4.

35. Shaw to Rogers, December 20, 1806, RGCM, no. 35, roll 4; Rogers to Smith, December 25, 1806, OL.

36. Smith to Shaw, January 26, 1807, LO.

37. Rogers to Shaw, January 28, 1807; Shaw to Rogers, January 29, 1807, RGCM, no. 35, roll 4; Abernethy, *Burr Conspiracy,* 195–98, 208–49.

38. RGCM, no. 35, roll 4; Smith to Rogers, August 11, 1807, LO. Rogers subsequently wrote to Surgeon James Wells about his testimony, and Wells replied. See Rogers to Wells, October 27, 1807; Wells to Rogers, October 28, 1807, ML.

39. Smith to Marshall, October 10, 1807, March 7, 1808, LO; Marshall to Smith, February 10, April 30, 1808, OL; Dr. William Ballard to Paul Hamilton, July 4, 1810, ML; Hamilton to Ballard, July 14, 1810, GLB.

40. Amos A. Evans to John Evans, February 13, 1809, War of 1812 Collection, William L. Clements Library, Ann Arbor, Mich.

41. Master Commandant David Porter to Master Commandant Philemon C. Wederstrandt, Commander, New Orleans Station, June 1, 1810, ML. According to Porter, the hospital was designed to accommodate only 14 patients.

42. Shaw to Hamilton, July 24, 1810, CL; Heermann to Hamilton, August 2, 1810; Heap to Hamilton, October 5, December 20, 1810; September 27, 1811, OL. One reason that Heap wanted to stay in New Orleans was that he married Margaret Porter of that city on January 23, 1810. See *Louisiana Gazette,* January 26, 1810. I am grateful to Richard Long of the Marine Corps Historical Center for this reference.

43. Brereton to Hamilton, May 17, 1811, OL.

44. Shaw to Hamilton, February 1, 1811, AF, roll 200.

45. Heermann to Hamilton, August 2, 1811, OL. Another medical officer who complained about inadequate pay was Surgeon's Mate William Barnwell. He said he could not buy the books he needed for his work. See Barnwell to Hamilton, July 31, 1811, OL.

46. *Louisiana Gazette,* May 16, 1811. The advertisement ran until the issue of July 3, 1811. Pierre Philippe de Marigny de Mandeville, a wealthy planter, land speculator, and state and local politician, subdivided the plantation of Bernard Marigny in 1805 and sold it. As the Faubourg Marigny it became the eighth district of New Orleans in 1810. See Clark, *New Orleans,* 281n.

47. Heap to Hamilton, September 27, 1811; Heermann to Hamilton, November 28, 1811, OL.

48. Heermann to Hamilton, August 2, November 28, 1811; Shumate to Hamilton, December 16, 1811, OL; Callahan, *List of Officers,* 497.

Chapter 6
Medical Care Ashore: Boston

1. Sources for this chapter, unless otherwise noted, are John W. Trask, *United States Marine Hospital, Port of Boston;* Richard H. Thurm, *For the Relief of the Sick and Disabled.*

2. *Annals of Congress,* 7th Cong., 1st sess., 261, 302–3, 721, 1372–74; *House Journal,* 7th Cong., 1st sess., 237–40; *Statutes at Large,* 2:192–93. In 1849, while arguing one of the Passenger Cases before the Supreme Court, Willis Hall observated: "A few years before the close of the last century, Congress set on foot a marine hospital fund for the relief of sailors. In 1802, it had accumulated to more than ninety thousand dollars. At this time Massachusetts and Virginia governed the Union. They concluded to divide the fund between them. Fifteen thousand dollars were appropriated to build a sailors hospital at Boston, and thirty-five thousand went to purchase an old hospital at Gosport, in Virginia." Philip R. Kurland and Gerhard Casper, *Landmark Briefs and Arguments of the Supreme Court of the United States: Constitutional Law* 3:365. Smith was arguing for the defendant in the case of Smith v. Turner.

The marine hospital at Norfolk was transferred to the United States on April 20, 1801. The $15,000 was appropriated by Congress to build the hospital at Boston on May 3, 1802. For Boston see *U.S. Statutes at Large,* 2:192–93. The law was passed on May 3, 1802.

3. Robert Smith to Samuel Brown, June 21, 1802, USND, *Barbary Wars,* 2:183.

4. Waterhouse to Benjamin Lincoln, February 9, 1803, Thurm, *For the Relief of the Sick and Disabled,* 111–13.

5. Charles Jarvis (1748–1807) was also a popular orator, a delegate to the state convention that ratified the federal Constitution, and a member of the state legislature until 1798.

6. Smith to St. Medard, February 17, 1804, LO.

7. Smith to St. Medard, March 15, 1804, LO.

8. Smith to St. Medard, March 21, 1804, April 19, 1804; Smith to Jarvis, May 12, 1804; Smith to St. Medard, May 12, 1804, LO; St. Medard to Smith, April 7, 1804, March 23, 1805, OL; USND, *Barbary Wars: Personnel and Ships' Data,* 53.

9. Wharton to Smith, August 27, 1805, Records of the U.S. Marine Corps, Letters Sent by the Commandant, RG 127, NA; Smith to Brown, September 3,

1805, GLB; Brown to Smith, September 13, 1805, ML; Smith to Brown, September 26, 1805, GLB.

10. Edwin C. Bearss, *Charlestown Navy Yard, 1800–1842,* 75–91.

11. Francis Johonnot, navy agent, to Smith, November 23, 1807, ML.

12. Gallatin to Lincoln, November 27, 1807, Letters of the Secretary of the Treasury to the Collector of Customs, Boston, M-178, roll 7, NA. Waterhouse to Smith, January 14, 1808, OL; Smith to Waterhouse, February 5, 1808, GLB; Gallatin to Lincoln, January 25, 1808, Letters from to the Collector of Customs, M-178, roll 7, NA.

13. Waterhouse to Smith, January 14, 1808, OL. James Sullivan, a Democratic-Republican, was governor of Massachusetts at this time. Eustis later became secretary of war.

14. Waterhouse to Jefferson, January 15, 1808, OL. Dr. Thomas Trotter (1760–1832) served in the Royal Navy from 1779 to 1802. In 1786 he published *Observations on the Scurvy,* and two years later he received his medical degree from the University of Edinburgh. He was now one of two physicians in the British navy with a regular medical degree. As physician of the fleet, he saw active service until he was injured in 1795; thereafter his duties were mainly on shore. Between 1796 and 1803 he published three volumes entitled *Medicina Nautica,* a collection of observations, case histories, and discussions of topics pertaining to naval medicine—except surgery. See Lloyd, ed., *Health of Seamen,* 214–15.

15. Waterhouse to Smith, January 27, 1808, OL. James Lloyd (1728–1810) studied medicine under Dr. William Clark of Boston, had two years' experience at Guy's Hospital in London as a dresser, and attended lectures by William Hunter and William Smellie. Returning to Boston, he built a large practice by applying his knowledge of midwifery and surgery. He served as surgeon at Castle William and was an advocate of the practice of general inoculation. Subsequently he was one of the incorporators of the Massachusetts Medical Society in 1781 and served as a councilor of the organization. Harvard conferred an honorary M.D. degree on him in 1790.

Samuel Danforth (1740–1827) graduated from Harvard College in 1758 and studied medicine under Dr. Rand, the elder. After working in Weston, Massachusetts, and Newport, Rhode Island, he returned to Boston, where he built a large and lucrative practice. In his work he relied on only a few powerful remedies, such as calomel, opium, ipecacuanha, and Peruvian bark. During the American Revolution he was a Loyalist. He was one of the original members of the Massachusetts Medical Society and served as its president from 1795 to 1798. Harvard awarded him an honorary degree in medicine in 1790.

John Warren (1753–1815) graduated from Harvard College in 1771 and studied medicine with his older brother, Joseph, who was subsequently killed in the Battle of Bunker Hill. Before the Revolution he practiced in Salem; and after his brother's death, he volunteered to serve as a private in the army but was appointed senior surgeon at the hospital established at Cambridge, Massachusets, for General George Washington's forces. Later he was senior surgeon of the army hospital on Long Island and at the General Hospital in Boston. In 1777 he left the army, and in addition to carrying out his hospital duties, he taught anatomy and surgery at Harvard. He is credited with having performed one of the first abdominal sections recorded in the United States. In his lifetime he was regarded as one of the leading surgeons in New England. See Howard A. Kelly and Walter L. Burrage, *American Medical Biographies*, 282, 710, 1193–95.

16. Waterhouse to Jefferson, January 15, 1808, OL.

17. Waterhouse to Smith, January 27, 1808, OL.

18. Ibid; Smith to Waterhouse, February 5, 1808, LO.

19. For these regulations see Thurm, *For the Relief of the Sick and Disabled*, 122–25.

20. Ibid.

21. Ibid.

22. Ibid.; Waterhouse to Benjamin Lincoln, June 29, 1808, Letters to the Collector of Customs, M-178, roll 7, NA.

23. Thurm, *For the Relief of the Sick and Disabled*, 124–26.

24. Waterhouse to Lincoln, July 19, 1808; Gallatin to Lincoln, August 28, 1808, Letters to the Collector of Customs, M-178, roll 7, NA.

25. Lincoln to Gallatin, June 16, 1808, Correspondence of the Collectors of Customs with the Secretary of the Treasury, M-178, roll 11, 199, NA; Gallatin to Lincoln, June 30, August 28, 1808, Letters to the Collector of Customs, M-178, roll 7, NA.

26. Gallatin to Dearborn, April 19, 1808, Letters to the Collector of Customs, M-178, roll 8, NA.

27. Waterhouse to Gallatin, July 13, 1809, cited in Thurm, *For the Relief of the Sick and Disabled*, 149–50.

28. Warner to Eustis, May 6, 1809, cited in Thurm, *For the Relief of the Sick and Disabled*, 140–42.

29. Nicholson to Smith, May 4, 1809, CL; Hamilton to Nicholson, July 12, 1809, LO.

30. Thurm, *For the Relief of the Sick and Disabled*, 149–50.

31. Madison to Dearborn, June 30, 1809; Gallatin to Dearborn, July 18, November 1, 1809; Waterhosue to Gallatin, July 13, 1809, cited in Thurm, *For the Relief of the Sick and Disabled*, 81–82, 148, 151, 181; Hamilton to David Townsend, September 28, 1811, GLB.

32. Hamilton to Waterhouse, July 21, 1809; Hamilton to Bates, July 21, 1809, GLB.

33. Bates to Hamilton, March 31, 1810, ML.

34. Bates to Hamilton, April 30, May 11, 1811, OL; Hamilton to Bates, May 6, October 29, 1811, LO.

35. Thurm, *For the Relief of the Sick and Disabled*, 183.

36. Ibid., 184–85.

37. Prescription Book of U.S. Marine Hospital at Charlestown, MS, 1816, vol. 2, RG 90, NA.

Chapter 7
Naval Health Care in the North and South

1. "Report of the Secretary of the Treasury, 1809," *Medical Repository* 11 (1811): 313–16.

2. Ibid.

3. Weems to Smith, April 13, 1805, OL; Robert Smith to Weems, April 17, 1805, LO. Weems's decision was the result of his being ordered to sea in July 1805, to which he could not respond because of illness. Then came the death of his father and the need to settle his estate, the responsibility for a 12-year-old sister, and Weems's desire to get married. See Weems to Smith, February 11, 1806, Resignations A–W, 1803–1825, RG 45, NA.

4. Smith to Aitken, July 19, 1805, LO; Aitken to Smith, February 5, 1806, OL; USND, *Barbary Wars: Personnel and Ships' Data*, 7:1, 18; Ewell to Smith, June 19, 1806, OL.

5. Ewell to Smith, July 15, July 18, August 22, 1806, OL; Smith to Ewell, August 6, 26, 1806, LO.

6. Ewell to Jefferson, May 17, June 26, July 4, July 15, August 28, 1806, Thomas Jefferson, Papers, microfilm, 1st ser., reel 36, LC; Ewell to Smith, July 15, 1806, OL; Smith to Ewell, February 25, 1807, LO.

7. Hunt to Smith, September 30, 1806, OL; Smith to Hunt, May 9, 1807, LO; Johnson to Smith, May 15, 1807; Osborne to Smith, May 16, 1807, ML; Hunt to Smith, May 17, 1807, OL; Smith to Marshall, July 6, 1807, LO; Marshall to Smith, July 8, 1807, ML; Smith to Cowdery, July 3, 1807, LO; Cowdery to Smith, July 22, 1807, OL.

8. Cowdery to Smith, August 7, 17, September 30, 1807, OL; Smith to Cowdery, August 24, September 25, 1807, LO; "Jonathan Cowdery," ZB File. For a sketch of Cowdery's life, see Pleadwell and Kerr "Jonathan Cowdery," 63–87, 243–68. Smith to Brown, August 11, 1807, LO. Brown was to have a short naval career. Appointed a surgeon's mate on August 11, 1807, he was promoted to surgeon on March 3, 1809, and ordered to the brig *Vixen*. The small quarters in that ship led him to resign later in that year.

9. Chauncey to Hamilton, May 22, 1810, CL; Smith to Chauncey, May 26, 1810, Letters to Commandants and Navy Agents, M-441, roll 1, NA.

10. Marshall to Hamilton, December 20, 1809, Navy Department Records, Subject File MA, RG 45, NA.

11. Ibid.; Marshall to Captain Charles Ludlow, March 29, 1813, OL.

12. Chauncey to Hamilton, December 20, 1810, CL.

13. Hamilton to Bassett, December 24, 1810, *ASP:NA*, 1:233–34; Hamilton to Marshall, March 7, 1811, LO.

14. Chauncey to Hamilton, August 18, 1810 with enclosure of a certificate from Surgeon Marshall, July 18, 1810, on Hatfield's duties, CL; Hamilton to Chauncey, August 24, 1810, Letters to Commandants and Navy Agents, M-441, roll 1.

15. Marshall to Hamilton, May 22, 1812 with enclosed letters of recommendation from Drs. Buchanan and Giles Smith, and from Richard Simmon, superintendent of the almshouse, May 18–20, 1812; Chauncey to Hamilton, June 5, 1812, ML; Hatfield to Hamilton, April 21, 1812, OL; Hamilton to Christie, July 10, 1812, LO. For a picture of health conditions in New York during these years, see John Duffy, *History of Public Health in New York City, 1625–1866*, 97–267. The other doctor to whom Chauncey referred was G. T. Hunt, apparently a civilian practitioner.

16. John Thomas Scharf and Thompson Westcott, *History of Philadelphia, 1609–*

1884, 2:1665–72; John F. Watson, *Annals of Philadelphia and Pennsylvania in the Olden Time,* 2:388–90.

17. Cutbush to Smith, July 29, 1807, OL; Harrison to Smith, April 18, 1808, ML.

18. F. L. Pleadwell, "William Paul Crillon Barton," *Annals of Medical History* 2 (1919):267–301; Barton to Charles Goldsborough, chief clerk, March 21, 1809, ML.

19. Goldsborough to Barton, April 3, 1809, GLB; Barton to Goldsborough, April 7, 1809, OL.

20. Barton, *Plan for the Internal Organization and Government of Marine Hospitals,* preface.

21. Hamilton to Barton, November 23, 1811, OL; Barton to Hamilton, November 27, 1811, LO. The officers to whom Barton referred were Surgeons Nicholas Harwood, Joseph New, Peter St. Medard, and George Davis.

22. Barton to Latrobe, Barton to Hamilton, December 26, 1811, OL; Benjamin Smith Barton to Hamilton, undated 1813, ML; Hamilton to Captain David Porter, January 6, 1812, LO.

23. Barton to Hamilton, July 11, 1811, OL; Barton to Rodgers, January 4, 28, March 16, 1812, John Rodgers Collection, NYHS.

24. In his book on marine hospitals, Barton later said that he had arrested several cases of scurvy in the United States by the liberal use of lime juice. He further tested its use as an antiscorbutic on his cruise in the *Essex* and urged that it be adopted for use in the navy. For the Royal Navy's experiments with lemons and limes, see Lloyd and Coulter, *Medicine and the Navy,* 3:293–328. For a recent analysis of the experiments, see Kenneth J. Carpenter, *History of Scurvy and Vitamin C,* 43–97. The Lords of the Admiralty authorized a daily allowance of three-quarters of an ounce of lemon juice per man in 1795, and there was a decline in scurvy cases after 1796. But the matter was still on an experimental basis in 1812.

25. U.S. Congress, *Annual Report of the Secretary of the Treasury, 1809,* 313–16. For general aspects of public health, see William Travis Howard, *Public Health Administration and the Natural History of Disease in Baltimore, 1797–1930.* On the early medical profession in Baltimore, see J. Thomas Scharf, *History of Baltimore City and County,* pt. 2, 729–37.

26. Robert Smith to Balfour, August 19, 1801, LO; Richmond C. Holcomb, *Century with Norfolk Naval Hospital, 1830–1930,* 111–12; U.S. Congress, *Annual Report of the Secretary of the Navy, 1809,* 313–16.

27. Surgeon John McReynolds's report on John Cassin to Secretary B. W. Crowninshield, June 25, 1817, CL.

28. Heermann to Hamilton, January 19, 1810, OL; Hamilton to Heermann, February 8, 1810, LO; Heermann to Hamilton, August 2, 1810, OL; Hamilton to Heermann, August 20, 1810, LO; Heap to Hamilton, December 20, 1810, OL.

29. Sinclair to Hamilton, July 5, 1810; Surgeon's Mate R. C. Edgar to Hamilton, August 6, 1810, OL.

30. Gassaway to Hamilton, August 24, 1812, ML.

31. Stark to Hamilton, August 3, 22, 28, 1810, OL; Hamilton to Stark, August 25, 1810, LO.

32. Stark to Hamilton, November 29, 1810, June 10, 1811, OL; Hamilton to Stark, August 25, 1810, LO.

33. Smith to Ingraham, November 24, 1808, GLB. This Dr. Aitken is not to be confused with Surgeon's Mate Hugh Aitken, who served in New York in 1805.

34. Hamilton to Ingraham, May 22, 1809, GLB.

35. McCormick to Hamilton, January 19, 1810, OL; Hamilton to McCormick, February 5, 1810, March 26, 1811; Secretary Hamilton to Charles Hamilton, April 2, 8, 1811, LO.

36. McCormick to Hamilton, March 30, 1810, OL.

37. Hamilton to Logan, April 2, September 13, 1810, LO; Logan to Hamilton, October 16, December 24, 1810, OL; Hamilton to Logan, January 4, 1811, LO.

38. Logan to Hamilton, April 4, May 13, 1811, OL; Hamilton to Logan, May 20, 1811, LO.

39. McCormick to Hamilton, July 27, 1811, OL.

40. Williams to Hamilton, August 28, 1811, ML.

41. Gwin Harris to Hamilton, September 7, 1811, OL; Hamilton to Harris, August 19, 1811, LO. On the career of Dr. Lemuel Kollock (1766–1823), see Edith D. Johnston, ed., "Kollock Letters, 1799–1850," *Georgia Historical Quarterly* 30 (1946) 220–25.

42. Harris to Hamilton, September 28, 1811, OL; Williams to Hamilton, November 21, 1811, ML.

43. Charles B. Hamilton to Secretary Paul Hamilton, October 4, 1811, March 21, 1812, OL.

Chapter 8
Washington, D.C.

1. Except as otherwise indicated, the sources of this chapter are the following records in the National Archives: OL, rolls 1–9; LO, rolls 5–9; ML, rolls 12, 40, 41; Navy Department Records, Letters from the Secretary of the Navy to Congress, vols. 1, 2, RG 45; and on the following printed works: USND, *Barbary Wars*, vols. 2, 3; *ASP:NA*, vol. 1; Karl Schuon, *Home of the Commandants;* Taylor Peck, *Round-Shot to Rockets; The Correspondence and Miscellaneous Papers of Benjamin Henry Latrobe*, ed. John C. Van Horne, vol. 3.

2. Robert Smith to Captain Thomas Tingey, March 16, 1803, USND, *Barbary Wars*, 2:374.

3. *U.S. Statutes at Large*, 2:297.

4. Thomas Ewell to Robert Smith, June 27, 1807, OL.

5. Smith to Ewell, April 21, 1807, LO.

6. Ewell to Smith, February 25, 1808, OL.

7. Edward Cutbush, *Preserving the Health of Soldiers and Sailors*, 89, 131–32.

8. Ibid., 225–26.

9. Ibid., 171.

10. *U.S. Statutes at Large*, 2:514, 544.

11. Ibid., 650–51.

12. Barton to Hamilton, October 15, 1811, OL.

Chapter 9
The War of 1812 at Sea

1. For background on the causes of the war and the war itself, see A. L. Burt, *United States, Great Britain, and British North America from the Revolution to the Establishment of Peace after the War of 1812;* Bradford Perkins, *Prologue to War;* Paul A. Varg, *Foreign Policies of the Founding Fathers;* Reginald Horsman, *Causes of the War of 1812;* Horsman, *War of 1812;* Benson J. Lossing, *Pictorial Field Book of the War of 1812;* Gilbert Auchinleck, *History of the War between the United States of America during the Years 1812, 1813, & 1814;* Harry L. Coles, *War of 1812;* J. Mackay Hitsman, *Incredible War of 1812;* John K. Mahon, *War of 1812;* J. C. A. Stagg, *Mr. Madison's War;* Donald R. Hickey, *War of 1812.*

On the naval aspects of the war, a most useful compilation is William S. Dudley, ed., *Naval War of 1812,* which covers from 1805 through 1813. An additional volume is planned. Indispensable secondary sources are Alfred T. Mahan, *Sea Power in Its Relation to the War of 1812;* Theodore Roosevelt, *Naval War of 1812.* Administrative developments are treated in Edward K. Eckert, *Navy Department in the War of 1812.*

Helpful biographical studies include Maloney, *Captain from Connecticut;* Paullin, *Commodore John Rodgers;* Long, *Nothing Too Daring;* Long, *Ready to Hazard;* Long, *Sailor Diplomat.*

Medical information is largely in manuscript form.

2. Rodgers to Hamilton, September 1, 1812, CL; Dudley, *Naval War of 1812,* 1:262–65. According to Paullin, *Rodgers,* 258, there were 300 cases of scurvy in the *United States* and the *Congress* alone.

3. Maloney, *Captain from Connecticut,* 191.

4. Ibid., 182. Maloney points out that Hull later collected $1,000 for Dunn and invested it in interest-bearing notes. He also helped get him a navy pension and found employment for him in navy yards for the remainder of his life.

5. H. Benjamin Bradburn, ed., "Medical Log of 'Old Ironsides,'" *Connecticut Medicine* 40 (1976):862–64; Amos Evans, *Journal Kept on Board the Frigate Constitution, 1812,* 374–77. The original "Medical Prescription Book Kept on Board the U.S. Frigate Constitution," by Surgeon Evans, is in the Historical Library of Yale University School of Medicine.

6. Evans, *Journal.*

7. Bradburn, "Medical Log," 866–68.

8. Crane to Hamilton, October 31, 1812, OL; Maloney, *Captain from Connecticut,* 199. Later Captain Archibald Henderson of the marines complained to the secretary that prisoners of the *Guerriere* were being held in the marine guardroom at the Boston Navy Yard. This was a source of inconvenience for the marines and discontent for the prisoners. Henderson asked that they be moved to a more secure place. See Henderson to Hamilton, December 19, 1812, ML. The men were later exchanged. A cartel ship is one commissioned in the time of war to convey prisoners for exchange between the belligerent powers. It carried only one gun for signal purposes, but no cargo, ammunition or implements of war and could not engage in any trading.

9. Mahan, *Sea Power*, 1:411–15; *Niles Weekly Register* 3 (1812):27; Dudley, *Naval War of 1812*, 1:537–41, 580–83; Master Commandant Jacob Jones to Hamilton, November 24, 1812, Letters Received by the Secretary of the Navy from Commanders, M-147, roll 4, NA.

10. Decatur to Hamilton, October 30, 1812, CL; Dudley, *Naval War of 1812*, 1:549–53, 615–16.

11. Lieutenant Glen Drayton to Hamilton, February 8, 1813, OL; Dudley, *Naval War of 1812*, 1:594–95.

12. Dudley, *Naval War of 1812*, 1:287, 640–49; *National Intelligencer*, March 9, 1814.

13. Amos Evans, Medical Prescription Book Kept on Board vs Frigate *Constitution*. Yale University School of Medicine, New Haven, Conn.

14. Lawrence to Jones, March 19, 1813, CL; Dudley, *Naval War of 1812*, 2:218–29.

15. Lieutenant George Budd to Jones, June 15, 1813, CL; Mahan, *Sea Power*, 2:126–47; Roosevelt, *Naval War of 1812*, 1:221–39; Dudley, *Naval War of 1812*, 2:335–47.

16. Hyde to Jones, February 14, 1814, ML.

17. Victor Hugo Paltsits, ed., "Cruise of the U.S. Brig *Argus* in 1813: Journal of Surgeon James Inderwick," *Bulletin of the New York Public Library* 21 (1917) 383–405. Inderwick replaced Surgeon William M. Clarke, who was sent ashore sick when the *Argus* sailed. When he recovered, Clarke was attached to the *John Adams* at New York.

18. Jones to Allen, June 5, 1813, CL; Roosevelt, *Naval War of 1812*, 1:249–56; Mahan, *Sea Power*, 2:216–19; *Niles Weekly Register*, 8:43; Paltsits, "Cruise of the U.S. Brig *Argus*," 383–405. For a discussion and refutation of British charges of malpractice on the *Argus*, see Ira Dye and J. Worth Estes, "Death on the *Argus*," *Journal of the History of Medicine and Allied Sciences* 44 (1989); 179–95.

19. Roosevelt, *Naval War of 1812*, 1:259–64; Mahan, *Sea Power*, 2:188–91; Lieutenant Edward R. McCall (second in command to Captain Isaac Hull), September 5, 1812, *ASP: NA*, 1:297; Hull to Jones, September 25, 1813, CL. McCall reported the *Boxer*'s losses as 20–35 killed and 14 wounded. But in Hull's report, the number is given as "67, exclusive of those killed and thrown overboard." Mahan notes that the number killed in the *Boxer* was evidently an exaggerated impression.

20. Captain David Porter, *Journal of a Cruise*; Porter to the Secretary of the Navy, July 3, 1814, CL.

21. Porter, *Journal of a Cruise*, 24–25, 27, 39.

22. Ibid., 40–43, 80, 150.

23. Ibid., 190–91, 202–4, 243–46.

24. Ibid., 39, 72, 99, 108, 143, 195–97, 219, 252–53, 451–52.

25. Ibid., chaps. 13, 14, and pp. 441–43.

26. Ibid., 447–94. Porter left Marine Lieutenant John Gamble in command of three prize ships at Nukahiva. His force consisted of three officers and 20 men, exclusive of six prisoners of war. Gamble was instructed to remain at the island for five and a half months, and if he did not hear from Porter by then, to seek the *Essex* at Valparaiso. If he did not find Porter there, he was authorized to dispose of the three prizes at that port and return to the United States. Three days after Porter

sailed, six men became sick on one of the prize ships, some suffering from dysentery and others from pains in the head and joints. In addition, one marine was recovering from a wound in his thigh. The weakened condition of the Americans encouraged the natives to attack. Four men were killed, including a midshipman; two others were wounded. Gamble was severely wounded in the heel and suffered from a fever. Three men deserted, and Gamble was faced with mutiny by his British prisoners. With a midshipman and six men, only two of whom were fit for duty, Gamble set sail for the Hawaiian Islands in a leaky prize ship, the *Sir Andrew Hammond.* In Hawaii, he took on nine men and had his ship captured by the HMS *Cherub.* Still suffering from his wound, Gamble had it dressed by the British surgeon. Subsequently, Gamble and other prisoners were landed in Rio de Janeiro. He returned home in a Swedish ship in August 1815. See ibid., 495–550.

27. Roosevelt, *Naval War of 1812,* 1:210–11; Ray to Secretary of the Navy, February 12, April 2, 1813, OL.

28. Roosevelt, *Naval War of 1812,* 1:243–44.

29. Ibid., 245–48.

30. Ibid., 2:8–9.

31. Ibid., 1:246–49; Angus to the Secretary of the Navy, July 30, 1813, OL.

32. Harold D. Langley, "Women in a Warship, 1813," *USNIP* 110 (1984):124–25.

33. Roosevelt, *Naval War of 1812,* 2:47–52.

34. Ibid., 47, 54.

35. Ibid., 55–61; Blakeley to the Secretary of the Navy, July 8, 1814, CL.

36. Roosevelt, *Naval War of 1812,* 2:35–40.

37. Ibid., 41–43; Donald G. Shomette, *War on the Patuxent, 1814.*

38. Pension file of David Townsend, no. 1451, NA.

39. Roosevelt, *Naval War of 1812,* 2:43–45. For additional accounts of the campaign against Washington and Baltimore, see Walter Lord, *Dawn's Early Light;* James Pack, *Man Who Burned the White House.*

40. Roosevelt, *Naval War of 1812,* 2:211–54. For additional information on the gulf campaign, see Wilburt S. Brown, *Amphibious Campaign for West Florida and Louisiana, 1814–1815;* Frank L. Owsley Jr., *Struggle for the Gulf Borderlands;* Charles B. Brooks, *Siege of New Orleans.*

41. Roosevelt, *Naval War of 1812,* 2:145–50.

42. Ibid., 165–77.

43. Ibid., 179–88.

44. Ibid., 188–89.

45. Surgeon Amos Evans to Commodore Charles Morris, April 9, 1846, War of 1812 Collection, W. L. Clements Library, Ann Arbor, Mich.; 35th Cong., 1st sess., S. Report 42, serial 938.

Chapter 10
The War of 1812 Ashore

1. Gilliland to Hamilton, March 3, 1812, OL; May 18, June 5, 1812, ML; Hamilton to Gilliland, April 16, June 13, 1812, LO.

2. Samuel Whittelsey to Granger, April 10, 1812, ML; William C. Whittelsey to Hamilton, October 8, 1812, OL; Hamilton to William C. Whittelsey, July 10, 1812, LO.

3. Merrill to Hamilton, July 18, 1812; Hamilton to Clarke, July 28, 1812; Hamilton to Ayer, December 29, 1812; Jones to Merrill, April 3, 1813, OL.

4. On the Portsmouth Navy Yard, see Maloney, *Captain from Connecticut,* chap. 9. For conditions in Portsmouth, see J. Worth Estes and David M. Goodman, *Changing Humors of Portsmouth.* In 1811, Portsmouth had a population of 6,973 and a death rate of 15.8 per 1,000. There are no statistics on the bills of mortality during 1812–17. That volume shows that Surgeon Thorn continued to practice in Portsmouth until his death in August 1827. Evidently he had a civilian practice in addition to his duties at the navy yard. He was appointed in 1806 and promoted in 1809.

5. For the impact of the war on New England, see Donald R. Hickey, *War of 1812,* 230–31; Marshall to Hamilton, May 22, June 6, 1812, ML; Hamilton to Christie, July 10, 1812, LO; Chauncey to Hamilton, June 5, 1812, ML. Samuel Jackson, whose request for an appointment as a surgeon's mate was not approved until July 10, 1812, applied to Marshall in June 1812 for the position of chief mate at the hospital. Accompanying his application was a certificate from an institution composed of "gentlemen of high professional respectability," according to Marshall. Despite this endorsement, Christie got the appointment, probably because of his experience in the almshouse. Later, when Christie was transferred to Sacket's Harbor, Jackson became the chief surgeon's mate under Marshall, and the latter argued that he should be paid as a hospital surgeon. See Marshall to Jones, July 14, 1813, OL.

6. Marshall to Hamilton, July 7, 1812; Mumford to Hamilton, July 8, 1812, ML.

7. Marshall to Hamilton, March 20, 1813, OL.

8. Lewis to Jones, October 31, 1813, ML; Jones to Clarke, March 13, 1813; Jones to Hamilton, March 13, 1813; Jones to Lewis, October 18, 1813, LO.

9. Muster Rolls of the Officers and Men Attached to the New York Navy Yard and to the Gunboat Flotilla Based at New York, 1813–15, Nimitz Library, U.S. Naval Academy, Annapolis, Md.

10. Marshall to Hamilton, July 22, 1812, OL; Hamilton to Marshall, August 4, 1812, LO. Later, Marshall made a trip to Washington to explain the system to Secretary Jones. See Marshall to Jones, May 29, 1813, OL; Jones to Marshall, June 4, 1813, LO.

11. Cutbush to Hamilton, July 6, 1812, OL.

12. Hamilton to Cutbush, July 9, 1812, LO. The secretary also assigned Surgeon William P. C. Barton to Cutbush as one of his surgeon's mates and promised to get him one more.

13. Cutbush to Hamilton, July 30, 1812, OL.

14. Hamilton to Cutbush, August 15, 28, 1812, LO; Cutbush to Hamilton, August 24, 1812, OL.

15. Hamilton to Whittelsey, October 21, 1812, LO; Whittelsey to Hamilton, November 11, 1812; Cutbush to Hamilton, November 16, 1812, OL; Hamilton to Cutbush, November 20, 1812, LO.

16. In June 1812, Cutbush inquired about the status of Dr. Barton, pointing out that he was then examining recruits for the army at a rendezvous and that Commodore Murray had no orders concerning him. Cutbush to Hamilton, June 29, 1812, OL; Hamilton to Cutbush, July 2, 1812 LO. The surgeon's uncle, Benjamin Smith Barton, wrote periodically to President Madison during the war, but there is nothing in surviving papers of Madison concerning Surgeon Barton. If there was an appeal to the president over the head of the secretary, it may have been made orally.

17. Cutbush to Hamilton, November 16, 1812, ML; Hamilton to Cutbush, November 20, 1812, LO.

18. Cutbush to Hamilton, November 16, 1812, ML.

19. Cutbush to Hamilton, January 4, 1813, OL; Jones to Commodore Murray, January 17, 1813, LO.

20. Jones to Barton, February 20, 1813, LO; Barton to Decatur, February 26, 1812, CL; Jones to Decatur, March 6, 1813; Jones to Barton, March 6, 16, 1813; Jones to Cutbush, March 17, 1813, LO; Decatur to Jones, March 26, 1813, CL.

21. Barton to Jones, May 10, 1813, OL; Benjamin F. Barton to Attorney General Richard Rush, June 3, 1813; Rush to Jones, June 6, 1813, ML; Jones to Barton, July 12, 1813, LO; Jones to Bainbridge, May 28, 1813, Letters Sent by the Secretary of the Navy to Commandants and Navy Agents, M-441, NA (hereafter cited as LSCNA); Jones to Heap, May 28, 1813, LO; Heap to Jones, July 20, 1813, OL.

22. Jones to Barton, July 28, 1813, LO; Barton to Jones, August 3, 1813, OL; Jones to Heap, July 28, 1813, LO; Thomas H. Gilliss for the accountant of the navy, September 10, 1813, Office of the Fourth Auditor, ML.

23. Heap to the Secretary of the Navy, April 25, 1814, OL. This was probably Charles M. Reese of South Carolina, who was commissioned as a surgeon on April 26, 1816.

24. Latrobe to Hamilton, June 25, 1812, ML.

25. Latrobe to the Secretary of the Navy, February 2, 1813; Latrobe to Secretary Benjamin Crowninshield, January 1, 1815, ML; William P. C. Barton, *Treatise Containing a Plan for the Internal Organization and Government of Marine Hospitals.*

26. For a brief account of the charges and countercharges between Ewell and Goldsborough and the public airing of them, see McKee, *Gentlemanly and Honorable Profession,* 17 and n. 46. Ewell asked Jones for permission to resign instead of being dismissed. Jones replied that Ewell's resignation would take effect when his accounts were settled. See Ewell to Jones, March 9, 1813, William Jones Papers, Uselma Clark Smith Collection, HSP; Jones to Ewell, May 5, 1813, Letters Sent by the Secretary of the Navy to Commandants and Navy Agents, M-441, NA. The matter of Ewell's account was still pending in December 1815.

27. Harrison to Hamilton, December 1812, ML. Huntt resigned on August 31, 1813.

28. Cutbush to the president, December 25, 1812, OL; Cutbush to Hamilton, December 25, 1812, ML; Jones to Cutbush, May 5, 1813, LO.

29. H. Huntt, "On the Epidemic," *Medical Repository,* 2d ser., 1 (1813):342–44.

30. Jones to Cutbush, September 1, 3, 6, 10, 14, 1814, LO; Cutbush to Jones, September 3, 5, 13, 1814, OL.

31. Cutbush to Commodore John Rodgers, president of Board of Navy Commissioners, May 2, 1815, Navy Department Records, Subject File, MA, RG 45, NA.

32. Cassin to the Secretary of the Navy, May 23, 1813, CL. Cassin's account of the Battle of Craney Island on June 22 is in his letter to Jones, June 23, 1813, CL. During this battle, Surgeon's Mate William Turk amputated two legs at the thigh. He complained to the secretary of the navy that the tourniquets that he took from the ship for this purpose were of poor quality and bent or broke when buckled. These tourniquets were acquired from the public medical store in Washington. More reliable tourniquets could be obtained in Philadelphia and other places in the country. See Turk to Jones, July 1, 1813, OL.

Surgeon Schoolfield was assigned to Norfolk in May 1812 to work under Surgeon Larkin Griffin, but he was paid only as a surgeon's mate. See Hamilton to Schoolfield, May 12, 1812, LO. Later, in August 1812, Surgeon Griffin was given a leave of absence for his health, and he died in November 1814. Schoolfield was acting surgeon from the time of Griffin's death until the end of the War of 1812. See Hamilton to Griffin, August 1, 1812, LO; Schoolfield to the Secretary of the Navy, February 27, 1815, OL.

33. Morrison to the Secretary of the Navy, September 15, October 5, December 11, 1812, February 8, 1813; Morrison to Jones, May 2, 10, 1813, OL; Hamilton to Morrison, October 16, 1812; Jones to Gautier, May 15, 1813, LO; Sailing Master John C. Mason to Jones, February 1, 1813; Morrison to Jones, June 1, 8, August 14, December 24, 1813, OL.

34. Logan to Hamilton, October 12, 1812, OL.

35. Thomas Mitchell to Jones, July 2, 1813, quoting a letter of Adams Bailey from the marine hospital of April 20, 1813, and endorsed in the Navy Department with information on Allison's death, ML.

36. Logan to Hamilton, November 20, 1812, OL.

37. Logan to Hamilton, October 12, 1812; Logan to Jones, February 1, 1813, OL.

38. Logan to Jones, February 1, 1813, May 10, 1813, and endorsement, OL.

39. Logan to Jones, December 31, 1814, OL; Captain David Porter to the Board of Navy Commissioners, August 1, 1817, LBNC, vol. 1, RG 45, NA; Jones to Logan, January 5, 1814, LO.

40. Baldwin to Jones, June 12, 1813, OL; Jones to Baldwin and Ray, March 11, 12, 1813; Jones to Captain Hugh Campbell, August 14, 1813, LO.

41. Baldwin to Jones, June 12, 1813; Grandison to Hamilton, December 20, 1812; Grandison to Posey, February 16, 1813, and endorsement, OL; Jones to Grandison, May 1, 1813, LO; Campbell to Jones, October 16, 1813, OL.

42. Sevier to Jones, June 7, 1813, ML.

43. Hamilton to Troup, October 17, 1812, LO; Grandison to Hamilton, December 2, 1812; New to Campbell, September 5, 1813; Campbell to Jones, October 16, 1813, OL.

Chapter 11
The War of 1812 on the Lakes

1. In addition to the sources listed in chap. 10, n. 1, useful information on the war on the lakes may be found in Max Rosenberg, *Building of Perry's Fleet on Lake*

Erie, 1812–1813; Morris Zaslow, ed., *Defended Border;* Pierre Berton, *Invasion of Canada, 1812–1813;* Berton, *Flames Across the Border, 1813–1814;* Alex R. Gilpin, *War of 1812 in the Old Northwest;* Harrison Bird, *War for the West, 1790–1813;* William Jeffrey Welsh and David Curtis Skaggs, *War on the Great Lakes;* special issue of *Journal of Erie Studies* 17 (1988) commemorating the 175th anniversary of the battle. For preparations on the lakes, see Dudley, *Naval War of 1812,* 1:278–343.

2. Chauncey to Buchanan, September 12, 1812, Chauncey Letterbook, NYHS.

3. Chauncey to Hamilton, November 17, 1812, Chauncey Letterbook, William L. Clements Library, Ann Arbor, Mich.

4. General Order, December 4, 1812, Chauncey Letterbook, Clements Library.

5. Chauncey to Buchanan, December 10, 1812, Chauncey Letterbook, Clements Library. The round trip to Albany was estimated at 25 days, but it included a side trip to New York so that Buchanan could visit his family over the Christmas holiday. In early February 1813, Buchanan was given another leave of 10–12 days to visit his family, provided it did not harm the public service. Presumably there were enough medical men to cover the sick cases. See Chauncey to Buchanan, February 4, 1813, Chauncey Letterbook, Clements Library.

6. Chauncey to Dodge, January 23, 1813; Chauncey to Jones, March 5, 1813, Chauncey Letterbook. Clements Library.

7. Chauncey to Jones, April 28, 1813, CL; in this letter, Chauncey reported the deaths of two midshipmen and "several" seamen. Chauncey to Jones, May 7, 1813, CL; Buchanan to Jones, Augusts 27, 1813, OL.

8. Chauncey to Jones, June 2, 1813, CL; Captain Richard Smith of the Marine Corps reported to his commandant in Washington that he had one man die a few days before the battle and than on June 11 there were 26 who were unfit for duty. He did not say how many of these had suffered wounds. Smith to Lieutenant Colonel Franklin Wharton, USMC, June 11, 1813, Letters Received, Commandant of the Marine Corps, RG 137, NA.

9. Herbert Fairlie Wood, "Many Battles of Stoney Creek," in Morris Zaslow, ed., *Defended Border,* 59–60; Chauncey to Jones, June 11, 1813, CL.

10. Chauncey to Jones, July 17, 21, 1813, August 19, 1813, CL.

11. Chauncey to Jones, August 4, 13, 1813, CL. For a survivor's account of the loss of the *Scourge,* see James Fenimore Cooper, *Ned Myers,* 77–100.

12. For pertinent documents see Dudley, *Naval War of 1812,* vol. 2, chap. 3.

13. Seebert J. Goldowsky, *Yankee Surgeon,* 12–13.

14. Ibid., 15, 19–21; Parsons to Hamilton, September 5, 1812, OL: Usher Parsons, "Diary Kept during the Expedition to Lake Erie," foreword, Usher Parsons Journals, Rhode Island Historical Society, Providence. (hereafter cited as Parsons, "Diary").

15. Goldowsky, *Yankee Surgeon,* 22–25; Parsons, "Diary."

16. Angus to Hamilton, December 1, 1812, OL; for Angus's injuries see Langley, "Respect for Civilian Authority," 23–37.

17. Goldowsky, *Yankee Surgeon,* 25–30; Parsons, "Diary."

18. Parsons, "Diary."

19. Ibid.

20. Ibid. One of the ailments common to the region was known as "Lake Fever." Mr. John W. Watkins of Tioga, New York, observed the effects of this disease in his settlement on Seneca Lake between 1795 and 1800 and wrote to Dr. Samuel Mitchell about it. Watkins described the symptoms as inflamed and very yellow eyes, a flushed face, pain in the back, head, limbs, and very severely in the breast, along with a sick stomach, dry skin, and constipation. Before the disease had run its course, the whole body turned yellow. It was Watkins's experience that as soon as the bowels were relieved and perspiration brought on, there was a quick recovery. In one extreme case where repeated clysters, calomel, and teas had no effect, the man was placed in a large cask of warm water. After the first immersion he began to perspire, and after the second the bowels were relieved and the man recovered. See John W. Watkins, "On the Disease Called Lake Fever," *Medical Repository* 3 (1800):359–61.

Surgeon Joseph G. Roberts later petitioned Congress for money for his services at Presque Isle because he was ordered by Perry to take charge of the hospital and thus missed the Battle of Lake Erie and the prize money. By the time the squadron left Erie in August, "a considerable number of patients, some of whom were dangerously ill," had been sent to the hospital at Erie. See Petition of Joseph G Roberts, September 12, 1814, U.S. Congress, House, *Journal,* 13th Cong., HR 13A-08.1, RG 233, NA.

21. Rosenberg, *Building of Perry's Fleet on Lake Erie, 1812–1823,* 21–52; Mahan, *Naval War of 1812,* 2:62–74. For pertinent documents see Dudley, *Naval War of 1812,* vol. 2, chap. 3.

22. Parsons, "Diary;" Goldowsky, *Yankee Surgeon,* 35–37; David Curtis Skaggs, "Joint Operations During the Detroit–Lake Erie Campaign, 1813," in William B. Cogar, ed., *New Interpretations in Naval History,* 126–28.

23. Parsons, "Diary;" Goldowsky, *Yankee Surgeon,* 37.

24. Usher Parsons, "Battle of Lake Erie, A Discourse Delivered before the Rhode Island Historical Society on February 16, 1853," and quoted in part in Goldowsky, *Yankee Surgeon,* 41–46; Parsons, "Diary." For a vivid account see Gerard T. Altoff, "Battle of Lake Erie," in William Jeffrey Welsh and David Curtis Skaggs, eds., *War on the Great Lakes,* 5–16; and Altoff's work based on the pension accounts of participants, *Deep Water Sailors, Shallow Water Soldiers.*

25. Parsons, "Diary;" Goldowsky, *Yankee Surgeon,* 46–61.

26. RGCM, case 193, roll 7.

27. William S. Dudley, "Commodore Isaac Chauncey and U.S. Joint Operations on Lake Ontario, 1813," in Cogar, *New Interpretations,* 146–53; Mahan, *Sea Power,* 2:274–328.

28. Chauncey to Jones, November 29, 1813, CL; Jones to Buchanan, February 15, 1813, LO.

29. Chauncey to Buchanan, December 13, 1813, Chauncey Letterbook, NYHS.

30. Chauncey to Jones, June 4, 5, 1814; Chauncey to Davis, June 28, 1814, Chauncey Letterbook, NYHS.

31. Property at Sacket's Harbor, July 15, 1815, Rodgers Family Collection, ser. 3A, LC.

32. Mahan, *Sea Power,* 2:354–82. For pertinent documents on naval activities

on Lake Champlain in 1813, see Dudley, *Naval War of 1812,* vol. 2, chap. 3; Macdonough to Jones, September 17, 10, 1814, CL.

Surgeon's Mate Gustavus Brown was assigned to Macdonough in May 1813. Surgeon William Caton, originally assigned to Sacket's Harbor, was transferred to Lake Champlain in January 1814. This created problems because Caton had been commissioned as a surgeon's mate after Brown and had been promoted to surgeon on the basis of his service under Chauncey at Sacket's Harbor. Brown respected Caton's ability but pointed out that prior to Caton's arrival he had performed all the medical duties in Macdonough's command without any assistance. To save his feelings about being superseded by a junior, Brown asked for a transfer to Washington. Instead, Caton seems to have become ill, Brown remained on the station, and he got some assistance from the army. See Brown to Jones, January 4, 1814, OL; Mary C. Gillett, *Army Medical Department, 1775–1818,* 173–74.

33. Except as otherwise indicated, this section is based on Anthony G. Dietz, "Prisoners of War in the United States during the War of 1812," Ph.D. diss. (Washington, D.C., American University, 1964).

34. Jones to Osborne; Jones to Whittelsey, April 29, 1813, LO.

35. Whittelsey to Jones, May 12, 1813, OL; Jones to Whittelsey, May 15, 1813, LO.

36. Whittelsey to Jones, July 27, November 24, 1813, OL; Log of the *Analostan,* RG 24, NA.

37. Roddis, "Naval and Marine Corps Casualties," 308. For the army's medical record in the War of 1812 and similar problems in determining casualties, see Gillett, *Army Medical Department,* 148–85. See also John W. Witt, "United States Marine Corps Deaths in Service, 1776–1925," 2 vols., an unpublished manuscript. Copy in Marine Corps Historical Center, Washington, D.C.

Chapter 12
Toward a More Professional Service

1. *U.S. Statutes at Large,* 3:202; Charles Oscar Paullin, *Paullin's History of Naval Administration, 1775–1911: A Collection of Articles Reprinted from the U.S. Naval Institute Proceedings,* 167, 173.

2. Field, *America and the Mediterranean,* 57–58, 104–5. This is the most comprehensive study of U.S. activity in the Mediterranean in the nineteenth century.

3. *U.S. Statutes at Large,* 3:321.

4. On the political and economic background of the panic, see Bray Hammond, *Banks and Politics in America from the Revolution to the Civil War,* 258–85. On the Missouri problems see Glover Moore, *Missouri Controversy, 1819–1821.* Naval aspects can be traced in Symonds, *Navalists and Antinavalists,* 219–31. On the panic itself, see Rothford, *Panic of 1819.*

5. Robert Erwin Johnson, *Thence Round Cape Horn,* 17–26.

6. Symonds, *Navalists and Antinavalists,* 220–21; Gardner W. Allen, *Our Navy and the West Indian Pirates;* Francis B. C. Bradlee, *Piracy in the West Indies and Its Suppression;* Richard Wheeler, *In Pirate Waters.*

7. Edward Baxter Billingsley, *In Defense of Neutral Rights.*

8. Symonds, *Navalists and Antinavalists,* 221–22; Harold D. Langley, "Robert F. Stockton," in James C. Bradford, ed., *Command under Sail,* 279–80; Peter Duignan and Clarence Clendenen, *The United States and the African Slave Trade, 1619–1862,* 20–29.

9. For biographical sketches of these secretaries, see Paolo E. Coletta, *American Secretaries of the Navy,* 1:101–40.

10. Cutbush to Commodore John Rodgers, president of the Board of Navy Commissioners, May 2, 1815, Navy Department Records, Subject File, MA, RG 45, NA; Cutbush to Jones, February 13, 1813, "Edward Cutbush," ZB File.

11. Cutbush to Crowninshield, January 29, 1815, OL.

12. Marshall to Crowninshield, February 24, 1815, OL; Crowninshield to Marshall, May 1, 18, 1815, LO; Crowninshield to Cutbush, Marshall, and Heap, May 29, June 14, 1815, LO.

13. Cutbush to Rodgers, May 2, 1815, Navy Department Records, Subject File MA, RG 45, NA.

14. Captain Samuel Evans and others to Crowninshield, May 1816; Captain William Bainbridge and others, December 13, 1816, U.S. Congress, Records of the Legislative Branch, Senate Committee on Naval Affairs, 16A-D9, RG 46, NA; Crowninshield to Charles Tait, January 23, 1817, Navy Department Records, Letters from the Secretary of the Navy to Congress, 2:460, RG 45, NA.

15. Marshall to Calhoun, January 6, 1817, *Senate Journal,* 14th Cong., 2d sess., NA.

16. *Annals of Congress,* 14th Cong., 2d sess., 30:442; Crowninshield to Charles Tait, January 23, 1817, *ASP:NA,* 1:443.

17. Rodgers to Crowninshield, January 22, 1817, LBNC.

18. Chidester to Parris, November 29, December 26, 1817; Chidester to Parrott, January 20, 1818, Records of the Legislative Branch, Senate Committee on Naval Affairs, 16A-D9, RG 46, NA; *Annals of Congress,* 15th Cong., 1st sess., 32:1794.

19. Crowninshield to Charles Tait, chairman of the Senate Committee on Naval Affairs, January 8, 1817, Navy Department Records, Letters from the Secretary of the Navy to Congress, RG 45, NA.

20. Crowninshield to Charles Tait, Chairman, Senate Naval Committee, February 8, 1817; Crowninshield to James Pleasants Jr., chairman, House Naval Committee, March 14, 1818, Letters from the Secretary of the Navy to Congress, RG 45, NA.

21. Thompson to the President of the Senate, December 29, 1819, *ASP:NA,* 1:617–18.

22. For an example of the Navy Department's usual reply, see Crowninshield to E. Leonard, May 28, 1817; Crowninshield to James W. Mason, March 3, 1817; B. Homans to Mordecai Morgan, September 19, 1818, GLB.

23. B. Homans to Henry Clay, October 8, 1818; John C. Calhoun, acting secretary, to Henry Clay, December 24, 1818, GLB; Callahan, *List of Officers,* 508.

24. B. Homans to Mordecai Morgan, September 19, November 11, 1818, GLB.

25. Harold and Margaret Sprout, *Rise of American Naval Power, 1776–1918,* 97.

26. Thompson to the Speaker of the House of Representatives, January 16, 1823, 17th Cong., 2d sess., H. Doc. 27, serial 76, 3; *ASP:NA,* 1:870.

27. Harris to Thompson, May 10, 1823, OL. The three surgeons were Leonard Osborne, William J. Barnwell Jr., and John H. Gordon. The mates were Benjamin Austin and John W. Peaco.

28. Thompson to Harris, May 19, 1823, LO; Harris to Thompson, August 26, 1823, OL; Rodgers to Harris, August 28, 1823, LO.

29. Ticknor to Thompson, April 16, 1823, OL.

30. *Annals of Congress,* 18th Cong., 1st sess., 41:831.

31. *ASP:NA,* 1:906–10.

32. Belt to Southard, January 28, February 12, 1824, OL: Southard to Belt, February 19, 1824, LO.

33. The case is reviewed in Southard's letter to President Monroe, February 13, 1824, Samuel Southard Letterbook, NYPL. Southard's orders to Phillips of September 23, November 24, 1823, and February 7, 1824, and his correspondence with Captain Creighton are in LO. Creighton said that it would be easy to seize Phillips and confine him on the ship, but he was unwilling to "Create any Excitement in the City." Creighton to Southard, February 6, 1824, CL.

34. Circular, Southard to all surgeons and surgeon's mates, December 12, 1823, LO.

35. Southard to Kennon, December 3, 1823, LO; Beattie to Southard, September 2, 1823, December 13, 1823, OL; Southard to Beattie, December 11, 13, 1823; Southard to Judson, December 30, 1823, January 6, 1824, February 10, 1824, LO; B. L. Lear [?] to Southard, January 22, 1824, ML.

36. Southard to Cutbush, Marshall, Barton, Harris, and Washington, May 31, 1824, LO.

37. Cutbush to Southard, June 10, 1824, OL.

38. Ibid.; Southard to Cutbush, June 17, 1824, LO.

39. Cutbush to Southard, June 10, 1824, OL.

40. Southard to Surgeon Thomas Harris and Lieutenant Commandant John D. Sloat, June 27, 1824, LO; USND, *Navy Register, 1826.*

41. Beers to Southard, December 28, 1824, OL; Southard to Beers, January 6, 1825, LO.

42. Harris to Southard, October 7, 1824, Samuel L. Southard Papers, box 11, published with permission of the Manuscripts Division, Department of Rare Books and Special Collections, Princeton University Libraries.

43. Charles Hay, chief clerk to Cutbush, November 23, 1824; Southard to Cutbush, Barton, Harris, and Washington, November 23, 1824; Southard to Imlay, March 25, 1825, LO; Harris to Southard, April 24, 28 [?], 1825, Southard Papers, box 14, Princeton University Libraries.

44. Harris to Southard, January 31, 1825, Southard Papers, Princeton University Libraries.

45. Chase to Parrott, February 16, 1825; Chase to Southard, March 24, 1825; Cornick to Southard, February 11, March 13, 1825, OL; Southard to Cutbush and others, March 23, 1825, LO. Cornick was promoted to Surgeon on May 2, and Chase on May 3, 1825.

46. Fiat Justitia, "The Navy," *National Gazette and Literary Register,* March 6, 1826. The Melville referred to was Henry Dundas, Lord Melville, the First Lord of the Admiralty.

47. *U.S. Statutes at Large,* 4:242.

48. *Niles Weekly Register,* April 28, 1827, 32, 146–47.

49. The petition or memorial was signed by Surgeons John A. Kearney, Thomas Harris, William P. C. Barton, and Henry W. Bassett, and Surgeon's Mates Charles Wayne, Mifflin Coulter, James M. Greene, G. W. Palmer, and Henry C. Pratt. The Senate version is printed in *ASP:NA,* 3:131–33. The memorial of the lieutenants is in ibid., 86–88.

The House version (same as the Senate's) is in Records of the Legislative Branch, House Committee on Naval Affairs, HR 20A-G13.2, RG 233, NA. On the Southard-Hayne relationship, see Harold D. Langley, "Robert Y. Hayne and the Navy," *South Carolina Historical Magazine* 82 (1981):311–30; *U.S. Statutes at Large,* 4:313–14.

50. *U.S. Statutes at Large,* 4:313–13.

51. Ibid., 330.

Chapter 13
Health Care and Hospitals, 1816–1829

1. Field, *America and the Mediterranean,* 58.

2. Crowninshield to McReynolds, April 7, 1815; Crowninshield to Decatur, April 8, 1815; Crowninshield to Chauncey, April 19, 1815, January 31, 1816, LO; Chauncey to Crowninshield, January 10, 1817; Chauncey to McReynolds, January 10, 1817, Chauncey Letterbook, NYHS.

3. Chauncey to the Governor of Minorca, January 22, 1817; Chauncey to George Erving, U.S. Minister to Spain, March 14, 1817; Chauncey to Captain John Shaw, January 22, 1817; Chauncey to Captain Charles Stewart, January 31, 1818, Chauncey Letterbook, Clements Library; Field, *America and the Mediterranean,* 105.

4. Field, *America and the Mediterranean,* 106–8.

5. Stewart to Thompson, June 1819, AF.

6. Thomas Brown to the Secretary of the Navy, May 4, 1820, AF; Thompson to Captain Jacob Jones, September 15, 1821, LO; Captain Jacob Jones to Thompson, November 26, 1821, AF; Field, *America and the Mediterranean,* 108–10.

7. Field, *America and the Mediterranean,* 108–12.

8. Enoch C. Wines, *Two Years and a Half in the Navy,* 1:116–17. Shortly before Wines's ship, the *Constellation,* left Port Mahon, the Spanish surgeon was transferred to a hospital on the Peninsula.

9. Goldowsky, *Yankee Surgeon,* 89–106. Parsons's medical journal of his cruise in the *Java* is in the Rhode Island Historical Society.

10. Harwood Family Papers, Green Library, Stanford University, Palo Alto, Calif. A log of the *Constitution* in the National Archives which begins on May 7, 1826 provides an opportunity to check Harwood's figures for most of the period during which he kept a record. While there is general agreement, there are 36 instances between June 1826 and May 1827 where his figures do not agree with those in the log. Usually he is off by only one or two, but in five cases the difference is between three and four. The log provides daily figures when Harwood has none,

but there are eight instances where there are no log entries but his journal records a daily total. On two days there is no entry in either source. Assuming that the log is generally accurate and using Harwood's entries when there are gaps, the daily average for the 13-month period when the two sources overlap is 13, and two deaths are recorded. A microfilm copy of the *Constitution's* log is M-1030, roll 3.

11. Captain John Rodgers to Secretary of the Navy, January 20, February 17, March 3, 1827, CL. The ship sailed with a complement of 916 including supernumeraries. According to the muster list of the *North Carolina*, 4 men died at Malta in January and February 1827, and another in March 1827 when the ship was at Port Mahon. For the impact of the ship's health record in Malta and proof of the value of vaccination, see Paul Cassar, *Medical History of Malta*, 253. According to Cassar, there were six deaths out of a crew of 950, but the muster list mentions the lazaretto in connection with only one death.

12. Thompson to Biddle, March 26, 1822, LO; Biddle to Thompson, July 24, 1822, OL; *Niles Weekly Register*, November 30, 1822, 23, 205–6; Long, *Sailor-Diplomat*, 99–100.

13. Maloney, *Captain from Connecticut*, 354–55; Long, *Sailor-Diplomat*, 101–5; Wainwright, *Commodore James Biddle*, 16–20. For a personal account of a bout with the fever, see Lieutenant Charles Gauntt, "Macedonian Journal," LC; for efforts to preserve the medical record see "Frigate Macedonian 1812," Yellow Fever Papers, College of Physicians, Philadelphia. The account of the investigation is in RGCM, no. 399.

14. Thompson to Porter, February 1, 1823, LO; Porter to Thompson, February 27, 1823 (misdated; should be March 17, 1823), CL; Thompson to Williamson, May 8, 1823, LO; Porter to Secretary of the Navy, August 11, 1823, CL; Thompson to Rodgers, Chauncey and Morris, August 29, 1823, LO; Long, *Nothing Too Daring*, 210, 215–16. The information about the exfoliation of the bone did not become known until Porter applied for a disability pension 15 years later and supported his statement with a letter from Surgeon Edmund L. DuBarry, who at the time of the incident was a surgeon's mate. See Long, *Nothing Too Daring*, 215. Smith Thompson resigned as secretary of the navy on August 31, 1823.

15. Southard to Porter, September 27, 1823; Southard to Harris, Washington, and Hoffman, September 23, 1823; Southard to Marshall, October 11, 1823, LO; Harris to General Thomas Cadwalader, October 5, 1823, Gratz Collection, HSP. Cadwalader was a major general in the Pennsylvania militia in the War of 1812 and later a director of the Second Bank of the United States.

16. Southard asked the army to transfer its barracks and fortifications at Barrancus to the navy. The army agreed and the transfer was made on May 24, 1825. Commodore Lewis Warrington in the *John Adams* entered Pensacola Bay on October 4, 1825, and landed his marines and refreshed his crew at the base. See *ASP:NA*, 2:99, 109–10; Edwin C. Bearss, *Fort Barrancas*, 62–65; *U.S. Statutes at Large*, 4:127; George F. Pearce, *The U.S. Navy in Pensacola*, 13–19.

17. Dillard to Harris, March 2, 1826, Yellow Fever Papers.

18. A series of articles on navy matters was published in the *New York National Advocate* under the pen name of Coram. In an article on January 12, 1826, Coram said that Rome's Pontine Marshes were salubrious in comparison with Thompson's

Island. Of Southard he said: "He saw, almost weekly, officers tottering into his office, emaciated, pale, and dubious of recovery, from diseases there [Thompson's Island] engendered, whom the humanity of the several commanders there had permitted to return home. Among them were all the medical gentlemen who had been stationed there, with the exception of those who made it a 'lasting habitation.' These officers were capable of making true statements; and they did so with great candour [sic], and with a fervor which marked them as humane men." See also Thompson to Hulse, May 12, 1823, LO; Warrington to Southard, September 12, 1827, LBNC.

19. Kennedy to Porter, November 4, 1824; Brodie to Barron, March 8, 1825, Barron Papers, Swem Library, College of William and Mary, Williamsburg, Va.

20. Wiesenthal to Southard, November 1, 1825, Barron Papers.

21. Claxton to Barron, November 28, 1828; Barron to Woodbury, January 25, 1834; Woodbury to Barron, January 27, 1834, Barron Papers; William Oliver Stevens, *Affair of Honor*, 173–75. In 1837 the House Committee on Naval Affairs reported a bill to compensate Barron, but it did not pass. Another House naval committee laid the bill on the table in 1841 as not being the proper subject for special legislation. For the Royal Navy's experience with ventilators, see Lloyd and Coulter, *Medicine in the Navy*, 3:72–73.

22. Morgan to Southard, December 10, 1824, OL. Apparently Southard did not reply to this letter.

23. Southard to Speaker of the House, March 6, 1826, Letters from the Secretary of the Navy to Congress, in response to the resolution of February 10, 1826, NA.

24. Southard's circular of May 26, 1826, was sent to the commanders of the navy yards at Portsmouth, Boston, New York, Philadelphia, Washington, and Norfolk; to naval commanders at Baltimore and Charleston and in the Mediterranean, the Pacific, and the West Indies; and to Captain James Biddle in the *Macedonian*, LO.

25. Page to Woolsey, May 27, 1829, John Rodgers Papers, ser. 3, vol. 9, LC; George Smith Blake, transcribed by Katherine McInnis, "When Smallpox Struck," *USNIP* 97 (1979):78–81.

26. Amos Evans Prescription Book, War of 1812 Collection, Clements Library.

27. Evans told the secretary that after years of arduous service he found that surgeons younger than himself received appointments to shore stations and hospitals. Some of these men had never served as mates or been to sea. Having thus been deprived of what he thought he was entitled to in the way of assignments that would allow him to support his family, he had requested the help of Captains Hull and Bainbridge to get a furlough, which the previous secretary had granted. This letter led to the revoking of his earlier orders for sea duty. See Evans to the Secretary of the Navy, March 29, 1821, OL.

28. Montgomery to Thompson, May 10, 1819, OL. I am grateful to Linda Maloney for calling this to my attention.

29. Hay to Dr. John Heap (father of the surgeon), January 22, 1824, GLB; S. D. Heap to the Secretary, December 21, 1825, Resignations of Officers, U.S. Navy, 1812–33, RG 49, NA; Callahan, *List of Officers*, 387.

30. Latrobe to Crowninshield, January 1, 1815, ML; Crowninshield to Charles

Tait, chairman, Senate Committee on Naval Affairs, January 8, 1817, Letters from the Secretary of the Navy to Congress.

31. Crowninshield to John Gaillard, president of the Senate, December 7, 1815; Crowninshield to the Speaker of the House, January 15, 1818, *ASP:NA*, 1:365–66, 451.

32. Crowninshield to the Speaker of the House, January 15, 1818; Crawford, Calhoun, and Crowninshield to the Speaker of the House, January 14, 1818, *ASP:NA*, 1:451–52.

33. Crowninshield to the Speaker of the House, January 15, 1818, *ASP:NA*, 1:451.

34. Smith Thompson to the Speaker of the House, January 14, 1819, *ASP:NA*, 1:609.

35. Cutbush to Crowninshield, May 25, 1818; Page to Crowninshield, August 23, 1818; Heermann to Crowninshield, August 23, 1818; Surgeon George T. Kennon to Crowninshield, May 29, 1818; Surgeon Charles Cotton to Crowninshield, May 17, 1818, *ASP:NA*, 1:610–13.

36. Trevett to Crowninshield, June 30, 1818; Marshall to the Secretary of the Navy, December 12, 1818; Logan to the Secretary of the Navy, June 10, 1818; *ASP:NA*, 1:613–14.

37. Pleasants to Rogers, February 10, 1819, LRBNC.

38. Rogers to Pleasants, February 13, 1819, *ASP:NA*, 1:653–54.

39. Smith Thompson, William H. Crawford, and John C. Calhoun, Commissioners of Navy Hospitals, to the Speaker of the House, December 21, 1821, *ASP:NA*, 1:744.

40. Southard to Daniel H. Miller, House Committee on Naval Affairs, January 31, 1829, 20th Cong., 2d sess., H. Rept. 61; Commissioners of Navy Hospitals to the House of Representatives, March 10, 1824, and enclosures, *ASP:NA*, 3:946–47.

41. *ASP:NA*, 3:14–15.

42. Southard to Michael Hoffman, Chairman of the House Committee on Naval Affairs, June 27, 1829, ibid., 299.

43. *U.S. Statutes at Large*, 4:31, 304, 360.

Chapter 14
Continuing Reform Efforts

1. W. Patrick Strauss, "John Branch," in Paolo E. Coletta, ed., *American Secretaries of the Navy*, 1:143–48.

2. W. Patrick Strauss, "Levy Woodbury," in Coletta, *American Secretaries of the Navy*, 1:151–53; Langley, *Social Reform*, 148–53, 227–32.

3. W. Patrick Strauss, "Mahlon Dickerson," in Coletta, *American Secretaries of the Navy*, 1:155–62; Langley, *Social Reform*, 103–9, 153–57.

4. W. Patrick Strauss, "James Kirke Paulding," in Coletta, *American Secretaries of the Navy*, 1:165–70; Langley, *Social Reform*, 153–57.

5. Branch to Logan, May 25, 1829, LO; Logan to Branch, May 23, 1829, Navy Department Records, Resignations, RG 45, NA.

6. Branch to Cutbush, June 6, 1829, LO; Cutbush to Branch, June 15, July 28, 1829; Branch to Cutbush, July 28, 1829, "Edward Cutbush," ZB File. Branch considered June 10, the day Cutbush met with him to appeal his order, as the date of his resignation.

7. Bradford to Barton, May 4, 1829, President's Naval Collection, F. D. Roosevelt Library, Hyde Park, N.Y.

8. American Seaman's Friends Society, *Sailor's Magazine* 1 (1829):156.

9. Ibid., 179.

10. *ASP:NA*, 3:469.

11. Ibid., 469–77; the replies are also printed in 21st Cong., 1st sess., H. Doc. 23, serial 195, vol. 1; Branch to the Speaker of the House, January 13, 1830, Navy Department Records, Letters from the Secretary of the Navy to Congress, 6, RG 45, NA.

12. 21st Cong., 1st sess., H. Doc. 22, serial 195, vol. 1; *Register of Debates*, 21st Cong., 1st sess., 6, pt. 1, 584–90; Langley, *Social Reform*, 225–69.

13. Woodbury, June 15, 1831, circular, LO; Langley, *Social Reform*, 227–28.

14. Heerman to Branch, January 18, 1830, OL.

15. Branch to Heerman, January 18, 1830, LO; Heermann to Branch, January 23, 1830, OL.

16. Barton to Bradford, August 20, 1830, Navy Department Records, Subject Files, MA-Hospital Administration, RG 45, NA.

17. Woodbury to Hayne, December 26, 1831, Records of the Legislative Branch, House Committee on Naval Affairs, HR 22A-D17.2, RG 233, NA; Woodbury's annual report, November 30, 1833, p. 26. One of the factors that probably contributed to the lack of support for the bill was the resignation of Senator Hayne on December 13, 1832, to become governor of South Carolina.

18. Woodbury to Harris, March 8, 1834, LO; Harris to Woodbury, March 12, 1834, OL; Woodbury to Washington, June 30, 1834, LO.

19. John Duffy, *Healers,* 143–46; Hull to Woodbury, January 6, 1834; Washington to Woodbury, September 10, 1834, Navy Department Records, Subject File, MS, box 189, NA.

20. Washington to Dickerson, October 4, 1834, OL.

21. Washington to Dickerson, January 7, 1834, Navy Records, Subject File, MA, box 2, NA.

22. Dickerson to Warrington, October 11, 1834, quoting Washington, LO.

23. Washington to Dickerson, May 4, 1835; Washington to John Boyle, acting secretary, May 29, 1835; May 28, 1836, OL; Boyle, to Washington, May 28, 1836, LO.

24. Harris to Woodbury, January 30, 1833, OL; *Senate Journal*, 24th Cong., 2d sess., S. Doc. 176 (serial 298).

25. Barton to Dickerson, February 13, 1838, OL.

26. William P. C. Barton, *Polemical Remonstrance;* Barton to Dickerson, March 8, 1838, OL; Dickerson to Barton, March 13, 1838, Mahlon Dickerson Papers, New Jersey Historical Society, Newark.

27. *Non Nauticus,* in *United States Gazette,* December 1839, an enclosure in an unsigned letter to Senator Samuel L. Southard, January 29, 1840, Southard Papers, box 68, Manuscripts Division, Department of Rare Books and Special Collections,

Princeton University Libraries. Paulding's report is printed in House Executive Document 39, 26th cong., 1st sess., 4–6.

28. Boyd to Paulding, January 12, 1839, Navy Department Records, Subject Files, MS-Epidemics, RG 45, NA.

29. The 1818 regulations relating to surgeons, surgeon's mates, hospital surgeons, and surgeons of the fleet, as well as to hospital ships, are printed in *ASP:NA*, 1:524–25, 534; Woodbury to Rodgers, October 1, 1831, LO.

30. Captain John Rodgers to Woodbury, October 1, 1831, LBNC, 4, RG 45, NA.

31. *U.S. Statutes at Large*, 4:516; U.S. Congress, *Annual Report of the Secretary of the Navy, 1833*, 38; for 1834, 3–4.

32. U.S. Congress, *Annual Report of the Secretary of the Navy, 1841*, 355–56.

33. *U.S. Statutes at Large*, 4:755.

34. *Senate Journal*, S. Doc. 10, 25th Cong., 3d sess., serial 338. The petition was signed by W. S. W. Ruschenberger, William Johnson, Samuel Moseley, Robert J. Dodd, Daniel Egbert, Amos A. Gambrill, and George Clymer. Of these, five began their naval careers in 1826, two in 1828, and four in 1829. Only Patton entered the service as a surgeon in 1831.

35. *Congressional Globe*, 25th Cong., 2d sess., 5:144.

36. U.S. Congress, *Annual Report of the Secretary of the Navy, 1830*, 188–89. Branch's report also contained information that the hospital at Sacket's Harbor, New York, was in a dilapidated state and totally unfit for use. Since there was no continuing naval need of the hospital or grounds, the Board of Navy Commissioners recommended that they be turned over to the Army. See John Rodgers to Branch, April 9, 1830, LBNC.

37. Chauncey to Branch, January 18, 1830, CL; Rodgers to Branch, February 2, 1831; Captain Charles Stewart, president of the Board of Navy Commissioners, to Woodbury, November 10, 1832, LBNC. According to the figures provided by Rodgers, the main building was estimated to cost $50,341.46, and each of the two side buildings, $26,194.57. Therefore, the total for the complete work should have been given as $102,731.60 instead of $102,750.

38. Elliott to Branch, February 4, 1830, CL.

39. Captain M. T. Woolsey to Branch, February 24, 1830, CL. In May 1829, Surgeon James Page reported to Woolsey that the "miserable huts that have been occupied as a temporary refuge for the sick" had become uninhabitable in warm weather and that there was a need for a hospital for 60–100 patients. See Page to Woolsey, May 27, 1829, John Rodgers Papers, ser. 3-A, vol. 9, LC. On the questions about repairs, see Rodgers to Branch, March 17, 1830, LBNC; Rodgers to the secretary of the navy, September 1, October 8, 13, 1830, LBNC.

40. *U.S. Statutes at Large*, 4:570; $20,000 was appropriated for the hospital at the Brooklyn Navy Yard, $25,000 for the one at Charlestown, Massachusetts, and $30,000 for Pensacola.

41. U.S. Congress, *Annual Report of the Secretary of the Navy, 1833*, 36.

42. Rodgers to Dickerson, March 16, 1836, LBNC. The board's estimates were broken down as follows: Chelsea, $19,380; Brooklyn, $30,500; Philadelphia, $30,000; Norfolk, $15,000; Pensacola, $58,000.

43. U.S. Congress, *Annual Reports of the Secretary of the Navy, 1839–1841.*

44. Ibid.

45. Naval medical officers to Andrew Jackson, undated but marked received February 8, 1837, OL.

46. Dickerson to Surgeon W. S. W. Ruschenberger, February 3, 1835, LO. A similar letter was sent to Surgeon William Plumbstead on March 19, 1835, LO.

47. Allan Millett, *Semper Fidelis*, 71–72; John K. Mahon, *History of the Second Seminole War*, 121–310.

Chapter 15
Health Problems, 1829–1842

1. Elliott to Branch, August 29, 1830, CL.

2. Chauncey to Branch, February 26, 1830; Barton to Ballard, March 10, 1830; an enclosure in Ballard to Branch, March 10, 1830, CL

3. Barton to Ballard, March 10, 1830, CL.

4. Ibid.

5. Ibid.

6. Ballard to Branch, April 3, 1830, CL, Barton to Branch, July 11, 1830, OL; William P. C. Barton, *Hints for Medical Officers Cruising in the West Indies*, 186, 203–05.

7. John Boyle, acting secretary, to Barton, July 13, 1830, LO; Barton to Ballard, July 15, 1830, Navy Department Records, Subject File, MS-Special Reports, box 189, RG 45, NA; Barton, *Hints for Medical Officers*, 202–4.

8. Barton to Branch, July 20, 1830, LO; Barton, *Hints for Medical Officers*, 176–85, 202–4.

9. Branch to Barton, August 23, 1830, LO; Branch to Bradford, August 10, 1830, Navy Department Records, Subject File, MA, RG 45, NA.

10. Barton, *Hints for Medical Officers*, 154, 195–98. The book was dedicated to Bradford.

11. Ibid., 10–11, 99–101.

12. Williamson to Bradford, July 3, 1830, Navy Department Records, Subject File, MA, RG 45, NA.

13. Barton to Bradford, August 10, 1830, Navy Department Records, Subject File, MA, RG 45, NA; Branch to Barton, September 2, 1830, LO; Barton to Bradford, September 9, 1830; Barton to Branch, September 30, 1830, OL.

14. Barton to Branch, October 22, November 22, 1830, OL.

15. Branch to Captain James Barron, February 15, 1831; Richmond C. Holcomb, *Century with the Norfolk Naval Hospital, 1830–1930*, 176.

16. Barton to Woodbury, June 10, 1833, OL; Acting Secretary John Boyle to Barton, June 12, 1833, LO.

17. Barton to Woodbury, December 16, 1833, OL; Woodbury to Barton, December 27, 1833, and enclosing the report of the Navy Commissioners, LO.

18. Dickerson to Barton, September 5, 1836, LO; Barton to Dickerson, September 6, 1836, OL; Robert Erwin Johnson, *Thence Round Cape Horn*, 48–51.

19. Rodgers to Woodbury, July 6, 1831, LBNC; Woodbury to the Board of Navy Commissioners, July 8, 1831, LO.

20. Barton to Paulding, June 1839, cited in Pleadwell, "William P. C. Barton," 290–91.

21. Bradford to Commodores Biddle and Elliott, June 23, September 3, 1829, LO; Sproston to Dodd, September 7, 1830; Dodd to Sproston, September 9, 1830; Sproston to Branch, October 26, 1830, OL.

22. Navy Department Records, Bureau of Medicine and Surgery, Hospital Tickets and Case Papers, RG 52, NA.

23. Barton to Branch, with an enclosure on Report of Patients in the U.S. Naval Hospital at Gosport, Va., December 14, 1830, December 18, 1830, OL.

24. Report of Patients from the U.S. Mediterranean Squadron on board the U.S. Ship *Lexington*, William N. Hunter, Esq., Commander, Hampton Roads Va., November 20, 1831, OL.

25. Return from the Hospital at Portsmouth, Va., for August 31, 1831; Quarterly Report of Diseases in the U.S. Ship St. Louis, April–June, 1830, Hospital Tickets and Case Papers, RG 52, NA.

26. Jonathan M. Foltz, "Medical Statistics of the U.S. Frigate *Potomac*," *New York Journal of Medicine* 1 (1843):189–207.

27. Constance Lathrop, "Vanished Ships," *USNIP* 60 (1934):949–51.

28. On the Wilkes Exploring Expedition see David B. Tyler, *Wilkes Expedition;* William Stanton, *Great United States Exploring Expedition of 1838–1842;* Herman J. Viola and Carolyn Margolies, eds., *Magnificent Voyagers;* Anne Hoffman Cleaver and E. Jeffrey Stann, eds., *Voyage to the Southern Ocean.* Wilkes's account is in his *Narrative of the United States Exploring Expedition During the Years 1838, 1839, 1840, 1841, 1842.* The letters of Wilkes to the secretary of the navy are collected in Records of the United States Exploring Expedition under the Command of Lt. Charles Wilkes, 1836–1842, M-75, NA. The manuscript journal of Surgeon Silas Holmes is in the Western Americana Collection, Beinecke Rare Book and Manuscript Library, Yale University, New Haven, Conn.

29. Holmes Journal.

30. Tyler, *Wilkes Expedition;* Stanton, *Great United States Exploring Expedition;* Viola and Margolies, *Magnificent Voyagers.*

Chapter 16
The Growth of Professionalism

1. USND, *Quasi-War,* 5:546–50.

2. USND, *Naval Regulations,* January 25, 1802, 16–17.

3. Woodbury to Dallas, January 24, 1832, LO; Dallas to Woodbury, February 26, 1832, CL; Woodbury to Dallas, March 13, 1832, LO; Bache to Dallas with enclosure, July 21, 1832, CL.

4. Woodbury to Commanders of Squadrons and Stations, March 27, 1834, LO.

5. Boyle to Dallas, April 1, 1831, LO.

6. For examples of men being vaccinated after 1815, see ante chap. 13–15.

7. Barton to Hamilton, November 9, 1811, OL; also, typescript copy in Navy Bureau of Medicine, Washington, D.C.

8. David S. Edwards Journal, David Shelton Edwards Papers, Armed Forces History Division, National Museum of American History, Smithsonian Institution.

9. Edward Cutbush, Thermometrical Journal, December 16, 1800–May 12, 1801, with letter of Cutbush to John Vaughan, librarian of the American Philosophical Society, July 10, 1801, American Philosophical Society Library, Philadelphia.

10. The article was in the form of a letter from Cowdery to Dr. Samuel L. Mitchell, May 10, 1809, and was published in *Medical Repository* 13 (1810):39–42.

11. Lewis Heermann, *Directions for the Medicine Chest.*

12. Barton, *Plan for Marine Hospitals*, 139–45; Pleadwell, "William P. C. Barton," 283–85.

13. Pleadwell, "William P. C. Barton," 285–86.

14. Thomas Harris, *Oration Delivered before the Philadelphia Medical Society, February 19, 1831;* Thomas Harris, "Case of Resection of the Elbow-joint," *Medical Examiner* 1 (1842):32–34, 38–39. In 1837, Harris published a biography of Commodore William Bainbridge. See Lewis H. Roddis, "Thomas Harris, M.D.," *Journal of the History of Medicine and Allied Sciences* 5 (1950):236–50.

15. Reynolds to Cutbush, July 6, 1825; Meehan to Cutbush, March 22, 1827, Edward Cutbush Papers, Library of Hobart and William Smith Colleges, Geneva, N.Y.

16. Usher Parsons, *Sailor's Physician;* Goldowsky, *Yankee Surgeon,* 150–52. It should be noted that while the Royal Navy began prescribing lemon juice as the best preventive of scurvy as early as 1795, Parsons was still adhering to the theory that acid was the proper therapy. This was understandable enough in the case of citrus fruits but not germane in the case of potatoes.

17. William S. W. Ruschenberger, *Three Years in the Pacific,* "Advertisement" preceding the introduction; Southard to Ruschenberger, July 10, 1827, Southard Letterbook, NYPL; Ruschenberger to Dr. Ward, May 21, 1889, William S. Ruschenberger Papers, Academy of Natural Sciences, Philadelphia.

18. Ruschenberger, *Three Years.*

19. Smith to New, November 8, 1805; Smith to Griffin, October 17, 1806, LO; Parsons to the Secretary of the Navy, January 30, 1818, OL.

20. Harris to Woodbury, January 30, 1833, OL.

21. Heermann to Smith, June 26, 1806, October 20, 1807, May 11, August 3, 1808, OL; Smith to Heermann, July 1, 1806; April 17, 1807, LO.

22. Goldowsky, *Yankee Surgeon,* 122–39; Frank Lester Pleadwell, "Usher Parsons (1788–1868)," *United States Naval Medical Bulletin* 17 (1922):436–41. For the introduction of the stethoscope in the United States, see Dale C. Smith, "Austin Flint and Auscultation in America," *Journal of the History of Medicine and Allied Sciences* 33 (1978):129–49.

23. Branch to Heermann, June 11, 1830, LO.

24. Pleadwell and Kerr, "Lewis Heermann," 142–45.

25. Philip A. Jordan, "Naval Surgeon in Paris, 1835–1836," *Annals of Medical History,* 3d ser., 2 (1940):526–36; 3 (1941):73–81.

26. For an account of the number of U.S. doctors who studied in Paris, see Russell M. Jones, "American Doctors and the Parisian Medical World, 1830–1840," *Bulletin of the History of Medicine* 47 (1973):40–65, 177–204. Jones has identified

222 American doctors who visited Paris during the decade of the 1830s, but virtually all were civilians. Of this total, 139 are known to have earned their M.D. degrees, most of them (54) from the University of Pennsylvania. Harvard was next (19), followed by the Medical College of South Carolina (14), the College of Physicians and Surgeons of New York (5), Transylvania University in Lexington, Ky. (4), and other medical schools (17).

There may have been a connection between these men and the doctors who later entered the navy. Of those known to have been in Paris, only Lewis Wolfley can be identified as a naval officer. But as Jones notes, it is impossible to know for sure just how many Americans studied in Paris because most did not take the diploma but attended lectures and visited clinics without paying the fees required for formal enrollment. Also, Americans paid for private instruction, but there are no records of the number. Depending on the duration of their leaves, naval medical officers were most likely to audit courses and visit clinics rather than take private instruction. For additional details of the influence of study in Paris, see Erwin H. Ackerknecht, *Medicine at the Paris Hospital, 1794–1848;* John Harley Warner, "Selective Transport of Medical Knowledge," *Bulletin of the History of Medicine* 59 (1985):213–31; Warner "Remembering Paris," *Bulletin of the History of Medicine* 65 (1991):301–25.

Chapter 17
Establishment of the Bureau of Medicine and Surgery

1. U.S. Congress, Annual Report of the Secretary of the Navy for 1840, passim; USND, *Navy Register 1840* (Washington, 1840).

2. Harry Bluff (Matthew F. Maury), "Scraps From the Lucky Bag, No. IV," *Southern Literary Messenger* 7 (1841):22–23.

3. Ibid.

4. U.S. Congress, *Annual Report of the Secretary of the Navy, 1840,* 22.

5. Ibid., *1841,* 353.

6. For background, see Langley, *Social Reform,* 229–38; *U.S. Statutes at Large,* 5:546.

7. *U.S. Statutes at Large,* 5:537.

8. Upshur to Dunbar, July 21, 1842, ML.

9. U.S. Congress, *Annual Report of the Secretary of the Navy, 1841,* 357; Claude H. Hall, *Abel Parker Upshur,* 136–37, 151.

10. *House Journal,* 27th Cong., 2d sess. (Serial 400), 343, 1231, 1454–44, 1470; *Senate Journal,* 27th Cong., 2d sess. (Serial 394) 405, 455, 548, 643, 645, 647–48, 654.

11. *U.S. Statutes at Large,* 5:579.

12. Pleadwell, "William P. C. Barton," 293.

13. During 1800–14, two-thirds of the navy's midshipmen came from the region between New York and Virginia, with Maryland, Virginia, and the District of Columbia contributing a little more than one-third of the total and New York, New Jersey, Pennsylvania, and Delaware supplying slightly less than one-third. See McKee, *Gentlemanly and Honorable Profession,* 59.

Bibliography

National Archives

General Accounting Office (formerly Treasury Department) Records. RG 217.

Letterbook of the Accountant of the Navy.
Letters Received by the Accountant of the Navy.
Records of the Fourth Auditor.

Legislative Branch Records.

U.S. House of Representatives. RG 233.
U.S. Senate. RG 46.

Marine Corps Records. RG 127.

Letterbooks of the Commandant of the Marine Corps.
Letters Received by the Commandant of the Marine Corps.

Navy Department Records.

Abstracts of Service of Naval Officers. Microcopy M-330.
Acceptances of Appointments by Officers. RG 45.
Area Files. M-625.
Board of Navy Commissioners. RG 45.
Bureau of Medicine and Surgery. RG 52.
Correspondence on Naval Affairs When the Navy Was under the War Department, 1794–98. M-739.
General Courts-Martial and Courts of Inquiry. M-273.
General Letterbook (Miscellaneous Letters Sent by the Secretary of the Navy). M-209.
General Orders and Circulars of the Secretary of the Navy. M-977.
Letters from the Secretary of the Navy to Commandants and Navy Agents. M-441.
Letters from the Secretary of the Navy to Congress. RG 45.
Letters of the Secretary of the Navy to Officers. M-149.
Letters Received by the Secretary of the Navy: Captains' Letters. M-125.
Letters Received by the Secretary of the Navy: Commanders' Letters. M-147.
Letters Received by the Secretary of the Navy from Officers below the Rank of Commander: Officers' Letters. M-148.
Miscellaneous Letters Received by the Secretary of the Navy. M-124.
Muster and Pay Rolls. RG 45.
Preble, George H. "History of the Boston Navy Yard, 1797–1874." M-118.
Resignations. RG 45.

Ships' Logs. RG 24.
Subject Files. RG 45.

State Department Records.

Despatches from the U.S. Consuls at Genoa. Microcopy T-64
Despatches from the U.S. Consuls at Gibraltar. T-206

Treasury Department Records.

Correspondence of the Secretary of the Treasury with Collectors of Customs. M-178.
Prescription Book of the U.S. Marine Hospital at Charlestown, Mass., 1816. RG 90.

Manuscripts

Adams, John. Papers. Microfilm, Massachusetts Historical Society, Boston. 1799–1800.
Barron, James. Papers. Swem Library, College of William and Mary, Williamsburg, Va.
Barry, John. Public and Private Correspondence of Commodore John Barry. John Sanford Barnes Collection. New York Historical Society, New York.
Biographical Information on American Navy Officers. Navy Operational Archives, Naval Historical Center, Washington Navy Yard, Washington, D.C.
Boyce, Thomas. Journal. New Jersey Historical Society, Newark.
Chauncey, Isaac. Letterbooks 1809–1815. New York Historical Society, New York.
———. Letterbooks 1812–1817. William L. Clements Library, Ann Arbor, Mich.
Clarke, William M. Journal. New York Public Library, New York.
Crabbe, Thomas. Journal Kept While on the *Hornet* [1815]. Library, U.S. Military Academy, West Point, N.Y.
Crowninshield, Benjamin W. Papers. Peabody Museum, Salem, Mass.
Cutbush, Edward. Thermometrical Journal, December 16, 1800–May 12, 1801, with letter of Edward Cutbush to John Vaughan, librarian of the American Philosophical Society, July 10, 1801. American Philosophical Society Library, Philadelphia.
———. Manuscripts. Josiah Trent Collection. Medical Center Library. Duke University, Durham, N.C.
———. Papers. Library of Hobart and William Smith Colleges, Geneva, N.Y.
Dale, Richard. Letterbook [1802]. Nimitz Library, U.S. Naval Academy, Annapolis, Md.
Dickerson, Mahlon. Papers. New Jersey Historical Society, Newark.
Dodd, Robert J. Papers. College of Physicians of Philadelphia Library, Philadelphia.
Dreer Collection. Historical Society of Pennsylvania, Philadelphia.
Du Barry, Beekman. Papers. Library, U.S. Military Academy, West Point, N.Y.
Edwards, David Shelton. Papers. Armed Forces History Division, National Museum of American History, Smithsonian Institution, Washington, D.C.

Evans, Amos. Medical Prescription Book Kept on Board U.S. Frigate *Constitution*. Yale Medical Library, Yale University, New Haven, Conn.

Foltz, Jonathan M. Papers. Franklin and Marshall College, Lancaster, Pa.

Gauntt, Lieutenant Charles. Macedonian Journal. Library of Congress, Washington, D.C.

Gillasspy, George.' Notebook. Rare Book Room, Van Pelt Library, University of Pennsylvania, Philadelphia.

Gratz Collection. Historical Society of Pennsylvania, Philadelphia.

Guillou, Charles Fleury Bienaimé. Papers, 1813–99. College of Physicians, of Philadelphia Library, Philadelphia.

Harbeck, Charles Thomas. Papers. Huntington Library, San Marino, Calif.

Harwood Family Papers. Green Library, Stanford University, Palo Alto, Calif.

Henry, Isaac. Papers. William R. Perkins Library, Duke University, Durham, N.C.

Holmes, Silas. Journal. Beinecke Library, Yale University, New Haven, Conn.

Horner, Gustavus. Papers. Library of Congress, Washington, D.C.

———. Papers. Alderman Library, University of Virginia, Charlottesville.

———. Papers. Virginia Historical Society, Richmond.

Jefferson, Thomas. Papers. Microfilm. Library of Congress, Washington, D.C.

Jones, William. Papers. Uselma Clark Smith Collection, Historical Society of Pennsylvania, Philadelphia.

Kearney, Lawrence. "Remarks on Board U.S. Brig Enterprise [1821]." Huntington Library, San Marino, Calif.

Log of the USS *Constitution* [1800–1801]. U.S. Naval Academy Museum, Annapolis, Md.

Morris, Charles. Papers. Chicago Historical Society, Chicago, Il.

Muster Rolls of the Officers and Men Attached to the New York Navy Yard and to the Gunboat Flotilla Based at New York, 1813–15. Nimitz Library, U.S. Naval Academy, Annapolis, Md.

Nicholson, J. B. Journal [1819–20]. Huntington Library, San Marino, Calif.

Orders and Regulations for the Government of the U.S. Ship *Washington*, 1817. Armed Forces History Division, Smithsonian Institution, Washington, D.C.

Parsons, Usher. Journals. Rhode Island Historical Society, Providence.

———. Papers. John Hay Library, Brown University, Providence, R.I.

Perry, Oliver Hazard. Papers. William L. Clements Library, Ann Arbor, Mich.

Pickering, Timothy. Journal [1800–1801]. Nimitz Library, U.S. Naval Academy, Annapolis, Md.

Preble, Edward. Papers. Library of Congress, Washington, D.C.

———. Collection. New England Historical and Genealogical Society, Boston.

President's Naval Collection. Franklin D. Roosevelt Library, Hyde Park, N.Y.

Ridgely, Charles O. "Remarks on Board the U.S. Frigate *Constitution* [1830]." Huntington Library, San Marino, Calif.

Rodgers, John. Papers. New York Historical Society, New York.

Rodgers Family. Papers. Library of Congress, Washington, D.C.

Ruschenberger, William S. W. Collection. American Philosophical Society, Philadelphia, Pa.

———. Papers, 1807–95. Academy of Natural Sciences, Philadelphia.

Rush, Benjamin. Manuscript Correspondence. Library Company of Philadelphia Collection, Historical Society of Pennsylvania, Philadelphia.

Sever, James. Papers. Library of Congress, Washington, D.C.

Shaw, John. Papers. Naval Historical Collection. Library of Congress, Washington, D.C.

Southard, Samuel L. Letterbook [1826–28]. New York Public Library, New York.

———. Papers. Princeton University Library, Princeton, N.J.

Spence-Lowell Collection. Huntington Library, San Marino, Calif.

Talbot, Silas. Papers. G. W. Blunt White Library, Mystic Seaport, Mystic, Conn.

Ticknor, Benajah. Papers. Yale University Library, New Haven, Conn.

Toner, Joseph M. Collection. Library of Congress, Washington, D.C.

War of 1812 Collection. Lilly Library, Indiana University, South Bend.

War of 1812 Collection. William L. Clements Library, Ann Arbor, Mich.

Washington, Bailey. Prescriptions [ca. 1810–54]. Armed Forces History Division, Smithsonian Institution, Washington, D.C.

Wiesenthal, Thomas. Medical and Surgical Journal on Board the Frigate *Java* [1816]. New York Historical Society, New York.

Woodbury, Levi. Papers. Library of Congress, Washington, D.C.

Yellow Fever Papers. College of Physicians, of Philadelphia Library, Philadelphia.

Printed Documents

Claiborne, William C. C. *Official Letterbooks of William C. C. Claiborne, 1801–1816*. Edited by Dunbar Roland. 6 vols. Jackson: Mississippi Department of Archives and History, 1917.

DePauw, Linda Grant, *et al.*, eds. *Documentary History of the First Federal Congress of the United States of America*. 11 vols. to date. Baltimore: Johns Hopkins University Press, 1972–.

Dudley, William S., ed. *The Naval War of 1812: A Documentary History*. 2 vols. to date. Washington, D.C.: GPO, 1985–.

Goldsborough, Charles W. *The United States Naval Chronicle*. Washington, D.C.: James Wilson, 1824.

Hamilton, Alexander. *The Papers of Alexander Hamilton*. Edited by Harold C. Syrett. 27 vols. New York: Columbia University Press, 1961–87.

Harris, Doris. *Distinguished Autographs Catalog No. 24*. Los Angeles: Doris Harris Autographs, December 1978.

Hening, William Waller, comp. *The Statutes at Large, Being a Collection of the Laws of Virginia*. 13 vols. Richmond, Va.: Samuel Pleasants Jr.,

Jefferson, Thomas. *The Papers of Thomas Jefferson*. Edited by Julian P. Boyd et al. 24 volumes to date. Princeton: Princeton University Press, 1950–.

Latrobe, Benjamin H. *Correspondence and Miscellaneous Papers of Benjamin Henry Latrobe*. Edited by John C. Van Horne. 3 vols. New Haven: Yale University Press, 1984–88.

Kurland, Philip R., and Gerhard Casper, eds. *Landmark Briefs and Arguments of the Supreme Court of the United States: Constitutional Law*. 81 vols. to date. Washington, D.C.: University Publications of America, 1975–.

Miller, Hunter, ed. *Treaties and Other International Acts of the United States of America, 1776–1863.* 8 vols. Washington, D.C.: GPO, 1931–48.

Palmer, William, ed. and comp. *Calendar of Virginia State Papers and other Manuscripts . . . Preserved . . . at Richmond.* 11 vols. Richmond, Va.: R. F. Walker, Publisher, 1875–93.

Rowland, Dunbar, ed. *The Mississippi Territorial Archives, 1798–1803.* Nashville, Tenn.: Brandon Printing Co., 1905.

U.S. Commerce Department. *Historical Statistics of the United States, Colonial Times to 1970.* 2 vols. Washington, D.C.: GPO, 1975.

U.S. Congress. *American State Papers: Documents, Legislative and Executive.* 38 vols. Washington, D.C.: Gales & Seaton, 1832–61.

———. *Annals of Congress. Debates and Proceedings in the Congress of the United States, 1789–1824.* 42 vols. Washington, D.C. Gales & Seaton, 1834–56.

———. *Annual Reports of the Secretary of the Navy, 1824–1842.* U.S. Navy Department Library, Washington, D.C.

———. *Congressional Globe, Containing the Debates and Proceedings, 1833–1842.* Washington, D.C., 1833–42.

———. House *Journal* 5th–27th Congresses, 1797–1842.

———. *Journals of the Continental Congress, 1774–1789.* Edited by Worthington C. Ford et al. 34 vols. Washington, D.C.: GPO, 1904–37.

———. *The Public Statutes at Large of the United States of America.* Compiled by Richard Peters. 8 vols. Boston: Little, Brown & Company, 1845–46.

———. *Register of Debates in Congress, 1825–1837.* 29 vols. Washington, D.C., 1825–37.

———. Senate *Journals,* 5th–27th Congresses, 1797–1842.

———. *U.S. Statutes at Large,* 1789–1842.

U. S. Navy Department. *Naval Documents Related to the Quasi-War between the United States and France.* 7 vols. Washington, D.C.: GPO, 1935–38.

———. *Naval Documents Related to the United States Wars with the Barbary Powers.* 7 vols. Washington, D.C.: GPO, 1939–45.

———. *Naval Regulations Issued by Command of the President of the United States of America, January 25, 1802.* Washington, D. C.: Way & Groff, 1802. Reprint, Annapolis, Md.: Naval Institute Press, 1970.

———. *Navy Register, 1819.* Washington, D.C.: Wade & Co., 1819.

———. *Navy Register, 1820.* Washington, D.C.: Davis & Force, 1820.

———. *Navy Register, 1822.* Washington, D.C.: Jacob Gideon, Printer, 1822.

———. *Navy Register, 1824.* Washington, D.C.: Gales & Seaton, 1824.

———. *Navy Register, 1826.* Washington, D.C.: Way & Gideon, 1826.

———. *Navy Register, 1832.* Washington, D.C.: F. P. Blair, 1832.

———. *Navy Register, 1835.* Washington, D.C.: B. Homans, 1835.

———. *Navy Register, 1840.* Washington, D.C.: Jacob Gideon Jr., 1840.

———. *Navy Register, 1841.* Washington, D.C.: Jacob Gideon Jr., 1841.

———. *Navy Register, 1842.* Washington, D.C.: Alexander & Barnard, 1842.

Wheelwright, Charles H. *Correspondence of Dr. Charles H. Wheelwright, Surgeon of the United States Navy, 1813–1862.* Edited by Hildegarde B. Forbes. Boston: Privately printed, 1958.

Books

Abernethy, Thomas Perkins. *The Burr Conspiracy.* New York: Oxford University Press, 1954.

Ackerknecht, Erwin H. *Medicine at the Paris Hospital, 1794–1848.* Baltimore: Johns Hopkins Press, 1967.

Allen, Gardner W. *Our Navy and the Barbary Corsairs.* Cambridge: Harvard University Press, 1905.

———. *Our Navy and the West Indian Pirates.* Salem, Mass., Essex Institute, 1929.

Allison, R. S. *Sea Diseases. The Story of a Great Natural Experiment in Preventive Medicine in the Royal Navy.* London: John Bale Medical Publications, 1943.

Altoff, Gerard T. *Deep Water Sailors, Shallow Water Soldiers: Manning the United States Fleet on Lake Erie, 1813.* Put-in-Bay, Perry Group, 1993.

Anderson, Roger C. *Naval Wars in the Levant, 1559–1853.* Princeton: Princeton University Press, 1952.

Auchinleck, Gilbert. *A History of the War between Great Britain and the United States of America During the Years 1812, 1813, and 1814.* Toronto, 1885. Reprint, Toronto and Redwood City, Calif.: Arms and Armour Press and Pendragon House, 1972.

Baker, William A. *A History of the Boston Marine Society, 1742–1967.* Boston: Boston Marine Society, 1968.

Barnes, William, and John Heath Morgan. *The Foreign Service of the United States, Origins, Development, and Functions.* Washington, D.C.: GPO, 1961.

Barton, William P. C. *A Polemical Remonstrance Against the Project of Creating a New Office of the Surgeon General of the United States: . . . .* Philadelphia: Privately printed, 1838.

———. *A Treatise Containing a Plan for the Internal Organization and Government of Marine Hospitals in the United States, Together With a Scheme for Amending and Systematizing the Medical Department of the Navy.* 2d ed. Philadelphia: Privately printed, 1817.

———. *Hints for Medical Officers Cruising in the West Indies.* Philadelphia: E. Littel, 1830.

Bearss, Edwin C. *Charlestown Navy Yard, 1800–1842: Historic Resource Study.* Boston: Boston National Historic Park, Mass., 1984.

———. *Fort Barrancas, Gulf Islands National Seashore, Florida.* Washington, D.C.: U.S. Department of the Interior, National Park Service, 1983.

Bemis, Samuel Flagg. *A Diplomatic History of the United States.* 5th ed. New York: Holt, Rinehart, & Winston, 1965.

Benes, Peter, ed. *Medicine and Healing: The Dublin Seminar for New England Folklife.* Boston: Boston University, 1992.

Berton, Pierre. *Flames across the Border, 1813–1814.* Boston: Little, Brown & Co., 1981.

———. *The Invasion of Canada, 1812–1813.* Boston: Little, Brown & Co., 1980.

Billingsley, Edward Baxter. *In Defense of Neutral Rights: The United States Navy in the Wars of Independence in Chili and Peru.* Chapel Hill: University of North Carolina Press, 1967.

Bird, Harrison. *War for the West, 1790–1813.* New York: Oxford University Press, 1971.

Blake, John Ballard. *Public Health in the Town of Boston, 1630–1882.* Cambridge: Harvard University Press, 1959.

Blane, Sir Gilbert. *Observations on the Diseases Incident to Seamen.* 3d ed. London: Murray & Highley, 1799.

Blanton, Wyndham B. *Medicine in Virginia in the Eighteenth Century.* Richmond, Va.: Garrett & Massie, 1931.

———. *Medicine in Virginia in the Nineteenth Century.* Richmond, Va.: Garrett & Massie, 1933.

Bradlee, Francis B. C. *Piracy in the West Indies and Its Suppression.* Salem, Mass.: Essex Institute, 1923. Reprint, Mystic, Conn.: Mystic Seaport, 1970.

Brant, Irving. *James Madison: Secretary of State, 1800–1809.* Indianapolis: Bobbs-Merrill Co., 1953.

———. *James Madison: President, 1809–1812.* Indianapolis: Bobbs-Merrill Co., 1956.

———. *James Madison: Commander in Chief, 1812–1836.* Indianapolis: Bobbs-Merrill Co., 1961.

Brooks, Charles B. *The Siege of New Orleans.* Seattle: University of Washington Press, 1961.

Brown, Wilburt S. *The Amphibious Campaign for West Florida and Louisiana, 1814–1815: A Critical Review of Strategy and Tactics at New Orleans.* Tuscaloosa: University of Alabama Press, 1969.

Buker, George E. *Swamp Sailors: Riverine Warfare in the Everglades, 1835–1842.* Gainesville: University Press of Florida, 1975.

Butt, Marshall W. *Early Portsmouth Physicians, 1761–1906: A Trial List with Brief Biographies.* Portsmouth, Va.: Portsmouth Academy of Medicine, 1969.

Butterfield, Lyman H., ed. *Letters of Benjamin Rush.* 3 vols. Princeton: Princeton University Press, 1956.

Cain, Emily. *Ghost Ships: "Hamilton" and "Scourge": Historical Treasure from the War of 1812.* Toronto: Beaufort Books, 1983.

Callahan, Edward W., ed. *List of Officers of the Navy of the United States and of the Marine Corps From 1775 to 1900.* New York: L. R. Hamersly & Co., 1901.

Callan, John F., and A. W. Russell. *Laws of the U.S. Relating to the Navy and Marine Corps.* Baltimore: John Murphy & Co., 1859.

Carpenter, Kenneth J. *The History of Scurvy and Vitamin C.* Cambridge: Cambridge University Press, 1988.

Cash, Philip, eds. *Medicine in Colonial Massachusetts, 1620–1820.* Boston: Colonial Society of Massachusetts, 1980.

Cassar, Paul. *Medical History of Malta.* London: Wellcome Historical Medical Library, 1964.

Cassedy, James H. *Medicine and American Growth.* Madison: University of Wisconsin Press, 1986.

Clark, John G. *New Orleans, 1718–1812: An Economic History.* Baton Rouge: Louisiana State University Press, 1970.

Clark, William Bell. *Gallant John Barry, 1745–1803.* New York: Macmillan Co., 1938.

Cleaver, Anne Hoffman, and E. Jeffery Stann, eds. *Voyage to the Southern Ocean: The Letters of Lieutenant William Reynolds from the U.S. Exploring Expedition, 1838–1842.* Annapolis, Md.: Naval Institute Press, 1988.

Clowes, William Laird. *The Royal Navy: A History from the Earliest Times to the Present.* 7 vols. London: Sampson, Low, Marston and Co., 1901.

Cogar, William B., ed. *New Interpretations in Naval History: The Eighth Sympo-sium of the U.S. Naval Academy.* Wilmington, Del.: Scholarly Resources, 1988.

Cohen, I. Bernard, ed. *The Life and Scientific and Medical Career of Benjamin Waterhouse: With Some Account of the Introduction of Vaccination in America.* 2 vols. New York: Arno Press, 1980.

Coles, Harry L. *The War of 1812.* Chicago: University of Chicago Press, 1965.

Coletta, Paolo, E. ed. *American Secretaries of the Navy.* 2 vols. Annapolis, Md.: Naval Institute Press, 1980.

Columbia University. *Columbia University Alumni Register, 1794–1931.* New York: Columbia University Press, 1932.

Cooper, James Fenimore. *History of the Navy of the United States of America.* 3 vols. in 1. New York: G. P. Putnam & Co., 1854.

Cordell, Eugene F. *Medical Annals of Maryland, 1799–1899.* Baltimore: Press of Williams & Wilkins Co., 1900.

Corner, George W. *Two Centuries of Medicine. A History of the School of Medicine, University of Pennsylvania.* Philadelphia: J. B. Lippincott Co., 1965.

Cowdery, Jonathan. *American Captives in Tripoli: or, Dr. Cowdery's Journal in Miniature Kept During His Late Captivity in Tripoli.* Boston: Belcher & Arm-strong, 1806.

Cunningham, Noble E., Jr. *The Process of Government under Jefferson.* Princeton: Princeton University Press, 1987.

Cutbush, Edward. *Observations on the Means of Preserving the Health of Soldiers and Sailors; and on the Duties of the Medical Department of the Army and the Navy: With Remarks on Hospitals and Their Internal Arrangement.* Philadel-phia: Fry & Kammerer, Printers, 1808.

Davis, Audrey, and Toby Appel. *Bloodletting Instruments in the National Museum of History and Technology.* Smithsonian Studies in History and Technology, no. 41. Washington, D.C.: Smithsonian Institution Press, 1979.

Davis, N. S. *Medical Education and Medical Institutions in the U.S.A., 1776–1867.* Washington, D.C.: U.S. Bureau of Education, 1877.

De Conde, Alexander. *The Quasi-War: The Politics and Diplomacy of the Unde-clared War with France.* New York: Charles Scribner's Sons, 1966.

Department of History, U.S. Naval Academy, eds. *New Aspects of Naval History.* Baltimore: Nautical and Aviation Publishing Co. of America, 1985.

Dobbins, Captain W. W., comp. *History of the Battle of Lake Erie (September 10, 1813) and Reminiscences of the Flagships "Lawrence" and "Niagara."* 2d ed. Erie: Ashby Printing Co., Publishers, 1913.

Duffy, John. *The Healers: A History of American Medicine.* New York: McGraw-Hill Book Co., 1976. Reprint, Urbana: University of Illinois Press, 1979.

———. *A History of Public Health in New York City, 1625–1866*. New York: Russell Sage Foundation, 1968.

Duignan, Peter, and Clarence Clendenen. *The United States and the African Slave Trade, 1619–1862*. Palo Alto, Calif.: Hoover Institution, 1963.

Dunglison, Robley. *A Dictionary of Medical Science*. 7th ed. Philadelphia: Lea & Blanchard, 1848.

Eckert, Edward K. *The Navy Department in the War of 1812*. Gainesville: University of Florida Press, 1973.

Egle, William H. *An Illustrated History of the Commonwealth of Pennsylvania Civil, Political, and Military, From the Earliest Settlement Until the Present Time*. Harrisburg, Pa.: De Witt C. Goodrich & Co., 1876.

Emmerson, John C., comp. *The Chesapeake Affair of 1807*. Portsmouth, Va.: Privately printed, 1954.

Estes, J. Worth. *The Changing Humors of Portsmouth: The Medical Biography of an American Town, 1623–1983*. Boston: Francis A. Countway Library of Medicine, 1986.

———. *Dictionary of Protopharmcology: Therapeutic Practices, 1700–1850*. Canton, Mass.: Science History Publications/USA, 1990.

Evans, Amos A. *Journal Kept on Board the Frigate "Constitution," 1812, by Amos A. Evans, Surgeon, U.S.N.* Reprinted from the *Pennsylvania Magazine of History and Biography* for William D. Sawtell. Concord: Bankers Lithograph Co., 1967.

Evans, Stephen H. *The United States Coast Guard, 1790–1915: A Definitive History*. Annapolis, Md.: Naval Institute Press, 1949.

Everest, Allan S. *The War of 1812 in the Champlain Valley*. Syracuse, N.Y.: Syracuse University Press, 1981.

Ewell, Thomas. *Conclusion of the Evidence of the Corruption of the Chief Clerk of the Navy Department*. Washington, D.C.: Privately printed, 1813.

———. *The Planter's and Mariner's Medical Companion*. 3d ed. Philadelphia: Andrew & Meehan, 1816.

Farnam, Henry W. *Chapters in the History of Social Legislation in the United States to 1860*. Washington, D.C.: Carnegie Institute, 1938.

Fenner, Frank, et al. *Smallpox and Its Eradication*. Geneva: World Health Organization, 1988.

Ferguson, Eugene S. *Truxtun of the "Constellation": The Life of Commodore Truxtun, United States Navy, 1755–1822*. Baltimore: Johns Hopkins Press, 1956.

Field, James A., Jr. *America and the Mediterranean World, 1776–1882*. Princeton: Princeton University Press, 1969.

Fleming, James Roger. *Meteorology in America, 1800–1870*. Baltimore: Johns Hopkins Press, 1940.

Fowler, William M., Jr. *Jack Tars and Commodores: The American Navy, 1783–1815*. Boston: Houghton Mifflin Co., 1984.

Gillett, Mary C. *The Army Medical Department, 1775–1818*. Washington, D.C.: GPO, 1987.

———. *The Army Medical Department, 1818–1865*. Washington, D.C.: GPO, 1987.

Gilpin, Alex. R. *The War of 1812 in the Old Northwest*. East Lansing: Michigan State University Press, 1958.

Goldberg, Isaac. *Major Noah: American-Jewish Pioneer.* New York: Alfred A. Knopf, 1937.

Goldowsky, Seebert J. *Yankee Surgeon: The Life and Times of Usher Parsons, 1788–1868.* Boston: Francis A. Countway Library of Medicine, 1988.

Gordon, Maurice Bear. *Aescualpius Comes to the Colonies: The Story of the Early Days of Medicine in the Thirteen Original Colonies.* Ventnor, N.J.: Ventnor Publishing, 1949.

Greeley, Augustus W. *Public Documents of Early Congresses.* Washington, D.C.: GPO, 1897.

Griffenhagen, George B., and James Harvey Young. *Old English Patent Medicines in America.* U.S. National Museum Bulletin 218, paper 10. Washington: Smithsonian Institution, 1959.

Griffin, Charles Carroll. *The United States and the Disruption of the Spanish Empire, 1810–1822: A Study of the Relations of the United States with Spain and with the Rebel Spanish Colonies.* New York: Columbia University Press, 1937. Reprint,: New York, Octagon Books, 1974.

Hall, Claude H. *Abel Parker Upshur, Conservative Virginian, 1790–1844.* Madison: State Historical Society of Wisconsin, 1964.

Hammond, Bray. *Banks and Politics in America from the Revolution to the Civil War.* Princeton: Princeton University Press, 1957.

Harrington, Thomas F. *The Harvard Medical School.* 3 vols. New York: Lewis Publishing Co., 1905.

Harris, Thomas. *An Oration Delivered Before the Philadelphia Medical Society, February 19, 1831.* Philadelphia: James Kay, Jr., & Co., 1831.

Heermann, Lewis. *Directions for the Medicine Chest.* New Orleans: John Morry & Co., 1811.

Heitman, Francis B. *Historical Register and Dictionary of the United States Army from Its Organization, September 29, 1789 to March 2, 1903.* Philadelphia: L. R. Hammersly, 1901.

Hitsman, J. Mackay. *The Incredible War of 1812: A Military History.* Toronto: University of Toronto Press, 1965.

Holcomb, Richmond C. *A Century with Norfolk Naval Hospital.* Portsmouth, Va.: Printcraft Publishing Co., 1930.

Hopkins, Donald R. *Princes and Peasants: Smallpox in History.* Chicago: University of Chicago Press, 1983.

Hopkins, Fred N., and Donald B Shomette. *War on the Patuxent, 1814: A Catalog of Artifacts.* Solomons, Md.: Calvert Marine Museum, 1981.

Horsman, Reginald. *The War of 1812.* New York: Alfred A. Knopf, 1969.

Hoxse, John. *The Yankee Tar: Authentic Narrative of Voyage and Hardships of John Hoxse, and Cruise of U.S. Frigate Constellation.* Northampton, Mass.: J. Metcalf, 1840.

Irwin, Ray W. *The Diplomatic Relations of the United States with the Barbary Powers, 1776–1816.* Chapel Hill: University of North Carolina Press, 1931.

Jacobs, James Ripley. *The Beginnings of the U.S. Army, 1783–1812.* Princeton: Princeton University Press, 1947.

Jensen, Merrill. *The New Nation: A History of the United States During the Confederation, 1781–1789.* New York: Alfred A. Knopf, 1950.

Johnson, Robert Erwin. *Thence Round Cape Horn. The Story of the United States Naval Forces on Pacific Station, 1818–1923.* Annapolis, Md.: Naval Institute Press, 1963.

Keevil, J. J, Christopher Lloyd, and Jack L. S. Coulter. *Medicine and the Navy, 1200–1900.* 4 vols. Edinburgh: E. & S. Livingstone, 1957–63.

Kelly, Howard A., and Walter L. Burrage. *American Medical Biographies.* Baltimore: Norman Remington Co., 1920.

Ketcham, Ralph. *James Madison: A Biography.* Paperback ed. Charlottesville: University Press of Virginia, 1990.

King, Lester S., ed. *A History of Medicine: Selected Readings.* London: Penguin Books, 1971.

Kiple, Kenneth F., ed. *The Cambridge World History of Human Disease.* New York: Cambridge University Press, 1993.

Langley, Harold D. *Social Reform in the U.S. Navy, 1798–1862.* Urbana: University of Illinois Press, 1967.

La Roche, René. *Yellow Fever Considered in its Historical, Pathological, Etiological and Therapeutical Aspects.* 2 vols. Philadelphia: Blanchard & Lee, 1855.

Lloyd, Christopher, ed. *The Health of Seamen: Selections from the Works of Dr. James Lind, Sir Gilbert Blane, and Dr. Thomas Trotter.* London: Navy Records Society, 1965.

Long, David F. *Gold Braid and Foreign Relations: Diplomatic Activities of U.S. Naval Officers, 1798–1883.* Annapolis, Md.: Naval Institute Press, 1988.

———. *Nothing Too Daring: A Biography of Commodore David Porter, 1780–1843.* Annapolis, Md.: Naval Institute Press, 1970.

———. *Sailor Diplomat: A Biography of Commodore James Biddle, 1783–1848.* Boston: Northeastern University Press, 1983.

Lord, Walter. *The Dawn's Early Light.* New York: W. W. Norton & Co., 1972.

Lossing, Benson J. *The Pictorial Field Book of the War of 1812.* New York: Harper Brothers, Publishers, 1869.

Mahan, Alfred T. *Sea Power in Its Relations to the War of 1812.* 2 vols. London: Sampson Low, Marston & Co., 1905.

Mahon, John K. *History of the Second Seminole War, 1835–1842.* Gainsville: University of Florida Press, 1967.

———. *The War of 1812: A Military History.* Gainesville: University of Florida Press, 1972.

Malcomson, Robert, and Thomas, Malcomson. *HMS "Detroit": The Battle for Lake Erie.* Annapolis, Md.: Naval Institute Press, 1990.

Malone, Dumas. *Jefferson the President: First Term, 1801–1805.* Boston: Little Brown & Co., 1974.

———. *Jefferson the President: Second Term, 1805–1809.* Boston: Little Brown & Co., 1974.

Maloney, Linda M. *The Captain from Connecticut: The Life and Naval Times of Isaac Hull.* Boston: Northeastern University Press, 1986.

Marks, Frederick W., III. *Independence on Trial: Foreign Affairs and the Making of the Constitution.* Baton Rouge: Louisiana State University Press, 1973.

Marti-Ibanez, Felix, ed. *Henry E. Sigerist on the History of Medicine.* New York: MD Publications, 1960.

————. *History of American Medicine: A Symposium.* New York: MD Publications, 1959.

Martin, Tyrone G. *A Most Fortunate Ship.* Chester, Conn.: Globe Pequot Press, 1980.

Masterson, Daniel M., ed. *Naval History: The Sixth Symposium of the U.S. Naval Academy.* Wilmington, Del.: Scholarly Resources, 1987.

McKee, Christopher. *A Gentlemanly and Honorable Profession: The Creation of the U.S. Naval Officer Corps, 1794–1815.* Annapolis, Md.: Naval Institute Press, 1991.

————. *Edward Preble: A Naval Biography, 1761–1807.* Annapolis, Md.: Naval Institute Press, 1972.

Millett, Allan R. *Semper Fidelis: The History of the United States Marine Corps.* New York: Macmillan Publishing Co., 1980.

Moore, Glover. *The Missouri Controversy, 1819–1821.* Lexington: University of Kentucky Press, 1966.

Norwood, William F. *Medical Education in the United States before the Civil War.* Philadelphia: University of Pennsylvania Press, 1944.

Owsley, Frank L., Jr. *Struggle for the Gulf Borderlands: The Creek War and the Battle of New Orleans, 1812–1815.* Gainesville: University of Florida Press, 1981.

Pack, James. *The Man Who Burned the White House: Admiral Sir George Cockburn, 1772–1853.* Annapolis, Md.: Naval Institute Press, 1987.

Palmer, Michael A. *Stoddert's War: Naval Operations During the Quasi-War with France, 1798–1801.* Columbia: University of South Carolina Press, 1987.

Parsons, Usher. *Battle of Lake Erie: A Discourse Delivered Before the Rhode Island Historical Society on February 16, 1853.* Palmyra, N.Y.: Benjamin T. Albro, Printer, 1854.

————. *The Sailor's Physician, Containing Medical Advice, for Seamen and other Persons at Sea, on the Treatment of Diseases, and on the Preservation of Health in Sickly Climates.* 2d ed. Providence, R.I.: 1824.

Paullin, Charles Oscar. *Commodore John Rodgers: Captain, Commodore, and Senior Officer of the American Navy, 1773–1838: A Biography.* Cleveland: Arthur H. Clark Co., 1910.

————. *Paullin's History of Naval Administration, 1775–1911.* Annapolis, Md.: Naval Institute Press, 1968.

Pearce, George F. *The U.S. Navy in Pensacola: From Sailing Ships to Naval Aviation (1825–1930).* Pensacola: University of West Florida Press, 1980.

Peck, Taylor. *Round-Shot to Rockets: A History of the Washington Navy Yard and the U.S. Naval Gun Factory.* Annapolis, Md.: Naval Institute Press, 1949.

Porter, David. *Journal of a Cruise.* New York: Bradford & Inskeep, 1815. 2d ed. New York: Wiley & Halsted, 1822. Reprint of combined eds., Annapolis, Md.: Naval Institute Press, 1986.

Pullen, Hugh F. *The "Shannon" and the "Chesapeake."* Toronto: McClelland & Stewart, 1970.

Ray, William. *Horrors of Slavery; or, the American Tars in Tripoli.* Troy, N.Y.: Oliver Lyon, 1808.

Reverby, Susan, and David Rosner, eds. *Health Care in America: Essays in Social History.* Philadelphia: Temple University Press, 1979.

Riley, James C. *The Eighteenth-Century Campaign to Avoid Disease.* New York: St. Martin's Press, 1987.

Risse, Guenter B. *Hospital Life in Enlightment Scotland.* Cambridge: Cambridge University Press, 1986.

Roddis, Louis H. *A Short History of Nautical Medicine.* New York: Paul B. Hoebner, 1941.

Roosevelt, Theodore. *The Naval War of 1812.* 3d ed. 2 vols. New York: G. P. Putnam's Sons, 1910.

Rosenberg, Max. *The Building of Perry's Fleet on Lake Erie, 1812–1813.* Harrisburg: Pennsylvania Historical and Museum Commission, 1950.

Rothford, Murray N. *The Panic of 1819.* New York: Columbia University Press, 1962. Reprint, New York: AMS Press, 1973.

Rothstein, William G. *American Physicians in the Nineteenth Century: From Sects to Science.* Baltimore: Johns Hopkins Press, 1972.

———. *American Medical Schools and the Practice of Medicine.* New York: Oxford University Press, 1987.

Runyan, Timothy J., ed. *Ships, Seafaring, and Society: Essays in Maritime History.* Detroit: Wayne State University Press, 1987.

Ruschenberger, William S. W. [An officer of the U.S. Navy pseudo.]. *Three Years in the Pacific; including notices of Brazil, Chile, Bolivia, and Peru.* Philadelphia: Carey, Lea & Blanchard, 1834.

Ruschenberger, William S. W. *Voyage Around the World; including the embassy to Muscat and Siam in 1835–37.* Philadelphia: Carey, Lea & Blanchard, 1838.

Rush, Benjamin. *Medical Inquiries and Observations: Containing an Account of the Bilious Remitting and Intermitting Yellow-Fever, as It Appeared in Philadelphia in the Year 1794.* Philadelphia: Thomas Dobson, 1798.

Rutland, Robert Allen. *The Presidency of James Madison.* Lawrence: University Press of Kansas, 1990.

Sabiston, David C., Jr., ed. *Davis-Christopher Textbook of Surgery: The Biological Basis of Modern Surgical Practice.* Philadelphia: W. B. Saunders Co., 1977.

Salvaggio, John. *New Orleans Charity Hospital.* Baton Rouge: Louisiana State University Press, 1992.

Sanford, Laura G. *The History of Erie County, Pa.* Philadelphia: J. B. Lippincott Co., 1862.

Scharff, John Thomas, and Thompson Westcott. *History of Philadelphia, 1609–1884.* 3 vols. Philadelphia: L. H. Everts & Co., 1884.

Schuon, Karl. *Home of the Commandants.* Rev. ed. Quantico, Va.: Leatherneck Association, 1974.

Shryock, Richard Harrison. *Medicine and Society in America, 1600–1860.* Ithaca, N.Y.: Cornell University Press, 1960.

————. *Medical Licensing in America, 1650–1965.* Baltimore: Johns Hopkins Press, 1967.

Sibley, J. L., Clifford K. Shipton, and Conrad Wright, eds. *Biographical Sketches of Those Who Attended Harvard College.* 17 vols. to date. Boston: Harvard University Press, 1873–.

Smelser, Marshall. *The Congress Founds the Navy, 1787–1798.* Notre Dame, Ind.: University of Notre Dame Press, 1959.

Sprout, Harold, and Margaret Sprout. *The Rise of American Naval Power, 1776–1918.* Princeton: Princeton University Press, 1939.

Stagg, J. C. A. *Mr. Madison's War: Politics, Diplomacy, and Warfare in the Early American Republic, 1785–1830.* Princeton: Princeton University Press, 1983.

Stanton, William. *The Great United States Exploring Expedition of 1838–1842.* Berkeley & Los Angeles: University of California Press, 1975.

Straus, Robert. *Medical Care for Seamen.* New Haven: Yale University Press, 1950.

Swanson, Neil H. *The Perilous Fight.* New York: Farrar & Rinehart, 1945.

Symonds, Craig L. *Navalists and Antinavalists: The Naval Policy Debate in the United States, 1785–1827.* Newark, Del.: University of Delaware Press, 1980.

Tenon, Jacques René. *Mémoires sur Les Hôpitaux de Paris.* Paris: P. D. Pierres, 1788.

Thompson, John D., and Grace Goldin. *The Hospital: A Social and Architectural History.* New Haven: Yale University Press, 1975.

Thurm, Richard H. *For the Relief of the Sick and Disabled: The U.S. Public Health Service Hospital at Boston, 1799–1969.* Washington, D.C.: GPO, 1972.

Trask, John W. *The United States Marine Hospital, Port of Boston.* Washington, D.C.: U.S. Public Health Service, 1940.

Tyler, David B. *The Wilkes Expedition: The First United States Exploring Expedition (1838–1841).* Philadelphia: American Philosophical Society, 1968.

USS *Constitution* Museum. *Naval Medicine in the Early Nineteenth Century.* Boston: Education Department, USS *Constitution* Museum, 1981.

Viola, Herman J., and Carolyn Margolis, eds. *Magnificent Voyagers: The U.S. Exploring Expedition, 1838–1842.* Washington, D.C.: Smithsonian Institution Press, 1985.

Wainwright, Nicholas B. *Commodore James Biddle and His Sketchbook.* Philadelphia: Historical Society of Pennsylvania, 1966.

Watson, John F. *Annals of Philadelphia and Pennsylvania, in the Olden Times; Being a Collection of Memoirs, Anecdotes, and Incidents of the City and its Inhabitants, and of the Earliest Settlements of the Inland Part of Pennsylvania, from the Days of the Founders.* 2 vols. Philadelphia: the author, 1857.

Watt, J., E. J. Freeman, and W. F. Bynum, eds. *Starving Sailors: The Influence of Nutrition upon Naval and Maritime History.* Greenwich: National Maritime Museum, 1981.

Welsh, William Jeffrey, and David Curtis Skaggs. *War on the Great Lakes: Essays Commemorating the 175th Anniversary of the Battle of Lake Erie.* Kent, Ohio: Kent State University Press, 1991.

Werner, Charles J. *Dr. Isaac Hulse, Surgeon, U.S. Navy, 1797–1856. His Life and Letters.* New York: Charles J. Werner, 1922.

Wheeler, Richard. *In Pirate Waters*. New York: Crowell Publishers, 1969.

White, Leonard D. *The Federalists: A Study in Administrative History*. New York: Macmillan Co., 1948.

———. *The Jeffersonians: A Study in Administrative History, 1801–1829*. New York: Macmillan Co., 1951.

———. *The Jacksonians: A Study in Administrative History, 1829–1861*. New York: Macmillan Co., 1954.

Wilkes, Charles. *Narrative of the United States Exploring Expedition During the Years 1838, 1839, 1840, 1841, 1842*. 5 vols. Philadelphia: Lea and Blanchard, 1845.

Williams, Ralph Chester. *The United States Public Health Service, 1798–1850*. Washington, D.C.: Commissioned Officers Association of the U.S. Public Health Service, 1951.

Wines, Enoch C. *Two Years and a Half in the Navy: or, Journal of a Cruise in the Mediterranean and Levant*. 2 vols. Philadelphia, 1832.

Zaslow, Morris, ed. *The Defended Border: Upper Canada in the War of 1812*. Toronto: Macmillan Co. of Canada, 1964.

Articles

American Seamen's Friend Society. *Sailor's Magazine* 1 (1829).

Anderson, Samuel. "An Account of Bilious Yellow Fever Which Prevailed on Board the United States Ship Delaware, in the Island of Curacao, From the Beginning of November 1799, Until the End of February, 1800." *Medical Repository* 5 (1802): 280–82.

Bell, Whitfield J. "Medical Practice in Colonial America." *Bulletin of the History of Medicine* 31 (1957): 442–53.

Blake, George Smith. "When Smallpox Struck." Transcribed by Katherine McInnis. *U.S. Naval Institute Proceedings* 97 (1979): 78–81.

Bluff, Harry [Matthew F. Maury], "Scraps From the Lucky Bag, No. IV." *Southern Literary Messenger* 7 (1841): 22–23.

Bradburn, H. Benjamin, ed. "The Medical Log of 'Old Ironsides.'" *Connecticut Medicine* 40 (1976): 859–68.

Bradley, George P. "A Brief Sketch of Origin and History of the Medical Corps of the U.S. Navy." *Journal of the Association of Military Surgeons of the United States* 10 (1902): 487–528.

Brings, Hans A. "Navy Medicine Comes Ashore: Establishing the First Permanent U.S. Navy Hospitals." *Journal of the History of Medicine and Allied Sciences* 41 (1986): 157–92.

Brown, Kenneth L. "Mr. Madison's Secretary of the Navy." *U.S. Naval Institute Proceedings* 73 (1947): 966–75.

Campbell, Harry J. "The Congressional Debate over the Seaman's Sickness and Disability Act of 1798: The Origins of the Continuing Debate on the Socialization of American Medicine." *Bulletin of the History of Medicine* 48 (1974): 423–26.

Cohen, Patricia Cline. "Statistics and the State: Changing Social Thought and

Emergence of a Quantitative Mentality in America, 1790 to 1820." *William and Mary Quarterly,* 3d ser., 38 (1981): 35–55.

Cook, Harold J. "Practical Medicine and the British Armed Forces after the 'Glorious Revolution.'" *Medical History* 34 (1990): 1–26.

Cowdery, Jonathan. "On the Efficacy of Alkalies to preserve Cleanliness and Health on ship-board, and on the Usefulness of Acid Fumigations for those purposes." *Medical Repository* 13 (1810): 39–42.

Cushman, Paul, Jr. "Benjamin P. Kissam: Naval Surgeon in the War of 1812." *Bulletin of the New York Academy of Medicine* 7 (1971): 50–66.

———. "Naval Surgery in the War of 1812." *New York State Journal of Medicine* 72 (1972): 1881–87.

———. "Usher Parsons, M.D. (1788–1868), Naval Surgeon in the Battle of Lake Erie." *New York State Journal of Medicine* 71 (1971): 2891–94.

Cutbush, Edward. "Case of Lumbar Abscess." *Medical Repository.* 5 (1802): 277–79.

Dye, Ira, and J. Worth Estes. "Death on the *Argus:* American Malpractice vs British Chauvinism in the War of 1812." *Journal of the History of Medicine and Allied Sciences* 44 (1989): 179–95.

Eaton, Leonard K. "Medicine in Philadelphia and Boston, 1805–1830." *Pennsylvania Magazine of History and Biography* 75 (1951): 66–75.

Estes, J. Worth. "Medical Skills in Colonial New England." *New England Historical and Genealogical Register* 134 (1980): 259–75.

———. "Naval Medicine in the Age of Sail: The Voyage of the *New York,* 1802–1803." *Bulletin of the History of Medicine* 56 (1982): 238–53.

———. "Patterns of Drug Usage in Colonial America." *New York State Journal of Medicine* 87 (1987): 37–45.

———. "The Practice of Medicine in Eighteenth Century Massachusetts: A Bicentennial Perspective." *New England Journal of Medicine* 305 (1981): 1040–47.

———. "Quantitative Observations of Fever and Its Treatment before the Advent of Short Clinical Thermometers." *Medical History* 35 (1991): 189–216.

Foltz, Jonathan M. "Medical Statistics of the U.S. Frigate *Potomac." New York Journal of Medicine* 1 (1843): 189–207.

Gallatin, Albert. "Report of the Secretary of the Treasury, 1809." Medical Repository 11 (1811):313–16.

Harmon, Judd Scott. "Marriage of Convenience: The U.S. Navy in Africa, 1820–1843." *American Neptune* 32 (1972): 264–76.

Harris, Thomas. "Case of Resection of the Elbow-Joint." *Medical Examiner* (New York) 1 (1842): 32–34, 38–39.

Hoyt, William D., Jr. "A Young Virginian Prepares to Practice Medicine, 1796–1800." *Bulletin of the History of Medicine* 11 (1942): 582–86.

Hudson, A. Edward, and Arthur Herbert. "James Lind: His Contribution to Shipboard Sanitation." *Journal of the History of Medicine* 11 (1959): 1–12.

Huntt, H[enry]. "On the Epidemic, as it Appeared Among Seamen and Marines, at the City of Washington." *Medical Repository,* 2d ser., 1 (1814): 342–44.

Johnston, Edith D., ed. "The Kollock Letters, 1799–1850." *Georgia Historical Quarterly* 30 (1946): 218–58, 312–56.

Jones, Russell M. "American Doctors and the Parisian Medical World, 1830–1840." *Bulletin of the History of Medicine* 47 (1973): 40–65, 177–204.

Jordan, Philip A. "A Naval Surgeon in Paris, 1835–1836." *Annals of Medical History,* 3d ser., 2 (1940): 526–36; 3 (1941): 73–81.

Korns, Horace Marshall. "A Brief History of Physical Diagnosis." *Annals of Medical History,* 3d ser., 1 (1939): 50–67.

Langley, Harold D. "Edward Field: A Pioneer Practitioner of the Old Navy." *Connecticut Medicine* 46 (1982): 667–72.

———. "Respect for Civilian Authority: The Tragic Career of Captain Angus." *American Neptune* 40 (1980): 23–27.

———. "Robert Y. Hayne and the Navy." *South Carolina Historical Magazine* 82 (1981): 311–30.

———. "Women in a Warship, 1813." *U.S. Naval Institute Proceedings* 110 (1984): 124–25.

Lathrop, Constance. "Vanished Ships." *U.S. Naval Institute Proceedings* 60 (1934): 949–51.

Louis, Elan Daniel. "William Shippen's Unsuccessful Attempt to Establish the First 'School for Physick' in the American Colonies in 1762." *Bulletin of the History of Medicine* 44 (1989): 218–37.

Mahew, Dean R. "Jeffersonian Gunboats in the War of 1812." *American Neptune* 42 (1982): 101–17.

Maps, James M. A Long Forgotten American Naval Cemetery [Port Mahon]." *American Neptune* 25 (1965): 157–67.

McKee, Christopher. "The Pathology of a Profession: Death in the United States Navy Officer Corps, 1797–1815." *War and Society* 3 (1985): 1–25.

———. ed. "Constitution in the Quasi-War with France: The Letters of John Roche, Jr., 1798–1801." *American Neptune* 27 (1967): 135–49.

Meiklejohn, A. P. "The Curious Obscurity of Dr. James Lind." *Journal of the History of Medicine and Allied Sciences* 9 (1954): 304–10.

Miller, Genevieve. "A Physician in 1776." *Journal of the American Medical Association* 236 (1976): 26–30.

Muller, Charles G. "Fabulous Potomac Passage." *U.S. Naval Institute Proceedings* 90 (1964): 85–91.

Packard, Francis B. "Medical Case Histories in a Colonial Hospital." *Bulletin of the History of Medicine* 12 (1942): 145–68.

Paltsits, Victor Hugo, ed. "Cruise of the U.S. Brig *Argus* in 1813: Journal of Surgeon James Inderwick." *Bulletin of the New York Public Library* 2 (1917): 383–405.

Paullin, Charles O. "Duelling in the Old Navy." *U.S. Naval Institute Proceedings* 25 (1909): 1155–97.

Pleadwell, Frank Lester. "Usher Parsons (1788–1868), Surgeon, United States Navy." *United States Naval Medical Bulletin* 17 (1922): 436–41.

———. "William Paul Crillon Barton, Surgeon United States Navy, A Pioneer in American Naval Medicine (1786–1856)." *Annals of Medical History* 2 (1919): 264–301.

———. "Edward Cutbush, M.D.: The Nestor of the Medical Corps of the Navy." *Annals of Medical History* 5 (1923): 337–86.

Pleadwell, Frank Lester, and W. M. Kerr. "Jonathan Cowdery, Surgeon in the United States Navy, 1767–1852." *United States Naval Medical Bulletin* 17 (1922): 63–87, 243–68.

———. "Lewis Heermann, Surgeon in the United States Navy (1779–1833)." *Annals of Medical History* 5 (1923): 113–45.

Pool, Eugene H., and Frank J. McGowan. "Surgery at New York Hospital One Hundred Years Ago." *Annals of Medical History*, n.s., 1 (1929): 489–539.

Ransom, John E. "The Beginnings of Hospitals in the United States." *Bulletin of the History of Medicine* 13 (1943): 514–39.

Roddis, Louis H. "Naval and Marine Corps Casualties in the Wars of the United States." *Military Surgeon* 99 (1946): 305–10.

———. "Naval Medicine in the Early Days of the Republic." *Journal of the History of Medicine and Allied Sciences* 16 (1961): 103–23.

———. "Thomas Harris, M.D., Naval Surgeon and Founder of the First School of Naval Medicine in the New World." *Journal of the History of Medicine and Allied Sciences* 5 (1950): 236–50.

Rooney, William E. "The Founding of the New Orleans Marine Hospital." *Bulletin of the History of Medicine* 25 (1951): 260–68.

———. "Thomas Jefferson and the New Orleans Marine Hospital." *Journal of Southern History* 22 (1956): 167–182.

Shippen, Edward. "Some Account of the Origin of the Naval Asylum at Philadelphia." *Pennsylvania Magazine of History and Biography* 7 (1883): 117–42.

Shryock, Richard H. "The Significance of Medicine in American History." *American Historical Review.* 62 (1956): 81–91.

Smith, Dale C. "Austin Flint and Auscultation in America." *Journal of the History of Medicine and Allied Sciences* 33 (1978): 129–49.

Tate, E. Mobray. "Naval Justice in the Pacific, 1830–1870: A Pattern of Precedents." *American Neptune* 35 (1975): 20–31.

Warner, John Harley. "Remembering Paris: Memory and the American Disciples of French Medicine in the Nineteenth Century." *Bulletin of the History of Medicine* 65 (1991): 301–25.

———. "The Selective Transport of Medical Knowledge: Antebellum American Physicians and Parisian Medical Therapeutics." *Bulletin of the History of Medicine* 59 (1985): 213–31.

Watkins, John W. "On the Disease Called Lake Fever of the Western Counties of the State of New York." *Medical Repository* 3 (1800): 359–61.

Newspapers and Periodicals

Aurora, General Advertiser. Philadelphia, 1797–98.
Baltimore Gazette. August 1827.
Carey's United States Recorder. Philadelphia, 1798.
Gazette of the United States. Philadelphia, 1797–98.
Louisiana Gazette. New Orleans, 1810–11.
Medical and Agricultural Register. Boston, 1806–07.

Medical Repository. New York, 1798–1820.
National Gazette and Literary Register. New York, 1826.
National Intelligencer. Washington, D.C., 1800–1842.
New York National Advocate. 1826–28.
Niles Weekly Register. Baltimore, 1811–49.
Providence Daily News. Providence, R.I., June 1834.
Southern Literary Messenger. Richmond, Va., 1830–42.
United States Telegraph. Washington, D.C., 1826–37.

Unpublished Materials

Carrigg, John J. "Benjamin Stoddert and the Foundation of the American Navy."
    Ph.D. diss., Georgetown University, 1953.
Dietz, Anthony G. "The Prisoners of War in the United States During the War of
    1812." Ph.D. diss., American University, 1964.
Richman, Allen M. "The Development of Medical Services in the United States
    Navy in the Age of Sail, 1815–1850." Ph.D. diss., University of Minnesota, 1973.
Rooney, William Eugene. "The New Orleans Marine Hospital, 1802–1861." M.A.
    thesis, Tulane University, 1950.
Smith, Dale Cary. "The Emergence of Organized Clinical Instruction in the Nine-
    teenth Century American Cities of Boston, New York, and Philadelphia." Ph.D.
    diss., University of Minnesota, 1979.
Tuleja, Thaddeus V. "A Short History of the New York Navy Yard." New York, 1959.
    Typescript.
West, James H. "A Short History of the New York Navy Yard." New York, 1941.
    Mimeographed.
Witt, John W. "United States Marine Corps Deaths in Service, 1776–1925." 2 vols.
    Spokane, Wash., 1986. Copy in Marine Corps Historical Center, Washington,
    D.C.

Index

Adams, Minister John, 1; President, 25, 27, 29, 44–45

Adee, Surgeon's Mate Augustus, 260–61

Algiers, 4, 5, 19, 80, 241, 242, 267, 272

Allen, Lt. William Henry, 151; Capt., 185–86

American Colonization Society, 244

American Philosophical Society, 339

American Seamen's Friend Society, 294

Anderson, Surgeon's Mate, 34, 68, 69

Angus, Lt. Samuel, 72, 76–77, 224–25

Antarctic, 327, 329, 331

Archer, Surgeon's Mate Starling, 50–51, 104

Armstrong, Surgeon's Mate John D., 177, 181

autopsies, 33, 281

Ayer, Surgeon Samuel, 186, 202

Bache, Surgeon's Mate Benjamin F., 260–61; Surgeon, 337

Bailey, Adams, 138–39

Bainbridge, Capt. William, 93, 95, 177, 181–86, 202, 267, 286

Balfour, Surgeon George, 23, 49, 54, 64–67, 105

Ballard, Capt. Henry E., 315–16, 322

Baltimore, Md., 16, 22, 23, 26, 154, 195, 214

Barbary pirates, 79

Barbary War, 80–87, 141, 160, 161, 163

Barney, Com. Joshua, 195, 213

Barnwell, Surgeon William, 109–12, 258, 338–39

Baron, Com. James, 277, 279, 294

Barron, Com. Samuel, 94, 95, 100, 101

Barry, Capt. John, 20–23, 27, 42, 54, 74

Barton, Benjamin Smith, 20, 150, 153, 209, 343

Barton, Surgeon William P. C., 150–53, 173, 207–10, 250, 263, 294–95, 297, 301–3, 312, 315–25, 338, 341–43, 357

Bassett, Rep. Burwell, 169–70

Bates, Dr. George, 137–38, 173

Beaumont, Dr. William, USA, 298–300

Belt, Surgeon's Mate William, 255–56

Biddle, Com. James, 243, 253, 274–75, 349

Birchmore, Surgeon's Mate William, 260–61; Surgeon, 326

Bladensburg, Battle of, 195, 213–14

Blane, Sir Gilbert, 53

bleeding, treatment by, 23, 64–67, 116, 272, 281, 341, 345

blockades, British, 198, 232

Board of Navy Commissioners, 241, 244, 250, 278, 287, 291–93, 296, 303–5, 308–10, 322–24, 352–53, 356

Bonaparte, Emperor Napoleon, 111, 175

Boston, Mass., 33, 74, 125–39, 183, 202

Boston Marine Society, 10, 125, 130–32

Boyd, Surgeon Thomas, 300, 304

Bradford, Richard H., 297, 319, 320

Branch, Sec. Navy John, 291, 297, 308–9, 315, 319, 321, 324

Brereton, Surgeon John A., 121–22, 213

Briggs, Dr. John P., USA, 236–37

Brown, Surgeon's Mate Gustavus, 237

Buchanan, Surgeon Walter W., 38, 50, 148, 210, 232, 233

Bullus, Surgeon's Mate John, 22, 24, 143, 144; Surgeon, 35, 50, 97, 105, 112, 161, 163, 164
Burr, Aaron, 117–19

Calhoun, Rep. John C., 248, 249; Sec. of War, 285
Canada, 175, 176, 219, 232
Carmick, Capt. Daniel, USMC, 112–17
cartel ships, 180, 202, 208, 237–38
casualties, naval and marine: Barbary War, 100; Quasi-War, 76–77; War of 1812, at sea, 176–84, 186, 188, 189, 192, 193, 198–200; —, on shore, 190, 196, 197, 205, 215–218; —, in Chesapeake Bay, 195; —, on the lakes, 221–223, 228–229, 236, 239; —, total, 240
Cathcart, James L., 86, 88, 95
Catlett, Surgeon's Mate Hanson, 34, 43–45, 71–72
Caton, Surgeon's Mate William, 221–22
Charity Hospital, New Orleans, 111, 114
Charleston, S.C., 157; care of seamen and marines in, 13, 157–59, 215–16, 218
Chase, Surgeon's Mate Charles, 262, 263
Chauncey, Capt. Isaac, 103, 145, 171, 219, 221, 226, 233, 267, 275, 308, 315–16
Chesapeake affair, 167, 169, 175
chloride of lime, use of, 323, 324
Christie, Surgeon's Mate Peter, 148–203
Claiborne, Camp, La., 112, 113
Claiborne, Gov. William C. C., 108, 111, 117
Clark, Consul Daniel, 110, 111
Claxton, Lt. Alexander, 180; Cmdr. 278–79
Cleghorn, Surgeon George, British Army, 272
cockpit, 41, 42, 58, 70, 189, 271, 294, 335

Columbia Medical School, N.Y., 185, 219
Commissioners of Navy Hospitals, 246–84, 285, 287
Cook, Surgeon's Mate, Andrew B., 204, 221, 222
convoys in Quasi-War, 27, 29
Coram (pseud.), 277
Cowdery, Surgeon's Mate Jonathan, 38, 51; Surgeon, 95–97, 98, 104, 144–45, 321, 325, 340, 348, 357
Crane, Lt. William M., 179, 180
Crowninshield, Sec. Navy Benjamin, 244–46, 250–51, 267, 284–86; Rep., 254
Cumberland Island, Ga., 159–60
Cutbush, Surgeon Edward, 36, 50, 51, 79, 86, 100, 101, 102, 150, 153, 167–73, 206–9, 211, 213–14, 239, 241, 244–46, 259, 275, 293–94, 339, 340, 342, 344

Dale, Capt. Richard, 25, 26, 81, 83, 84
Dallas, Sec. Treas. Alexander, 210, 284
Dandridge, Dr. William, 160, 216
Danforth, Dr. Samuel, 131, 132, 380 n15
Davis, Surgeon George, 50, 88, 97, 105, 153, 173, 233
Dearborn, Gen. Henry, 130, 135, 137, 139, 221
Decatur, Capt. Stephen, Sr., 25, 47, 70–71
Decatur, Lt. Stephen, Jr., 93, 94, 104, 105, 151, 154, 156; Capt. 180, 181, 190, 192, 198, 205, 209, 241, 267, 278, 342
Derne, capture of, 95, 101
Dickerson, Sec. Nav. Mahlon, 292, 300–301, 302, 303, 310, 313, 350
Directors of Marine Hospitals, duties of, 16–17
Dodd, Surgeon Robert, 323, 324
drunkenness, 44, 61
duels, 86–87, 105, 173

Eaton, Consul William, 81, 84, 88, 95, 101

Elliott, Commander Jesse D., 227; Capt., 309, 315, 316

Embargo Act, 134, 141, 157, 176

Estes, J. Worth, M.D., 106

Eustis, Dr. William, 130, 131; Sec. War, 136

Evans, Surgeon's Mate Amos, 119, 123; Surgeon, 177, 178, 179, 181, 182, 281, 282

Ewell, Surgeon Thomas, 143, 144, 164, 166, 167, 173, 206, 210, 211

Fiat Justitia (pseud.), 263

Field, Surgeon's Mate Edward, 62, 63, 72

flogging, 47, 48, 54, 63, 306

Florida, 276, 277, 337; purchase of, 269; Seminole War in, 292; Spanish-held, 176. *See also* Pensacola, Fla.

Foltz, Asst. Surgeon Jonathan, 301, 325–26

Fox, Asst. Surgeon John L., 329, 331–33

France: and Louisiana, 111; problems with, 6–7, 11, 19; revolution in, 5, 19; treaties with, 2, 19, 29, 48, 80, 150; undeclared war with, 19–27

Francis I, Emperor of Austria, 268

Franklin, Minister Benjamin, 1, 109

Galapagos Islands, 186–87

Gallatin, Rep. Albert, 15; Sec. Treas., 80, 110, 111, 134, 135, 137, 139, 203

Gamble, Cmdr. Thomas, 282, 283

Gamble, Lt. John M., USMC, 189, 386–87

Gibraltar, 80, 81, 83, 84, 86, 87, 89, 97, 99, 104, 268, 270, 271

Gilchrist, Passed Asst. Surgeon Edward, 328, 329

Gillasspy, Surgeon George, 20, 22, 37, 42, 49, 150

Goldsborough, Charles W., 112, 114, 115, 173, 211, 214, 247

Gordon, Surgeon John H., 262, 263

Great Britain, 80; benefits to seamen, 17; blockade of U.S. ports, 202; Greenwich hospital, 8, 9, 15; hospitals for seamen, 8, 9, 12, 15; relations with U.S., 166–67, 176, 312

grog. *See* liquor ration

Guillou, Asst. Surgeon Charles F. B., 329, 331, 333

gunboats, 95, 102, 116, 117, 141, 158, 159, 171, 201, 202, 203, 204, 208, 215, 216, 217, 223, 235, 341

Halifax, Nova Scotia, 180, 184, 202, 204, 239, 240

Hamilton, Sec. Nav. Paul, 136, 137, 138, 146, 153, 154, 155, 156, 158, 159, 169, 170, 171, 201, 204, 205, 206, 208, 210, 284, 285, 341, 342

Hamilton, Sec. Treas. Alexander, 10–11, 126

Hamilton, Surgeon's Mate Charles B., 158, 159, 160, 204

Harris, Surgeon's Mate Benjamin G., 51, 70–71

Harris, Surgeon Thomas, 180, 252, 253, 254, 276, 294–95, 298, 301, 303, 312, 342, 343, 356; school of, 253, 261, 262, 346–47

Harrison, Gen. William H., 227, 230; President, 293, 306, 353

Harrison, Surgeon's Mate John, 211, 213, 214, 239

Harvard College, 125, 128, 136

Harvard Medical School, 127, 130

Harwood, Midshipman Andrew, 273–74

Havana, Cuba, 74, 274, 275, 316, 317

Hayne, Senator Robert Y., 265, 297

Heap, Surgeon Samuel D., 104, 120, 123, 209, 210, 246–47, 269, 282, 283, 284

Heermann, Surgeon's Mate Lewis, 38, 39, 51; Surgeon, 93, 94, 104, 120, 121, 122, 123, 156, 198, 294, 295, 296, 340–41, 347–49

Henry, Surgeon's Mate Isaac, 23, 24, 34, 43, 58

Hermonine, HMS, mutiny in, 45

Higginson, Stephen, 24, 34, 74

Hoffman, Surgeon Robert K., 262, 263, 276

Holmes, Asst. Surgeon Silas, 227–29, 332

Horner, Asst. Surgeon Gustavus, R. B., 317, 352

hospitals, naval: at Black Rock, N.Y., 224, 225, 226; at Boston, 128–29, 130–32, 136–37, 138, 179, 309–11; at New Orleans, 115, 117, 119; at New York, 142–48, 171, 172, 204, 309–11; at Norfolk, 155–56, 275, 289, 310, 320–21; at Pensacola, 308–11; at Philadelphia, 150–51; at Port Mahon, Minorca, 267, 268, 269, 270, 273, 274; at Portsmouth, New Hampshire, 312; at Presque Isle, 226–27, 230; regulations for, 171–73, 247; reports on, 250, 285, 286, 310; at Sacket's Harbor, 219, 221, 235; Senate bill on, 286, 287; at Spermacati Cove, Sandy Hook, 20; at Syracuse, Sicily, 101; at Washington, D.C., 210–14, 162, 163, 169–70, 312

hospitals for seamen: act establishing, 16; bill for, 9–13; at Jamaica, 59; in New England, 142, 143; at New Orleans, 108–11, 119, 120, 122–23; at New York, 142, 143, 145–46; at Norfolk, 8; at Philadelphia, 148–50

Hoxse, Seaman John, 59, 75

Hull, Lt. Isaac, 95; Capt., 177, 179, 204, 275, 282, 300

Hulse, Surgeon Isaac, 277

Huntt, Surgeon's Mate Henry, 211, 212

Inderwick, Surgeon James, 185–86

inoculation, 33, 103, 125, 273

Jackson, Gen. Andrew, 196; President, 244, 291, 305, 312–13

Jacques, Surgeon's Mate Gershom, 50, 104

Jarvis, Dr. Charles, 128, 129, 130

Jefferson, Minister Thomas, 1, 4, 137, 161; Sec. State, 2, 3, 4; President, 48, 80, 81, 88, 89, 94, 108, 109, 110, 112, 135, 141, 143, 144, 163

Jenner, Dr. Edward, 33

Jones, Lt. Jacob, 118; Master Commandant, 180; Capt., 269

Jones, Sec. Nav. William, 203, 205, 209, 210, 211, 213, 214, 215, 216, 217, 241, 245

Judson, Surgeon Elnathan, 258, 343

Kearney, Surgeon John A., 199, 313

Kennedy, Cmdr. Edmund P., 277, 278

Key West. *See* Thompson's Island, Fla.

Lake Borgne, La., battle of, 195, 196

Lake Champlain, N.Y., 232, 236; battle of, 235

Lake Erie, 219, 223, 225, 232; battle of, 228; casualties, 228–29; Black Rock, naval force at, 223; building U.S. squadron on, 222, 227; Presque Isle, naval force at, 227

Lake Ontario, 219, 232; attack on Kingston, 221; attack on Sacket's Harbor, 222, 232, attack on York, 221–22; seamen and marines at Sacket's Harbor, 221; sick in Chauncey's command, 232; Stony Creek, battle at, 222

Latrobe, Benjamin H., 153, 210, 284

Lawrence, Capt. James, 183–84

Le Chevalier, Surgeon's Mate Oliver, 216

Leghorn, Italy, 6, 81, 84, 86, 89

lemon juice, 327, 338, 342

lime juice, 65, 70–71, 154, 329, 342

limes, 187, 342

Lincoln, Collector of Customs Benjamin, 125, 134, 135

Lind, Dr. James, 53, 67, 340, 368 n1, 370 n30

liquor ration, 156, 169, 292, 294–95, 318, 342, 354
Little Belt incident, 175
Livingston, Rep. Edward, 13–14
Lloyd, Dr. James, 131, 132, 380 n15
loblolly boy, 21, 47, 54, 103
Logan, Surgeon George, 158, 159, 215, 216, 286, 293
Louisiana, 110, 111, 112, 114, 197, 268

McCormick, Surgeon Daniel, 157, 159
Macdonough, Commodore Thomas, 235, 236, 273
McHenry, Sec. War James, 21, 126
McReynolds, Surgeon John D., 267, 271
Madison, Sec. State James, 108; President, 135, 137, 175, 203
Malta, Island of, 81, 87, 88, 89, 99, 104, 274
Marine Barracks, Washington, D.C., 163; care of sick at, 165, 166
Marine Hospital Fund, 142, 149, 160, 169, 171, 284–89
Marine Hospitals, 16, 108–9, 125–27, 132–33, 135, 149, 155–56, 177, 284
Marshall, Surgeon Samuel L., 37, 45, 46, 50, 51, 122, 144, 145, 146, 172, 173, 203, 204, 205, 206, 246, 247, 248, 258, 262, 286
Marshall, Surgeon Thomas, 50, 63, 102, 103, 105, 119
Massachusetts Medical Society, 125, 128
Maury, Lt. Matthew F., 352–54
medical officers, navy: animosity toward, 45; care of medicines and instruments, 118, 146, 161, 163–64, 165, 166, 337; court martials of, 42–48; duties of, 5, 85, 86, 122, 123, 128, 143, 168–69, 335–36, 337, 339; examination of, 204, 253, 255, 258, 259, 261–64, 266, 269, 347; liquor ration, 294–95; number of, 49–51, 105, 169, 240, 245–46, 251, 312–13, 351; pay, 5, 123, 167, 245, 247–49,

252, 253, 255, 263–66, 306–8, 342; private practice of, 114, 122, 338; professional improvement of, 168, 252–53, 335–50; rank of, 245, 247, 248, 250, 265–66; rules and regulations for, 85–86, 171–73, 244, 247, 304–6, 335; sea duty, 49, 104, 115, 118, 256–58, 293, 303–4, 313; statistics on place of acceptances, 49–51, 240, 358, 376 n59; study in Europe, 155, 347–50; surgeon general and medical bureau, 250, 296–304
medical practice, naval: in the Barbary War, 79–106; at Beaufort, S.C., 215; at Boston, 126–39, 202; at Charleston, S.C., 158–59, 210, 215, 216, 218; in the *Constitution*, 273–74; at Cumberland Island, Ga., 159, 160; in the *Franklin*, 268–69; in the *Java*, 271–73; in the *Macedonian*, 274–75; at New Orleans, 100, 112–23; at New York, 142–46, 204–5; at Norfolk, 155–56, 202, 275–310; at Philadelphia, 150–51; at Pisa, Italy, 269; at Portland, Maine, 202; at Port Mahon, Minorca, 270–71, 273, 274; at Port Petre, Ga., 217; in the Quasi-War, 20, 23, 34–39, 53–77; at Sacket's Harbor, N.Y., 219, 221, 222, 224, 232, 233, 235; at St. Mary's, Ga., 217; at Savannah, Ga., 217; at Sunbury, Ga., 217–18; at Thompson's Island, Fla., 276–77; in the *United States*, 268; in the War of 1812, 176–240; at Washington, D.C., 213–14; at Wilmington, N.C., 215
medical purveyor, 164, 205–6, 251, 305
medical schools, European and American, 29
medical supplies and surgical instruments, 25, 26, 49, 113, 150, 161, 164, 202, 205, 206, 246, 251–52, 265, 296, 298, 301, 303–5, 321–23, 329, 337, 390 n32
medical treatments, 31, 32

medicine chest, 11, 20, 143, 215, 221, 224

Mediterranean Squadron, 242, 267, 286, 301, 348, 350

mental cases, 3, 69–70, 134, 142, 354

Mercer, Rep. Charles, 253–54

Miller, Surgeon Robert, 187–88

Mitchell, Rep. Samuel Latham, 128, 130

Monroe, President James, 243, 251, 252, 255, 257, 275, 342

Montgomery, Surgeon's Mate, 188, 282, 283, 284

Morgan, Surgeon's Mate Mordecai, 252, 279; Surgeon, 303

Morocco, 2, 80, 86

Morris, Com. Richard V., 84, 85, 87, 88, 89, 97, 100

Morris, Lt. Charles, 178; Capt., 275

Morrison, Surgeon's Mate E. D., 214, 215

Mullowny, Lt. John, 21, 22, 29, 72

Murray, Capt. Alexander, 27, 28, 62, 86, 87, 151, 206, 207, 208, 210

Naples, Italy, 89, 103, 267–68

Naval Asylum, Philadelphia, 288, 310, 312, 351

Naval Hospital Fund, 171, 249–50, 284–89, 308, 354

navy accountant, 113, 115, 136

navy yards: Boston, 127, 141, 202, 274, 275, 285, 351; New York, 24, 127, 141, 205, 219, 279, 280, 285, 351; Norfolk, 24, 127, 141, 274, 351; Pensacola, 351; Philadelphia, 127, 141, 206, 208, 285, 342, 351; Portsmouth, N.H., 24, 127, 141, 351; Washington, D.C., 127, 141, 161, 162, 163, 206, 210, 211, 239, 241, 285, 298, 301, 351–52

New Castle, Del., 76, 207, 245

New Orleans, La., 107–23, 195, 196, 197, 237

Newport, R.I., 61, 74, 273

New York City, 13, 24, 74, 171, 203, 204

Nicholson, Capt. Samuel, 24, 35, 130, 136

Noah, Surgeon's Mate Mordecai, 256–57; Surgeon, 279

Non-Intercourse Act, 141, 157, 176

Non Nauticus (pseud.), 303–4

Norfolk, Va., 8, 24, 76, 90, 155, 156, 214, 276, 320, 321

Nukahiva, Marquesas Group, 186, 188

nurses, 114, 126, 133, 166, 190–92, 320

Osborne, Surgeon's Mate Leonard, 238, 239, 240

Pacific Squadron, 242

Palmer, Asst. Surgeon James C., 328, 329, 333

Parrott, Rep. John F., 249, 262, 263

Parsons, Surgeon's Mate Usher, 223, 224, 225, 226, 227–31; Surgeon, 271, 344–45, 348

Paulding, Sec. Nav. James K., 293, 303, 304, 306, 315, 319, 356

Peaco, Surgeon's Mate John W., 259, 260, 261

Pennsylvania, Univ. of, 20, 29, 210, 343

Pennsylvania Hospital, Philadelphia, 74, 76, 150, 151, 243

Pensacola, Fla., 276, 277, 337; hospital at, 277, 280, 308–9, 310, 311, 315, 317, 349

pensioners, navy, 246, 285, 287

Perry, Lt. Oliver H., 180–81, 223, 227, 231; Capt., 271, 272

Philadelphia, Pa., 6, 20, 37, 149, 343, 354; care of sick sailors in, 13, 21, 74, 76

Phillips, Surgeon's Mate Manuel, 256, 257

Physick, Dr. Philip Syng, 69, 282

Pinckney, Rep. Thomas, 12, 13

pirates: of Algiers, 80; in West Indies, 274

Porter, Lt. David, 103; Capt., 152, 153,

186, 188, 189, 208, 275, 276, 278, 342
Port Mahon, Island of Minorca, 84, 267, 268, 269, 270–71, 273, 274, 349
Preble, Capt. Edward, 63, 64, 89, 90, 93, 94, 95, 96, 97, 99, 103
Presque Isle, Pa., 223, 226
Puerto Rico, 7, 27

Quackenbos, Surgeon's Mate George C., 116, 118

Ray, Surgeon's Mate Hyde, 190, 217
Read, Surgeon John K., Jr., 49, 105
Read, Surgeon William, 24, 34, 60
Ringgold, Lt. Cadwalader, 329, 332
Roberts, Surgeon's Mate Joseph, 225, 231, 232
Rodgers, Lt. John, 87, 89, 95, 96, 102; Com., 106, 145, 146, 175, 176, 177, 180, 342; President, Board of Navy Commissioners, 244, 247, 248, 253, 270, 275, 287, 293, 309
Rogers, Surgeon William, 112–19
Ruschenberger, Asst. Surgeon William S. W., 345; Surgeon, 346, 352
Rush, Dr. Benjamin, 20, 21, 23, 25, 64, 67, 68, 69, 72, 73, 108, 148
Rush, Surgeon John, 25, 49, 67, 68

Sacket's Harbor, N.Y., 219, 221, 222, 223, 224, 232, 233, 235, 255
sailors, distressed American, 3, 7, 11, 27
St. Mary's, Ga., 157, 158, 192, 216, 217
St. Medard, Surgeon Peter, 35, 50, 51, 89, 90, 91, 92, 105, 128, 129, 153
Salter, Surgeon Thomas B., 269, 283
Santo Domingo, 7, 63, 111
Savannah, Ga., 217, 239
Schoolfield, Surgeon Joseph J., 156, 214
Seminole War, Second, 292, 313, 314
Sever, Capt. James, 62, 63
Sewall, Rep. Samuel, 12–15
Shannon, Surgeon Richard C., 46, 69

Shaw, Master Commandant, John, 75, 102, 115, 117, 118, 119, 120, 122; Capt., 155, 268
Sickles, Surgeon J. Frederick, 327, 328
Sigourney, Midshipman James B., 190, 196
slave trade, 244, 354
Smith, Sec. Nav. Robert, 80, 88, 94, 97, 104, 115, 116, 117, 119, 128, 129, 130, 143, 144, 150, 157, 161, 163, 164, 347
Southard, Sec. Nav. Samuel L., 244, 255, 256, 258–65, 276, 277, 278, 279, 288, 289, 293, 337, 344, 345; Senator, 304
Spain, 4, 107, 110, 243; U.S. relations with, 267–70, 276
Spence, Navy Agent Keith, 116–17
Spermacati Cove, Sandy Hook, N.J., 204, 205
Sprosten, Asst. Surgeon George S., 323, 324
Starke, Surgeon Robert B., 51, 151, 153, 156–57
stethoscope, 348, 350
stewards, hospital, 166, 245, 246, 320
Stewart, Capt. Chas., 199, 268, 269
Stoddert, Sec. Nav. Benjamin, xix, 25, 26, 27, 34, 61, 64, 74, 75, 76, 127, 161, 247
stoves in ships, 55, 168, 340
Strong, Surgeon's Mate Joseph C., 49, 73, 75, 150
Sullivan's Island, S.C., 157, 158, 215, 216
Sweden, 2, 6
Syracuse, Sicily, 94, 99, 100, 102

Thompson, Sec. Nav. Smith, 244, 250, 251, 252, 253, 274–75, 284
Thompson's Island, Fla., 243, 275, 276, 277
Ticknor, Surgeon's Mate Benajah, 253, 260, 261
Tingey, Capt. Thomas, 161, 162, 165, 166, 212, 214

Tisdale, Surgeon's Mate Nathaniel, 50, 104
Toulon, France, 84, 87
Trevett, Surgeon Samuel R., 286
Tripoli, 5, 80, 81, 88, 89, 93, 94, 95, 102, 242
Trotter, Dr. Thomas, 131
Truxtun, Capt. Thomas, 22, 23, 24, 26, 42, 54, 55, 63, 74, 84
Tunis, 5, 80, 81, 88, 242
Turner, Navy Accountant Thomas, 75, 115, 171
Turner, Surgeon William, 61, 105

Upshur, Sec. Nav. Able P., 306, 333, 353–54, 356
U.S. Army, 112, 313
U.S. Congress, 3, 4, 5, 7, 11, 12, 16, 17, 24–25, 26, 162, 169, 242, 309–12
U.S. Consuls, 2–3, 7, 11
U.S. Department of State, 87, 238
U.S. House of Representatives, 11, 12–15, 286, 294, 303
U.S. Marine Corps, 26, 106, 112–13, 115, 116, 117, 169, 298
U.S. Marines, 128, 129, 143, 169, 298, 313
U.S. merchant marine, 79, 80
U.S. Navy Department, 5, 17, 19, 24–26, 85, 112, 206, 215, 223, 255, 264, 275, 284, 285, 291–93, 300–302, 354, 356, 360
U.S. President, 6, 20, 25, 137, 143, 144, 163, 253, 291, 293, 353
U.S. Senate, 4–5, 248, 286–87
U.S. Treasury Department, 5, 10, 16, 26, 125, 127, 171, 288
U.S. War Department, 5, 20, 21, 114

vaccination, 130, 131, 272, 273, 274, 279, 286, 327, 328, 338
Valpariso, Chile, 188, 242
Van Buren, President Martin, 293, 312, 353
venereal disease, 71, 118, 133, 138, 143, 207, 271, 282, 283, 328, 329

venereal fee, 71, 207, 249, 342, 371 n39
ventilation of ships, 40, 41, 42, 55, 56, 168, 274, 277, 278, 279, 317, 340

Warner, Dr. John G., 136, 380, 381 n15
War of 1812, 175–240
warrant officers, 162, 189
Warren, Dr. John, 131, 132
Warrington, Capt. Lewis, 193, 199, 300
Warrington, Com. Lewis, 243
warships, British: HMS *Guerriere*, 177, 200; HMS *Macedonian*, 180, 185
warships, French: *La Vengeance*, 29, 58, 59, 75, 76; *L'Insurgente*, 35, 56, 57, 58
warships, U.S.: *Adams*, 85, 86, 89, 211, 212; *Alligator*, 192, 200, 244; *Argus*, 95, 101, 104, 176, 185, 215; *Baltimore*, 37, 43; *Brandywine*, 315, 318, 320; *Carolina*, 196, 197; *Chesapeake*, 63, 85, 86, 88, 89, 138, 144, 145, 167, 169, 183, 184, 185, 186; *Congress*, 37, 61, 62, 63, 94, 176, 235, 239; *Constellation*, 5, 19, 22, 23, 24, 34, 40, 42, 49, 50, 54, 56, 58, 63, 64, 68, 73, 75, 76, 79, 85, 86, 87, 92, 94, 104, 161, 189, 190, 207, 242, 294; *Constitution*, 5, 19, 24, 40, 41, 42, 90, 92, 102, 103, 177, 179, 180, 181, 182, 183, 186, 199, 202, 227, 273, 274; *Cyane*, 256, 257; *Delaware*, 25, 26, 27, 34, 68, 69; *Eagle*, 47, 235, 236; *Enterprise*, 75, 81, 85, 87, 88, 89, 102, 103, 104, 158, 186, 274; *Essex*, 40, 61, 63–64, 81, 85, 86, 92, 94, 102, 151, 152, 153, 156, 186, 188, 189, 208, 209; *Essex Jr.*, 186, 189; *Etna*, 118, 119, 192; *Franklin*, 117, 268, 269; *Ganges*, 25, 37, 60, 67, 71, 72, 73; *General Greene*, 26, 40, 60, 162; *Grampus*, 280, 301; *Guerriere*, 195; *Hornet*, 95, 104, 157, 176, 183, 186, 190, 192,

199, 258, 274, 277–78; *Insurgente,* 77; *Intrepid,* 93, 94; *Java,* 271–72, 286, 300; *John Adams,* 37, 85, 87, 88, 94, 99, 103, 201, 224; *Lawrence,* 227, 228, 229, 230; *Macedonian,* 242, 274, 190, 192; *Montezuma,* 27, 29, 34, 72; *Nautilus,* 95, 104, 156, 179, 180; *New York,* 85, 87, 88, 89, 90, 99, 211; *Niagara,* 228; *North Carolina,* 274; *Peacock,* 193, 199; *Pennsylvania,* 292; *Philadelphia,* 38, 51, 70, 93, 94, 95, 99; *President,* 49, 81, 83, 84, 94, 100, 175, 176, 192, 198; *Retaliation,* 67, 74; *Richmond,* 37, 60; *Saratoga,* 232, 235, 236; *Scammel,* 37, 46, 69; *Siren,* 93, 102; *Spark,* 269, 274; *United States,* 19, 20, 22, 24, 27, 37, 73, 74, 151, 156, 176, 180, 190; *Wasp,* 131, 180, 193, 200, 207

Washington, D.C., 90, 127, 163, 210, 211, 212, 213, 239, 284

Washington, President George, 2, 4

Washington, Surgeon Bailey, 186, 239, 258, 276, 298, 300–303

Washington Navy Yard, 161, 162, 163, 165–66

Waterhouse, Dr. Benjamin, 33, 34, 127–28, 130–37

Watkins, Surgeon's Mate Tobias, 34, 44, 154

Webb, Surgeon Charles, 47, 48, 50

Weems, Surgeon's Mate Nathaniel T., 90, 91; Surgeon, 143

Wells, Surgeon James, 50, 105, 115, 116, 117, 120

Welsh, Dr. Thomas, 125, 132

West India Squadron, 243, 309, 314, 315, 337

West Indies, 7, 27, 243, 244, 278, 279, 294, 310, 315, 344, 349

Wharton, Lt. Col. Franklin, Commandant, USMC, 129, 157, 165

Whittelsey, Surgeon's Mate Samuel, 201, 207, 208, 210, 238, 239

Whittle, Assistant Surgeon John S., 329, 331

Wiesenthal, Surgeon's Mate Thomas, 258, 259, 278

Wilkes Exploring Expedition, 292, 293, 326, 333

Wilkes, Lt. Charles, 326, 327, 328, 329, 331

Wilkinson, Gen. James, 117, 118

Williamson, Surgeon Thomas, 275, 320, 321

Windship, Surgeon Amos, 35, 43

Wolcott, Sec. Treas. Oliver, 125, 126

Wolfley, Asst. Surgeon Lewis, 349–50

Woodbury, Sec. Nav. Levi, 279, 295, 297, 301, 305, 310, 322–23, 337; Sec. Treas., 292

yellow fever, 22, 23, 60–61, 68–69, 77, 111, 112, 120, 149, 275–76, 277–79, 344

York, Upper Canada, 221, 222

Library of Congress Cataloging-in-Publication Data

Langley, Harold D.
    A history of medicine in the early U.S. Navy / Harold D. Langley.
        p.   cm.
    Includes bibliographical references and index.
    ISBN 0-8018-4876-8 (alk. paper : hc)
    1. Medicine, Naval—United States—History—19th century. 2. United
States. Navy—Medical care—History—19th century. I. Title.
    [DNLM: 1. United States. Navy. 2. Naval Medicine—history—United
States. VG 123 L283h 1995]
VG123.L36 1995
359.3'45'0973—dc20
DNLM/DLC
for Library of Congress   94-31383

Lightning Source UK Ltd.
Milton Keynes UK
UKHW010752030120
356267UK00003B/247/P